THEMES AND PERSPECTIVES IN NURSING

THEMES AND
PERSPECTIVES
IN
NURSING

Edited by

Keith Soothill, Christine Henry
and Kevin Kendrick

Centre for Health Research, Lancaster University

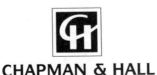

CHAPMAN & HALL

London · New York · Tokyo · Melbourne · Madras

Published by Chapman & Hall, 2–6 Boundary Row, London SE1 8HN

Chapman & Hall, 2–6 Boundary Row, London SE1 8HN, UK

Chapman & Hall, 29 West 35th Street, New York NY10001, USA

Chapman & Hall Japan, Thomson Publishing Japan, Hirakawacho Nemoto Building, 7F, 1-7-11 Hirakawa-cho, Chiyoda-ku, Tokyo 102, Japan

Chapman & Hall Australia, Thomas Nelson Australia, 102 Dodds Street, South Melbourne, Victoria 3205, Australia

Chapman & Hall India, R. Seshadri, 32 Second Main Road, CIT East, Madras 600 035, India

First edition 1992

© 1992 Keith Soothill, Christine Henry and Kevin Kendrick

Typeset in 10 on 12 point Sabon by Columns Design and Production Services Ltd, Reading
Printed in Great Britain by Hartnolls Ltd, Bodmin, Cornwall

ISBN 0 412 43990 5

A catalogue record for this book is available from the British Library

Library of Congress Cataloging-in-Publication data available

Contents

Contributors   vii

Acknowledgements   ix

Preface   x

PART I   *PERCEPTIONS OF NURSING*   1

1   Nursing and doctoring: where's the difference?   4
   Lesley Mackay
2   The media representation of the nurse: 16
   the implications for nursing   *Joanne Holloway*
3   Nursing, advertising and sponsorship: some ethical   41
   issues   *Ruth Chadwick*
4   NHS nursing: vocation, career or just a job?   56
   Brian Francis, Moira Peelo and Keith Soothill
5   Conceptions of the nature of persons by doctors,   75
   nurses and teachers   *Christine Henry*

PART II   *EDUCATION*   89

6   The nurses' reformation: philosophy and pragmatics   91
   of Project 2000   *Kevin Kendrick and Anne Simpson*
7   Interpersonal and therapeutic skills in the 'New   101
   Curriculum' for nurse education   *Tom Chapman and
   Helen Fields*
8   Performance indicators and changing patterns of   114
   accountability in nurse education   *Ruth Balogh*
9   Professional conceptions of mental illness and   138
   related issues   *Glen Pashley*

PART III   *CLINICAL*   155

10   Patient advocacy in nursing   *Paul Witts*   158
11   Assessing the stress in persons with cancer: 181
   an exploration of the main perspectives of stress in
   relation to their psychological care   *Liz Hanson*

12 Conceptions of care   *Helen Ellis*   196
13 Nursing wastage from the nurses' perspective   214
    Catherine Williams, Jon Barry and Keith Soothill
14 Difficulties in provision of care for the elderly by   231
    auxiliaries – implications for the new support worker
    Emily Griffiths
15 Considerations of personhood in nursing research: 245
    an ethical perspective   *Kevin Kendrick*

PART IV   *MANAGEMENT*   259

16 Managing nurse wastage   *Jon Barry, Keith Soothill*   261
    and Catherine Williams
17 Nurse supply modelling   *David Worthington*   276
18 Angels in red? patterns of union membership   293
    amongst UK professional nurses   *Paul Bagguley*
19 Nurses and the prospects of participative   310
    management in the NHS   *Stephen Ackroyd*

Index   331

Contributors

Mr Stephen Ackroyd is an organizational consultant and Lecturer in the Management School, Lancaster University.

Dr Paul Bagguley is Lecturer in the Department of Social Policy and Sociology, University of Leeds.

Ms Ruth Balogh was Research Officer on the project to develop performance indicators for the English National Board for Nursing, Midwifery and Health Visiting and is currently a freelance research and evalaution consultant.

Mr Jon Barry is Research Officer, Centre for Applied Statistics, Lancaster University.

Dr Ruth Chadwick is Director of the Centre for Applied Ethics, University of Wales College of Cardiff.

Dr Tom Chapman is Principal Lecturer in the Department of Applied Social Sciences, Edge Hill College of Higher Education.

Ms Helen Ellis is a course teacher in the Department of Post Basic and Continuing Education, Preston and Chorley School of Nursing.

Ms Helen Fields is Assistant Director of Nurse Education, Sefton School of Health Studies.

Mr Brian Francis is Assistant Director, Centre for Applied Statistics, Lancaster University.

Ms Emily Griffiths is staff nurse on a continuing care ward, Ulverston Hospital, Cumbria, and postgraduate in the Department of Applied Social Science, Lancaster University.

Ms Liz Hanson is a former staff nurse at Weston Park Hospital, Sheffield, and is currently Visiting Lecturer, School of Health and Community Studies, Sheffield City Polytechnic.

Professor Christine Henry is Dean of the Faculty of Health, Lancashire Polytechnic.

Ms Joanne Holloway is a former staff nurse and former student at Lancaster University studying psychology and sociology.

Mr Kevin Kendrick is Senior Lecturer in Health Care Ethics, Lancashire Polytechnic.

Dr Lesley Mackay is Senior Research Fellow in the Department of Applied Social Science. Lancaster University.

Ms Glen Pashley is Senior Lecturer in Curriculum Development in the Faculty of Health, Lancashire Polytechnic.

Dr Moira Peelo is Research Associate, Department of Applied Social Science, Lancaster University.

Ms Anne Simpson is Principal of the Lakeland College of Nursing and Midwifery.

Professor Keith Soothill is Professor of Social Research in the Department of Applied Social Science, Lancaster University.

Ms Catherine Williams is Lecturer in the Department of Nursing and Health Studies, St Martin's College, Lancaster.

Mr Paul Witts is Senior Lecturer in the Department of Nursing in the Faculty of Health, Lancashire Polytechnic.

Dr David Worthington is Lecturer in Operational Research and Operations Management, the Management School, Lancaster University.

Acknowledgements

Many people have assisted, both directly and indirectly, in bringing this collaborative project to fruition. To everyone we extend our thanks. In particular, we much appreciate the willingness of our contributors to act on the suggestion of Moira Peelo that any royalties accruing from the book should go to a fund administered by the Centre for Health Research at Lancaster University. The object of the fund is to assist nurses to carry out research. Hence, any success that this book achieves will help — albeit in a small way — some nurses to develop their research ideas. We hope that everyone who has supported us in various ways feels that the venture has been worthwhile.

Keith Soothill
Christine Henry
Kevin Kendrick

Preface

The delivery of effective health care is a major priority for the nursing profession and nurses must therefore confront issues related to all aspects of health and health care reform. A priority is to develop appropriate texts which will not only complement the rapid changes in nursing education, but also encourage confidence in appraisal and allow students of nursing and the qualified practitioner to sensitively utilize their critical skills.

The transfer of nursing education to the higher education sector is occurring in different ways on a national and international level. This emphasizes a variety of changes, such as new opportunities in nursing and midwifery career structures, the advancement of nursing research, professional practice and accountability. The positive aspect lies with providing a confident nurse practitioner for the 1990s and beyond. This text therefore presents significant issues and themes which directly relate to the 1990s, and the significant changes, such as perceptions of nursing, education, clinical professionalism and management.

Keith Soothill
Christine Henry
Kevin Kendrick

PART I

Perceptions of Nursing

Perceptions of nursing, both from within the profession and by those viewing the profession from the outside, are crucial ingredients in understanding the present standing of nurses. What soon becomes evident is the complexity of the messages being conveyed. Nursing seems to be in a state of flux: important changes are currently taking place, and other fundamental shifts are very much on the horizon. However, this is not something new within nursing and, as Brian Francis and his colleagues note in this volume (Chapter 4), the classic paper of Whittaker and Olesen (1964)* points to how the legend of Florence Nightingale, widely accepted as the culture-heroine of the nursing profession, has many faces and many functions. The differing interpretations of the Nightingale legend reflect prevailing ideologies within nursing, and each generation claims something specific from the Florence Nightingale legend as its own, so 'to some women it projects the face of traditional womanhood, to others it shows how traditional femininity could be combined with a career'. Today various other models of nursing are emerging and there seems little doubt that the Nightingale legend will be reinterpreted yet again to match emerging perceptions of the nursing profession.

Previous work on nursing has tended to consider the profession in isolation but, whatever else they do, nurses must interact with a whole range of other professional groups as well as the lay persons who are their patients. A crucial area where much difficulty is experienced is in the relationships between doctors and nurses. In brief, the relationship between doctors and nurses is both complicated and contradictory. Thus, for example, nurses

* Whittaker, E. and Olesen, V. 1964. The faces of Florence Nightingale: functions of the heroine legend in an occupational sub-culture. *Human Organisation* 23(2): 123–30.

may sometimes find the behaviour of doctors leaves a lot to be desired and yet nurses often greatly value the approval of doctors. Failures to understand or appreciate their distinctive roles as well as recognizing the difficulties under which the other works may adversely affect patients, both directly and indirectly.

While the problem of adequate communication and working relations between nurses and doctors has long been recognized as a serious one for the NHS, there has been little systematic study of the issue. As part of a major study of this area, Lesley Mackay focuses in Chapter 1 on the different perceptions which these two – still essentially gendered – occupations hold of each other. While it is a fact that in hospitals the jobs that nurses and doctors do often overlap, it is surprising, therefore, that the descriptions of the 'good nurse' and the 'good doctor' given by doctors and nurses are so different. Part of the explanation seems to lie in the way that doctors and nurses contrast the content of the work which they do. Many doctors seem to have unflattering attitudes towards the work of nurses; and nurses' demands for patient-orientated doctors appear to go unheard. Curiously, nurses and doctors, it seems, are seeking a mirror image of their own skills in their ideal doctors and nurses.

While many of the public will in the course of their lives have first-hand experience of the ministrations of nurses, for most of the time the powerful images of nursing displayed in the media will have a more immediate impact. Hence, it is increasingly being recognized that the way in which nurses are portrayed in the media has important implications in general for the status of nursing in society. Joanne Holloway (Chapter 2) identifies four main stereotypes – the angel, the handmaiden, the battle-axe and the sex symbol – which underpin detrimental images of nursing. She relates these stereotypical representations to an underlying ideology which in turn has an historical basis in society.

Holloway stresses that it is important that nursing continues to recognize the relevance of campaigning against detrimental images, stereotypes and representations, but makes two points which are often overlooked. First, it is crucial that nursing takes account of the contribution it has itself made over the years to the perpetuation of the ideology behind these images. Secondly, there needs to be greater recognition of the positive effect that appropriate media images can have. So, for example, Holloway notes how there has been a progression from the notion of 'nurse' being totally encapsulated within the notion of 'woman' to the current representations which emphasize more fully nurses as workers.

Ruth Chadwick (Chapter 3) tackles another issue of contemporary concern. As the current trend in health care provision moves more towards a market-based system, this produces some problems for nurses. In particular, Chadwick considers the ethical issues involved in advertising by nurses, which in turn raises questions about the wearing of logos on uniforms, advertising in the health care environment, and commercial sponsorship. The specific focus is on the appropriateness or otherwise of the recent statement by the United Kingdom Central Council for Nursing, Midwifery and Health Visiting (UKCC) on these issues. In fact, Chadwick examines and then challenges the applicability, in the health care context, of the standard justifications of advertising.

Brian Francis, Moira Peelo and Keith Soothill (Chapter 4) maintain that the demand for higher pay for nurses has provided a narrow focus for widely expressed concern about the National Health Service in recent years. Their work shows how nurses are not a homogeneous group; instead they have differing attitudes to the NHS and to nursing. The authors' use of a probabilistic clustering technique known as latent class analysis identified four groups with very different perceptions of nursing. They argue that, to meet the nursing demands of the future, we need to come to terms with meeting the needs of *each* of these various groups of nurses.

Part I concludes with a focus by Christine Henry on conceptions of the nature of persons. This contribution indicates how philosophical approaches may be helpful in seeking to understand what is meant by the concept of the person. This discussion is a prerequisite before Henry goes on to suggest that a better comprehension of the concept is necessarily central for good health care. In examining the ethical and educational implications of the various conceptions leading to some recommendations for the education of nurses, doctors and teachers, this chapter provides a useful platform for Part II on education.

CHAPTER ONE

Nursing and doctoring: where's the difference?

Lesley Mackay

Introduction

In recent research into nurses' recruitment and wastage, the relationship between doctors and nurses has often been reported to be unsatisfactory (e.g. Mackay 1989). Nurses, and in particular junior nurses, spoke of being ignored by doctors. Some doctors wouldn't even look at a student nurse or an enrolled nurse. When these doctors wanted information, only a staff nurse or a sister would do. It became apparent that patient care must suffer when communication between doctors and nurses could not take place because a nurse didn't have enough stripes on her cap. Not only does patient care suffer but valuable time and energy are wasted looking, or waiting, for the 'right' nurse to talk to. When communication between members of the health care team is poor, everyone suffers. Inter-professional relationships between all members of the health care team are important. But none is more important than that between nurses and doctors.

Despite the critical importance of inter-professional relationships in hospitals, it is an area which has not been researched systematically. Yet it is through the 'sieve' of the hospital that all health care professionals proceed. The relationships encountered within the hospital are likely to be replayed or at least reflected in the relationships between health care workers in the community.

At Lancaster University we decided to undertake research into inter-professional relations between doctors and nurses in hospitals. We have received funding from the Economic and Social

Research Council to carry out the investigation. Once the pilot survey had been conducted and our ideas clarified, we conducted fieldwork in five locations in Scotland and England which included teaching and non-teaching hospitals. As little research has been undertaken in this area, our investigation is very much exploratory in nature. Our aims have been to provide a 'map' of the working relationships between nurses and doctors – the difficulties and the successes in day-to-day working relations.

We have conducted interviews with 25 nurses and 25 doctors at each location. The nurses interviewed were staff nurses or sister/charge nurses. The doctors were house officers, senior house officers, registrars, senior registrars and consultants. We chose to concentrate on five main specialties: general medicine, general surgery, psychiatry, medicine for the elderly, and intensive care. In keeping with the exploratory nature of the research, we used semi-structured interviews.

Ideal types

In previous research into nurse recruitment and wastage (Mackay 1989), we asked nurses about their conceptions of the 'good nurse'. From nurses at the top to those newly embarking on nursing, there was broad agreement on the attributes of the good nurse. We wished to investigate this area further. How did the description of a doctor's ideal nurse compare with that of a nurse? What was the 'good doctor' like? Did nurses and doctors have similar views as to their ideal doctor?

Nurses' and doctors' views regarding ideal types of the good nurse and the good doctor are built up from a variety of sources. The socialization that takes place during training ensures that the views of the newcomers soon come to reflect those of older colleagues. In our previous research we found surprising similarity between the views of first-year nursing students and nursing officers as to the attributes that made a 'good nurse'. (For an interesting discussion of socialization of nurses, see Conway 1983, and for a personal view of the socialization of a doctor, see Marinker 1974.) Personal experience and knowledge are combined with stereotypes from the mass media. (The way in which nurses are portrayed in the electronic media is reported by Kalisch and Kalisch 1986, and see Chapter 2 in this volume. For a view of the way the medical profession is presented in the media, see Karpf 1988.)

The notion of a 'good nurse' and a 'good doctor' is implicit in many of the opinions and attitudes of doctors and nurses. The notion serves as a benchmark for their own and the other group's behaviour at work. To some extent, it is a standard against which members of one's own and the other group are measured. We asked both nurses and doctors to describe 'the good nurse' and 'the good doctor'. For ease of reporting only, nurses will be referred to as female and doctors as male. (It is worth noting, however, that although half of all medical students are now female this has not yet altered the assumption of nurses in general conversation that doctors are male.)

'The good nurse': *the nurses' view*

For nurses, the 'good nurse' is caring and sensitive to the needs of patients. The aspects emphasized by nurses centre on the way a nurse relates to her patients: the need to be genuine, understanding, patient, kind. The good nurse will listen and communicate well. She will be approachable and she will have time to talk. At the same time the good nurse has to be assertive and to remain calm whatever the circumstances. For the most part, the attributes of the good nurse are personal characteristics. While such attributes can be developed, they cannot be learned. (Gamarnikow 1978 points to the similarities between the 'good nurse' and the 'good woman'.)

The emphasis which nurses place on 'character' may be a reflection of the continuing influence of Florence Nightingale (see Baly 1986 for an appreciation of the influence of Florence Nightingale). Nightingale stressed the importance of the personal character of the nurse rather than training or skills. In her view, the good nurse was kind, compassionate and patient. Such a nurse is born not made. (For discussions of the dynamics regarding the image of the nurse, see Ehrenreich and English 1973 and Salvage 1985.) As the good nurse cannot be 'made', the value set upon training and the development of skill is not great. I have argued elsewhere that nurses do not sufficiently value their training and the skills they develop (Mackay 1989).

'The good nurse': *the doctors' view*

For doctors, the 'good nurse' is competent at her job: she knows about her patients, she will anticipate problems and she will use her initiative. While it is important for a good nurse to be sensitive to the needs of patients, it is even more important for her to act as a first line of defence for doctors. The good nurse will act as the doctor's 'eyes and ears' on the ward in his absence and be someone on whom he can rely. And doctors are often absent from the ward. The good nurse will be willing and able to contribute information towards patient management. At the same time, the good nurse will ensure that doctors are not 'pestered' unnecessarily or thoughtlessly. Doctors are in a position of considerable dependence on the judgements of nursing staff as, for example, when to summon the doctor.

'The good nurse': *differences of opinion*

An important difference in the descriptions of the good nurse given by doctors and nurses is that relating to 'skill'. Although some nurses mention the need for the good nurse to be competent and good at her job, the emphasis is on character rather than on skills. For medical staff, character is secondary to competence. Competence means that a nurse knows when a patient needs attention; she can take decisions; she knows what she's doing, and the ward runs smoothly. At the same time, competence comes through experience and through knowledge. It is an attribute which can be acquired. Thus, while nurses appear to maintain a belief that nurses are 'born not made', doctors value the skills which are acquired through training. It is worth noting in passing that nurses, in explaining why they took up nursing, frequently say that it is 'something I always wanted to do'. Doctors, on the other hand, often mention that they entered medicine because they had the requisite number and grades of 'A' levels or that they were encouraged to enter medicine by their schools. In other words, nurses' reasons for their career choice tend to focus on some idea of vocation while doctors' choices focus on academic attainment.

It is noteworthy that doctors emphasize the skill aspect, the learned component, of work activity. They, after all, go through extensive training in which the level of their knowledge and skill becomes all important. Primarily, doctors are trained as scientists. A glance at any prospectus for a British medical school will illustrate the importance of the scientific perspective. An emphasis on the scientific is made at the expense of an emphasis on a sense of vocation. For admission to medical school, academic attainments appear to be all important. However, the thrust of this comment does need qualifying in the light of Johnson's (1971) persuasive research which has shown that type of school and medical family connections are particularly important in selecting medical students. It appears that relatively little scrutiny is given to the personal characteristics of potential doctors. From the prospectuses of UK medical schools it also appears that few doctors receive more than a token input during their training regarding interpersonal relations. Yet it is these interpersonal relations on which nurses place so much weight. There appears to be a fundamental difference in the orientations of those who recruit and train in medicine and nursing.

Given the processes of socialization, it is not surprising that both doctors and nurses emphasize the attributes which are valued within their own occupation. Correspondingly, nurses and doctors attach less value to the attributes valued in the other occupation.

'The good doctor': *the nurses' view*

Nurses' evaluations of the 'good doctor' centre repeatedly on the way patients are treated. The good doctor does not rush patients, he will spend time talking with them and he will listen carefully to what they have to say. He will take time to tell patients what is being planned for them with regard to their treatments. The good doctor also needs to be a listener – to nursing staff as well as to patients. Indeed, the good doctor seeks, and listens to, advice from nurses. He consults nurses, treating them as equals and he is receptive to their opinions. A few nurses, but they are a minority, mention the need for a doctor to be competent and to know what he is doing. Again, for nurses, the emphasis is upon interpersonal skills rather than on skills as a medical practitioner. (That is not to say that a bad or incompetent doctor is tolerated by nurses.)

'The good doctor': *the doctors' view*

Doctors' evaluations of the good doctor mainly focus on the level of skill. The good doctor should, above all, be competent at his job. At the same time he should be inquisitive, decisive, and not too 'businesslike' with patients. Similarly, the good doctor should be approachable and willing to spend time with patients.

'The good doctor': *differences of opinion*

In comparing the views of nurses and doctors, there was a clear difference in the priorities regarding the good doctor. Nurses emphasized doctors' 'approach' to patients; doctors emphasized the skills required. Although nurses very much value the doctor who seeks their advice and uses their experience, this aspect was only occasionally mentioned by doctors.

As noted earlier, nurses and doctors particularly value attributes in the other group which are valued within their own occupation. Yet if these ideals were achieved and doctors, say, were to increase the importance they accorded to interpersonal skills, it would negatively affect nurses' claims to have a distinctive competence which sets them apart, and is worthy of respect, from doctors.

The attributes valued by doctors and nurses underline a difference in perception as to priorities in hospital health care that has considerable implications in the current debates. Nurses, on the one hand, emphasize 'getting to know the patient as a person', while doctors emphasize 'getting to the root of the problem' with the aim of correctly and speedily diagnosing 'the problem'. While the medical profession focuses on the biophysical, nursing focuses on the illness, 'a concept referring to the broader subjective experiences and practical difficulties faced by patients' (Campbell-Heider and Pollock 1987). The medical profession would argue, quite rightly, that the primary concern of the patient is the diagnosis and cure of the problem for which the patient was admitted. Nursing staff would argue, again quite rightly, that, in order to treat a patient effectively, many different aspects of the patient ought to be taken into consideration. The tension between the two perspectives is highlighted in decisions about when to stop 'active treatment' of patients. Thus, nurses often say that doctors want to pursue treatment 'to the bitter end', while they would prefer some patients to be left to die in peace and with dignity.

Doctors say that they have a duty to do everything they can to save life and that nurses do not have to bear the final responsibility for patients' lives.

The difference between what nurses do and what doctors do

The doctors and nurses we interviewed were asked to 'describe the difference between what a nurse does and what a doctor does'. The question was aimed at obtaining descriptions of the relation between nursing and medicine. The question essentially asks for a contrast to be made between the roles. And, to state the obvious, it is a question which emphasizes differences rather than similarities. This is an important point because in quite a number of areas the tasks of nurses and doctors, especially junior doctors, overlap.

This task overlap between (junior) doctors and nurses is not often mentioned when doctors and nurses are asked to describe the differences in their work. On the few occasions that the blurring of roles between nurses and doctors was mentioned, it was primarily from doctors and nurses working within psychiatry.

'The difference': *the doctors' view*

Doctors' descriptions of the difference focus on the central role that doctors see themselves as occupying: doctors give the orders; doctors diagnose and prescribe; doctors have the final say. Nurses are seen by doctors as obeying the doctor's orders, administering the treatment, and undertaking 'basic care'. Primarily it is a power relationship which is being described by these doctors. The doctor has the power: he prescribes, he initiates, he decides and he orders.

'The difference': *the nurses' view*

In the nurses' descriptions of the difference, they use the same words as the doctors. For example, 'doctors decide what nurses are going to do'; 'they (doctors) decide what needs doing and we

do it'; 'doctors prescribe and nurses carry it out'. As with the
doctors' descriptions, there is an explicit acceptance of a power
relationship: the one giving orders, the other following orders.
Campbell-Heider and Pollock (1987) comment: 'nurses accept the
notion that only a physician can diagnose a health problem; they
rely on the physician for decision-making and reflect passive-
dependent behaviours; the doctor is reinforced as the "captain";
and the whole process is so subtle that the rationale for this
behaviour is actually distorted.'

'The difference': *a comparison*

The caring role and the practical role which nurses carry out are
mentioned often by both doctors and nurses. But doctors make
little mention of the close relationship that nurses enjoy with
patients, while nurses quite often refer to this aspect. Thus, nurses
will refer to 'looking after the whole patient' or being 'involved
with everything to do with the patient'. Some nurses describe
themselves as being 'the patient's advocate', but this role was not
mentioned by the doctors (for a summary of the arguments
relating to this role see Castledine 1981 and Chapter 10 in this
book). At the same time, nothing about the doctor's relationship
with the patient was ever mentioned by either nurses or doctors.

The nurse's role is often viewed in extremely limited terms by
doctors. Thus nurses look after the 'basic functions' of patients –
give patients their food; wash the patients. Some doctors
emphasize the importance of the basic work, pointing out that
nurses give continual, 24-hour care and that nurses have an
intimate contact with patients that doctors lack. Yet, again and
again, the lack of decision-making power is implicit in the doctors'
comments. Nurses 'act out what we say'; they 'administer the
prescribed treatment'; and they 'facilitate our work'. The nurse's
role here is one of support. It is not one of equivalence. Only
occasionally does a doctor refer to teamwork in describing the
difference between what nurses and doctors do.

The stark division between doctors ordering and nurses obeying
is less clear cut for those nurses who see their role as prescribing
nursing care. In the view of these nurses, nursing has a distinct
area of expertise which is not under the direction of the medical
profession. (The presence of two conflicting ideologies in nursing
– nurses as autonomous professionals and nurses as subordinates

to doctors – has been commented on elsewhere – Devine 1978.)
Doctors did not mention any such distinct or discrete area of
competence of nursing staff.

Discrepancies between the two questions

The descriptions of the good nurse and doctor contrast with the
perceptions of differences between what nurses and doctors do.
The good nurse who uses her initiative is simultaneously seen by
some doctors simply as being involved in carrying out basic care.
The doctor who describes nurses as doing bedpans and washing
patients also wants the good nurse to 'pick up what he's missed'.
Doctors who stress the centrality of their own diagnostic role and
their direction of the activities of nursing staff, at the same time
want the good nurse to be 'capable of assessing patients'. Thus, in
response to one question, there is a denial of the need for nurses to
be skilled, yet, in response to the second question, the high value
placed on a skilled nurse is asserted. Why? One possible answer is
in the great disparity in pay, status and career prospects of doctors
in comparison with nurses. Thus, doctors may need to defend that
disparity by maintaining the high level of skill required by
doctors and the relatively low level of skill required to be a nurse.
Yet, in the actual working situation, the reality is that doctors
depend extensively on nurses for information. Nurses who lack in
skill and expertise are likely to cause doctors a great deal of
additional and unnecessary work.

It is worth noting that nurses are aware of undertaking
diagnoses, as when, for example, they are taking decisions about
calling a doctor to see a patient. Doctors are aware of this aspect
of the nurse's role, but its importance is played down. There is an
acceptance, say, that nurses undertake basic assessments of
patients, but less attention is given to the 'intuitive' decision taken
by a nurse to call a doctor because the patient is 'not right'. In
fact, the experience which is required in reaching 'intuitive'
decisions appears not to be recognized by doctors and to be
insufficiently recognized by nurses. Nevertheless, these diagnoses
are essentially interim diagnoses only. The fact that they can
contribute to saving life is another matter. There is a widespread
recognition amongst nurses (and doctors) that doctors take the
final and the ultimate decisions and responsibility for the care of

patients. (The dominance of doctors can be illusory; see Stein 1967 and Hughes 1988.)

Some nurses, while describing the directing and ordering role of doctors, also see the good doctor as one who treats nursing staff as equals and/or who is prepared to work as part of a team. It is difficult to see how a group which is seen to bear the final responsibility for patients can realistically be expected to treat as equal a group which carries out their orders. It is also difficult to see the current relationship between doctors and nurses as being other than unequal. After all, the majority of these nurses and doctors attest to the decision-making role of the medical profession and the need for nurses to carry out doctors' orders. This is not, however, to say that these nurses see themselves in the role of 'handmaiden'. Indeed, such a label is abhorred by most nurses.

It appears that both doctors and nurses, in describing the good nurse and the good doctor respectively, set out an ideal which mirrors their own activites. Yet, in describing the differences in the work roles, the work of nurses is simplified by doctors. Similarly, the unilateral decision-making role of doctors is emphasized. At the same time, the division between nurses and doctors is enlarged, in denial of the interdependent nature of the relationship between doctors and nurses. The need for the nurse to act as 'the eyes and the ears' of the doctor, for her to undertake some level of diagnosis and for her to make decisions and initiate action are ignored in the contrasts between roles. It seems that, when pressed, doctors seldom make reference to ideas of teamwork or of working together as equals. This is nothing new. As Mackie (1984) has noted: 'Despite the doctor's dependence on a reliable surrogate, he has until recently refused to acknowledge the registered nurse either as a member of an emerging discipline with a unique contribution to the nation's health or even as a junior partner within his authority.'

Conclusion

Essentially, the questions about the good doctor and the good nurse and about the difference between what each does have probed the attitudes of nurses and doctors to one another. And it is worth noting that many of the difficulties and conflicts which doctors and nurses report in everyday working relationships centre on the attitudes displayed to one another. The difficulties reported regarding attitudes may well be a reflection of the contradictory nature of these attitudes. It seems that nurses want doctors to exhibit the characteristics of the good nurse and doctors want nurses to exhibit the characteristics of the good doctor.

The comments regarding the good nurse and the good doctor are perhaps more revealing of the subjects whose opinions were sought than of the objects they described. Nurses and doctors are sensible in setting a high value on their own skills. However, in seeking to find a reflection of one's own skills in the work of another group, there is an implicit denial of that other group's contribution. Doctors are not as good at their interpersonal skills as nurses. Nurses are not diagnosticians or decision-makers regarding medical treatment. Each group has its own sphere of competence, to which greater recognition needs to be given by the other. Neither, as one doctor and one nurse pointed out, can work on their own. The current irony, however, is that doctors seem to want nurses to be like doctors and, similarly, nurses want doctors to be like nurses. This is not a helpful way forward. Perhaps some of the tensions encountered in working together could be overcome if the special contribution which each group has to make was more fully recognized.

Acknowledgements

The author is a member of the team on the ESRC project (Grant Number R000 23 1394) at Lancaster University on the inter-professional relations of doctors and nurses. The team is grateful to the various health authorities concerned for their help and support in this work.

References

Baly, M. E. 1986. *Florence Nightingale and the Nursing Legacy*, London: Croom Helm.
Campbell-Heider, N. and Pollock, D. 1987. Barriers to physician-nurse collegiality: an anthropological perspective. *Social Science and Medicine* 25(5): 421–5.

Castledine, G. 1981. The nurse as the patient's advocate – pros and cons. *Nursing Mirror*, 11 November, 153(20): 38–40.

Conway, M. E. 1983. Socialization and roles in nursing. *Annual Review of Nursing Research* 1: 183–208.

Devine, B. A. 1978. Nurse-physician interaction: status and social structure within two hospital wards. *Journal of Advanced Nursing* 3: 287–95.

Ehrenreich, B. and English, D. 1973. *Witches, Midwives and Nurses: a history of women healers*. New York: Feminist Press.

Gamarnikow, E. 1978. Sexual division of labour: the case of nursing. In A. Kuhn and A. Wolpe (eds), *Feminism and Materialism*. London: Routledge & Kegan Paul.

Hughes, D. 1988. When nurse knows best: some aspects of nurse/doctor interaction in a casualty department. *Sociology of Health and Illness* 10(1): 1–22.

Johnson, M. L. 1971. A comparison of the social characteristics and academic achievement of medical students and unsuccessful medical school applicants. *British Journal of Medical Education* 5(4): 260–3.

Kalisch, P. and Kalisch, B. 1986. A comparative analysis of nurse and physician characters in the entertainment media. *Journal of Advanced Nursing* 11: 179–95.

Karpf, A. 1988. *Doctoring the Media*. London: Routledge.

Mackay, L. 1989. *Nursing a Problem*. Milton Keynes; Open University Press.

Mackie, L. 1984. Chapter in A. Duncan and G. McLachlan (eds), *Hospital Medicine and Nursing in the 1980s: Interaction between the professions of medicine and nurse*. London: Nuffield Provincial Hospitals Trust.

Marinker, M. 1974. Medical education and human values. *Journal of the Royal College of General Practitioners* 24: 445–62.

Salvage, J. 1985. *The Politics of Nursing*. London: Heinemann.

Stein, L. 1967. The doctor–nurse game. *Archives of General Psychiatry* 16: 699–703.

CHAPTER TWO

The media representation of the nurse: the implications for nursing

Joanne Holloway

Introduction

The representation of 'the nurse' within media depictions is increasingly being considered an issue of great concern. The way in which nurses are portrayed is believed to have implications in general for the status of nursing in society.

Most of the literature around this topic emerges from the United States. The main protagonists are Kalisch and Kalisch (1983, 1986, 1987), who have particularly concentrated on the historical changes of media representations of the nurse and the implications these images have for nursing. In the United Kingdom, the nursing press has been the body which has given the highest profile to this issue. In 1983, the *Nursing Times* ran the 'Public Image of the Nurse' campaign and currently, on alternate weeks, it runs a page ('Synapse' and 'Media Watch') where readers are encouraged to send in examples of 'negative images' of the nurse. In practical terms an exercise such as this is useful in raising awareness, providing a forum for debate and defining what is objected to (Betterton 1987).

However, a simple advocation of more 'positive' or 'real' images of nursing is problematic. The media, certainly in their fictional form, do not directly set out to recreate reality. More broadly, the media are not simply a mirror of the world. As Kappeler (1986: 3) highlights (with particular reference to pornography): 'Representations are not just a matter of mirrors, reflections, keyholes. Somebody is looking at them through a complex array of meanings and conventions.' For these kinds of reasons there will be a consideration of the meaning and ideology behind the way in which nurses are portrayed in the media and not so much concern with notions of positive and negative images.

Media, in this context, will be defined in their broadest terms. This not only includes aural, visual and written media associated with contemporary society, but also will incorporate the way in which these transmitters of ideas are utilized historically – how, for example, texts concerning the history of nursing identify and concentrate on particular historical events and ignore others (Salvage 1985). This creates a history of nursing which is used to perpetuate a particular ideology about the status and role of nursing both in society and within nursing itself. In brief, therefore, the representations of the nurse within the media will be seen to be only part of a wider discourse which overall defines and forms the social status of nursing.

An important element within this wider discourse is the fact that the vast majority of nurses are women or, more specifically, nursing is seen as a female occupation. Hence, the way in which nurses are represented has common ground with the way that women are represented within the media in general.

The issue of nursing's public image and its relation to representations produced in the media is certainly important. As Kalisch and Kalisch (1986: 193) note: 'an understanding what image power is, how it is acquired, how it can be lost and how it affects resource allocation decisions could well determine whether nursing will move forward or be left behind in the coming decade.' The issue of 'public image' is also emphasized by Austin *et al.* (1985), who advocate that nursing needs to obtain a better understanding of its present 'image' in order to progress.

Ideology and stereotypes

Four stereotypes

The detrimental images which have been highlighted by the nursing press largely fall into four main stereotypes – the angel, the handmaiden/non-entity, the battle-axe and the sex symbol. These stereotypes are important not only because nurses themselves feel that these stereotypes are detrimental, but also because they are particularly well defined in terms of popular images within the visual and/or written media.

The notion of stereotype often implies a fixity in image (Betterton 1987), but the way in which nurses are represented in the media will be shown to be changing. It will be argued that these changes in the way in which nurses are represented in the media come not so much from nursing striving for more 'positive' or 'realistic' images of itself, but from changes within nursing. These changes are ones which involve nursing asserting its strength and importance with regard to the role it plays in health care. Current shifts in nursing practice offer a challenge to the stereotypes which suggest that the nursing role is 'passive' and is of less importance to health care than the medical profession.

At this stage three points are relevant. First, the particular way in which nurses are represented in the media supports and reinforces a general belief system in society about the status and role of nurses. Secondly, in recognizing the media as one element of a larger discourse of perception formation, an analysis of the meaning and messages behind these images will enhance a greater understanding of the factors which contribute to nursing's status. This issue is of particular importance when nursing is attempting to instigate change. The third point is that many campaigners actively campaign to eliminate detrimental images of nurses. Action such as this remains important, although not sufficient. In order that there is an effective challenge to the way in which the nurse is represented in the media, there needs to be a greater understanding of the structures which support the ideology within which these representations are embedded.

What is the ideology behind the stereotypical images?

The ideology behind the media representation of the nurse is epitomized by four stereotypical images and their derivatives. These images will be seen to incorporate particular meanings which are related to the underlying ideology. Thus, these images will be seen to be one way by which the ideology itself is transmitted.

It will be argued that these stereotypical images in the media arise from an ideology which is two-fold and paradoxical. Thus, the meaning entrenched within these images forms part of an ideology which informs that, first, nurses are women (this helps to maintain secondary job status) and secondly, but paradoxically, nurses have potential 'power/control' over individuals' lives which in patriarchal terms must be reduced. This latter aspect particularly relates to the vulnerability of the male patient with respect to the female nurse.

It is useful to consider what exactly is meant by ideology in this context. For this purpose it is useful to use Hall's analysis (in Bridges and Brunt 1981) of the concept of ideology. Hall (1981: 31) argues first that (with reference to racism) 'ideologies do not consist of isolated and separate concepts, but in the articulation of different elements into a distinctive set or chain of meanings'. A second important point which Hall raises relates to the unconscious aspect of ideology. In other words, not only do the ideas purveyed from within an ideology become seen as 'common sense' but also, as Hall notes (1981: 31), 'ideologies are not the product of individual consciousness or intention. Rather we formulate our intentions *within ideology*'. Thus, this notion of ideology is complex, yet in everyday terms is thought to reflect commonsense beliefs. These concerns highlight the entrenched nature of this ideology within representations of the nurse.

The very fact that the ideology itself incorporates a paradoxical duality necessitates a complex set of images to reflect both aspects in the maintenance of the status of nursing and to undermine nurses' potential control.

From image to stereotype

An 'image' can be defined as a particular set of ideas which, whether heard, seen or read, conjures up a particular visual image or group of images. In specific terms, such images lead to a particular attitude about nursing. These images do not exist in isolation, nor are they necessarily ends in themselves. These images are part of our culture (Kuhn 1982).

Stereotyping involves the assimilation of social information into mental representations. The assimilated material is dependent on information formed from the individual's experience in various social settings. From these mental representations the individual is able to make broad assessments of the 'normal' activities of groups predominantly based around sex, race, job role and age (Kaler *et al.* 1989). Thus, the formation of stereotypes is a socially constructed process and the categories which result are based on societal norms.

The most important implication of stereotyping in this context is that of sex stereotyping. Many occupations besides nursing have stereotypes associated with them (Gallagher 1987), but, according to Kaler *et al.* (1989: 85), 'Sex stereotyping has been accused of preventing the public from viewing the nurse as an educated professional; it instead has created the vision of the nurse as, first and foremost, a woman'. Stereotyping from this point of view maintains the association between nursing and women. This association is obviously in reality quite true (although this does not necessarily mean it must always be so). However, in terms of the ideology, the association of nursing with femaleness is only part of this message.

'Good' nurse and 'bad' nurse

The four stereotypes, which are seen to encapsulate the meanings of the ideology, can be incorporated within a dichotomy of 'good' nurse, 'bad' nurse. Thus, the angel and the handmaiden stereotypes conform to notions of 'goodness' and battle-axe and sex symbol conform to notions of 'badness'. While this polarization of good and bad meanings within one ideology increases the complexity of this ideology, it is necessary to facilitate its dual purpose of maintaining the status quo and of undermining the threat of the potential power of female nurses to 'normal' patriarchal relations. It is relevant when Muff (1982) highlights the fact that notions of women simultaneously representing 'supreme good and basest evil' were endemic within ancient mythology. Being embedded in history in this way makes such a dichotomy and such stereotypes even more entrenched.

Each of the stereotypical images will now be considered in turn.

Nurses as angels

The association of 'nurse' with 'angel' is a common occurrence in the media. It is an association which in contemporary contexts is particularly connected with the press, but it also has had visual depictions within television and film. The image itself is associated with particular attributes, that is, those which define the nurse as virtuous, dedicated and altruistic.

Within the context of television, there have been such occurrences as the title *Angels* (1976–1983) for a hospital-based soap opera, which highlights the 'normality' of the nurse/angel association. The main visual representation of the angel-type nurse has been most associated with turn of the century Hollywood films (Kalisch and Kalisch 1987). This particular depiction of nurses in the First World War was popular in the 1920s. Kalisch and Kalisch (1987: 52) identify a common thread to all the war films starring nurse characters: 'Not only is the nurse portrayed as noble and courageous – a veritable martyr to German evil – but the nursing identification assures that she dies with all her redeemed virtue.' The importance of these films was related to their support of the 'war effort', showing that women could play an important role. However, as Kalisch and Kalisch (1987: 5) note, 'The nursing identification provided an effective way to mask the novelty of female independence with traditional female values'.

More recently – at a time when nurses were striking over the state of the NHS and pay – an analysis of the *Nursing Times* during 1988 revealed many references to the notion of angels or to the attributes implied by this image. Thus, referring to the strike in February 1988 on the London radio station (LBC) there were headlines such as 'The Striking Angels' and 'Nurses' Halos Remain Intact', and in the provincial press headlines of 'Fallen Angels on the Picket Line' (*Nursing Times*, 10 February 1988).

The notion of 'angels' was used by newspapers in trying to overcome the dilemma of whether or not to support a nurses' strike. This was seen as a particular problem because the nurses were generally enjoying public sympathy. The problem was reconciled by newspapers sympathizing with the reasons for the action, but not supporting strike action (Vousden 1988). Hence, headlines such as 'Fallen Angels' have a complex message to carry. Certainly, the notion of 'angel' contains within it ideas of what it is to be a 'good' nurse, a tradition in the media which had been embodied in many of the images of the early Hollywood films.

Nurse as handmaiden/non-entity

Handmaiden and non-entity images have been grouped together as they both imply similar ideas about nursing.

The type of media representation in which nurses are depicted as handmaiden or non-entity are endemic within television and film. These representations tend to occur in any situation which focuses on the medical role. Handmaiden images depict nurses in such situations as: following doctors' orders, assisting doctors and appearing to have no autonomy of their own. Similarly, non-entity images relate to the depiction of nurses as purely background features – for example, walking the corridors or answering telephones and not generally participating in nursing activities.

The image has been particularly evident since the 1960s when hospital soap dramas became popular. An export from the United States, *Dr Kildare*, epitomized this. In *Dr Kildare*, medical treatment and the character of Dr Kildare were central to the plot. There were many nurses in the background who were a routine part of the programme, yet whose characters and roles were seriously undeveloped. According to Kalisch *et al.* (1983: 193), 'unexamined and unemphasized, these nurses nevertheless have exerted a tremendous influence on the audience perception of the role of nursing in the contemporary hospital routine'.

The handmaiden/non-entity image is also reflected within health documentaries. A *40 Minutes* production shown in 1989 about open heart surgery performed on a baby reflected this. Great emphasis was placed on the surgeon's role, with very little emphasis on the nurses' role in providing pre-operative care to child and parents. Similarly, post-operative care in the Intensive Care Unit tended to concentrate on medical intervention in nursing care.

With these images nurses are seen to be not only subservient to doctors, but also 'controlled by them'. So, for example, mentioning the pay award, the *Wrexham Evening Leader* (22 April 1988) commented: 'The 15.3% pay award for nurses is just what the doctor ordered' (*Nursing Times*, 6 July 1988, p. 23).

These images convey the message not only that nurses are subservient to doctors, but, more particularly, that in terms of patient recovery the nurses' role is of secondary importance to that of the doctors. The study of Kalisch and Kalisch (1986: 185) stresses that 'the contribution of the nurse to health care as portrayed in the entertainment media has been distinctly under-played, and conversely the role of the physician has been presented in an exaggerated, idealistic, and heroic light'.

The implications of the meanings transmitted within the angel and the handmaiden image have similar intentions. Entrenched within both images are notions of the maintenance of the status quo. This is achieved in two ways, first by offering no challenge to the status quo and secondly (and relatedly) by assuming a secondary job status of nursing to the medical profession.

Nurses as sex symbols

The image of the nurse which specifically emphasizes her sexuality is a newer image, yet one which has been around from the 1950s and was still prominent in the 1980s (Kalisch *et al.* 1983). This image ultimately focuses on the nurses' appearance and is utilized in a range of media, epitomized visually from the 'Barbara Windsor' nurse of the *Carry On* films to pornographic images. The fact that the sex-symbol image covers such a wide spectrum of images, from the flirtatious to the pornographic, is an indication of the diversity of forms which this representation takes. All of the representations though emphasize the nurse's sexual availability as a woman.

In terms of the representation of nurses, an emphasis on sexuality is a method of creating a 'meaning' which defines that nurses' appearances are more important than the job that nurses do. Thus, nurses' 'value' is attained not through their work but through such attributes as appearance and sexual availability.

The 'popularity' of the representation of sexual availability is evident across a wide range of media genres. The soap opera *The Young Doctors* particularly highlights the concentration on sexual availability and appearance. Thus, the nurses tend to be attractive and slim with immaculate hair and makeup. Their flirtatiousness and sexuality are emphasized by tight-fitting and short uniforms.

Within popular films this image is often in evidence. Thus, in *Carry On* films, for example in *Carry On Nurse*, Barbara Windsor plays a nurse who is depicted as sexy, brainless and flirtatious with doctors and patients. This image is made more potent by the fact that 'her sexy nurse is interchangeable with all the other dumb blonde charaters she portrays' (Salvage 1985: 22). Thus, a close association is maintained between nurse and femininity.

Nurse as battle-axe

This stereotype is mostly applied to nurses who are older and who have developed their careers within nursing (i.e. they tend to have reached 'matron' status, as it continues to be referred to within the media). These 'battle-axe' nurses are portrayed as having an authoritarian, autocratic and uncompromising attitude, which is vented on junior nurses, doctors and also patients.

The 'battle-axe' nurse is most often depicted in film, particularly comedy. The most familiar example can again be seen in the *Carry On* films. In *Carry On Doctor*, for example, there is the matronly figure played by Hattie Jacques. Here the matron is portrayed as a person who has authority and control over the lives of everyone from patient to doctor. She is uncompromising in the wielding of her power. Yet ultimately she is undermined by being made a fool of.

Similarly, the character of 'Big Nurse' in *One Flew Over the Cuckoo's Nest* revenged herself on men by making the patients' lives a misery (Muff 1982). According to Kalisch and Kalisch (1987), the depiction of Nurse Ratched is of a woman who has a maternal attitude to her patients and does seem to care, yet has an obsessive–compulsive personality needing to control the lives of her patients totally.

The meaning incorporated within this stereotype relates to two important elements: first, the fact that the nurse has progressed in terms of career and, secondly, that she is unmarried (most of these representations are of single women).

This particular image is problematic as it does not allow nurses any critical, evaluative or analytical skills in their work. Thus, there is a need to impose rigorous tasks, rules and regulations so that there is no need for the nurse to think for herself.

The implications of this stereotype again can be related to stereotypes of women. By failing to get married, the woman has undermined patriarchal, societal norms. As well as this, such an image works in collaboration with the sex-symbol stereotype by undermining 'the nurse' in order to reduce the threat or the potential power which the nurse may have in relation to the vulnerability of the (male) patient.

The ideology and the representations

The meanings and implications characterized within the four identified stereotypical representations of the nurse need to be related to the underlying ideology. Despite the paradoxical nature of the ideology, there is a 'common thread' of nursing being a female occupation. Research by Austin *et al.* (1985) has revealed that the concepts of 'nurse' and 'feminine' are associated in people's minds. Both of them were perceived as good and active, yet both were seen as having very little power.

Further research in the United States by Kaler *et al.* (1989) aimed at seeing how the public rated nursing in relation to other professions based on certain personality attributes concluded (p. 87) that 'The public image of the nurse continues to focus on those characteristics consensually endorsed as being feminine'. The study also revealed that nurses rated highly on helping skills and concern for others. From this it can be suggested that nursing is a 'metaphor for all things feminine' (Fagin and Diers 1983). In fact, the representations of nurses in the media in their stereotypical form reinforce the association of nursing with women's work.

The implication of such a relationship is indicated in 'Women's Issues' (1989): 'The popular myth of nursing as women's work means that training is given low priority, pay remains low and nurses' status is kept low.' So the juxtaposition of nursing (and its 'female' attributes) with medicine (associated with higher status and authority) – the persisting stereotype of angel and hand-maiden/non-entity – means that the secondary job status of nurses compared with doctors remains unchallenged through a portrayal of servility, passivity and little power. The inequality in this relationship is further exemplified by the fact that doctors are given what Karpf (1988a) refers to as 'legitimating power'. Thus, the media tend to attribute 'objective' knowledge to doctors, while nurses continue to be associated with the 'feminine realm of caring' (Karpf 1988a: 17). In consequence, these associations undermine nurses' contributions to health care both verbally and practically.

The second aspect of the ideology relates to a situation which could potentially undermine patriarchal relations, i.e. the potential power relation of the female nurse over the patient (particularly referring to male patients). Thus, as Bologh (1979) notes, the patient (male) is undermined not only through illness, but also by his dependence on a woman (nurse). Bologh highlights this argument by using the example of get well cards. In these cards the potential power of nursing is undermined in two possible ways. The first way is through reducing the nurse to a sex object, because, as Bologh (1979: 146) notes, 'The depiction of the nurse as a sexual object may have the effect of boosting the male patient's status as a dominant, hence potent male at a time when his potency is questionable'. The other way of undermining the nurse is through depicting the nurse as powerful, but as an inflictor of discomfort. Thus, the derogatory battle-axe image can be seen as 'determined to inflict physical discomfort or pain on the vulnerable patient' (Bologh 1979: 146). Thus, the potential imbalance is restored by means of the derogatory representations of sex symbol and battle-axe.

Such messages portrayed through the media have implications for nursing. While not arguing for any direct effects transmitted by the media, or ignoring the way in which the audience (as individuals) read and internalize the complexity of meanings by which nurses are portrayed in the media, it must be reasserted that the media form part of the wider discourse which disseminates particular ideas and knowledge about the status of nursing. However, the specific argument proposed here is that the ideology under consideration affects nursing by maintaining the status quo and inhibiting change.

This approach is in contrast to a tendency, for example by Kalisch and Kalisch, to argue in terms of a direct relationship between the way in which nurses are represented in the media and the way (for instance) in which nurses perceive themselves. In brief, Kalisch and Kalisch (1986) argue that the media images directly cause the nurse to have a 'negative' self-image about her job role.

Gallagher (1987) has attempted to challenge such a view by using a questionnaire survey to discover whether there is a relation between nurses' self-image, ideal self-image and media representations. The results revealed that the media did not influence nurses' own self-perception and that self-image did not relate closely to media image, suggesting 'the limited effect of the media image of the nurse as a factor in affecting self-concept change in nurses' (Gallagher 1987: 676).

However, questionnaire analysis is a problematic means of dealing with the notion of 'media effects'. In order to acknowledge the complexity of the functioning and location of media in society, it is more realistic to perceive the media's contribution in terms of a particular working of societal beliefs. Thus, in terms of 'self-image' of nurses, the influence of media representations depends not only on the perceptions of the individual nurse, but also on the internalization of the other messages in society which shape what it is to be a nurse. In particular, there are the contributing factors of the socialization of girls/women in society which is reflected within the stereotype of the angel. As Salvage (1985: 21) notes: 'Many nurses like this image of themselves, and fail to see that it has become a substitute for positive action to improve their pay and conditions.'

In a wider context, the implications of the ideology encompassed by these representations also has relevance at a political level. Indeed, Kalisch and Kalisch (1987: 187) argue that the way in which the media portray nursing forms the basis of policy making:

> If policy makers and their constituents are consistently exposed to images that depict the nurse as merely an unintelligent hand maiden to the physician, then they are much less disposed to pass legislation that gives nurses more autonomy in their practice or to allocate sufficient resources to advance the role of the nurse in health care.

The lack of recognition of their worth is emphasized in particular when nurses as health 'professionals' are not consulted over important documents which directly relate to health issues. The most recent example of this was highlighted by the exclusion of the Chief Nursing Officer from the government-oriented NHS policy board (Salvage 1989b).

Factors contributing to the media representation of the nurse

How particular images come to be represented in the media requires a broader assessment of the location of the media within society. Here it will be argued that the media represent certain ideas, beliefs and knowledge within society. The media do not create these ideas, but neither do they merely reflect. An added complexity is the role which nursing itself has played in emphasizing certain attributes both publicly and through the socialization of nurses within the hospital institution, which has contributed to the maintenance of these images. Thus, both society (in general) and nursing (in particular) will be seen to contribute to the way in which nurses are represented in the media.

An historical assessment of the progress of nursing reveals that the meanings incorporated within the four media stereotypes have a historical basis within society.

So the undermining of nurses as carers and healers is not just a contemporary concern, but has a historical basis. Similarly, the highlighting of the association between nursing and sexual availability, for example, can be seen to have a long history in undermining women's skills. Between the fourteenth and seventeenth centuries, when witches were persecuted for their blasphemous healing skills, one of the criteria for persecution was the association between witches and sexuality. The medieval church wa a misogynist's heaven. Women were perceived as sexual beings and, as pleasure in sex was influenced by the devil, women were condemned: 'In the eyes of the church, all the witch's power was ultimately derived from her sexuality. Her career began with sexual intercourse with the devil' (Ehrenreich and English 1973: 12).

The representation of nurses in the media as doctors' handmaidens or, alternatively, of nursing being of secondary status to medicine has its precursor in the emergence of the male medical profession during the nineteenth century. The role of the healer was taken over by men when the prestige, monetary gain and potential power of the curing skill was realized. The curing skills of men were then positively portrayed by establishing a theoretical and scientific base. Women continued to operate as carers, in the home and subsequently in the hospitals as medical assistants (Ehrenreich and English 1973). The creation of this dichotomy led to the embodiment of women's natural role as carers and ultimately as nurses while the scientific logical role of men was that of medic. From this perspective it can be seen that the origins of the medical profession accompanied by the undermining of women's work in society perpetuated the handmaiden image of the nurse.

Cultural and societal influences are thus important in maintaining particular ideologies. Nursing itself has also collaborated within this process. Salvage (1985) argues that the 'acceptable' face of nursing has been enforced through the socialization and education of nurses. In particular, Salvage (1985: 33) notes:

The authorised version of history that nurses have been given emphasises assumptions and activities which reinforce the status quo, and deliberately avoids or conceals historical evidence of discontent and pressure for change in power relation or working conditions.

This perspective on the history of nursing notes how certain events are emphasized, both within nursing and within society. So, as Salvage (1985) argues, while the work of such nurses as Florence Nightingale is well known, what is certainly not common knowledge is the fact that during the early 1920s there were important strikes by nurses for better pay and conditions. Yet, even Nightingale's story has had imposed upon it a particular reinterpretation. Thus, emphasis remains on her martyr-like devotion rather than on her forward-thinking attempts to remove the control of nursing from the medical profession by striving for nursing autonomy in an attempt to remove the handmaiden image.

Nursing may implicitly perpetuate the ideology behind the representations in the media. Indeed, nursing often utilizes these very images to hide behind. Thus, Salvage (1985: 27) notes that the angel or handmaiden images may be stereotypes which are easier to conform to than to challenge – 'hiding behind them may help to avoid the problems and the pain of relating to patients and clients as equals and as adults'.

Studying the media

It is tempting to leave the discussion at a theoretical level but there needs to be a consideration of how the ideology is perpetuated and possibly modified. Hence, we now focus for analysis on three recent examples of nursing portrayed on television – a documentary, Stitching up the NHS, and two soap operas, Young Doctors and Casualty – and consider these with regard to the existence of stereotypical images of nursing.

STITCHING UP THE NHS

This documentary, televised on 28 August 1989 on Channel 4, set out to assess the effects of the government White Paper on the future of the NHS. The programme specifically considered the effects of the White Paper on community services, but also contemplated the issues of competition and opting out for hospitals wanting to self-govern.

The White Paper has important implications for nurses. The

effects of these proposals have the potential for creating particular problems for hospital nurses by, for example, the need for hospitals to compete for patients. This situation has the potential for creating a conveyor-belt approach to health care.

In fact, the medical perspective dominated not only over other health professionals (particularly nurses) but over patients too. In this programme, not only were nursing issues not discussed, but nursing opinion on more general matters was also absent. Out of a total of 30 people interviewed, 16 were doctors and 3 were nurses. The latter were all senior nurses (a spokesperson for the Royal College of Nursing, a Community Nursing Officer and the chairperson of the Health Visitors' Association). All three spoke articulately, yet no nurse working at 'grass roots' level in the community or in the hospital was interviewed. This contrasts dramatically with medical opinion, which ranged from medical student to consultant.

This kind of documentary implicitly contributes to the maintenance of the current status of nursing. This programme is important not so much in terms of the way in which it portrays nurses at work, but more in its explicit emphasis on the legitimization of the medical contribution to the discussion and its consequent undermining of nursing's 'voice'.

YOUNG DOCTORS

This soap opera set in a general hospital in Australia is a daytime 'soap' which is screened two to three afternoons a week. Its concern is mainly with the lives of the doctors and nurses and other hospital staff rather than with their roles within the hospital and on the wards. Of particular relevance is the fact that, in a small *Nursing Times* survey, 17 per cent of those interviewed felt that *Young Doctors* was the most unflattering portrayal of nurses in the media (*Nursing Times*, 28 January 1987, p. 22).

The stereotypes in this programme are of both the handmaiden/non-entity and the sex-symbol variety. The handmaiden stereotype is particularly evident in doctor/nurse working relationships. Nurses spend much of their time fetching and carrying, answering the telephone or passing on messages for doctors. The non-entity stereotype is perpetuated by nurses often appearing behind the reception desk and performing general administrative duties.

The theme of romance and relationships is prevalent and in particular predominates between doctors and nurses. This reveals in general a romanticization of the doctor/nurse relationship. The notion of romance, whether overt or not, is always implicitly suggested by the sexualization of nurses with regards to their appearance. This is epitomized by the line of one of the doctor characters in the programme commenting on the fact that he would not mind matron's job: 'imagine having the final say with all those sexy little nurses' (*Young Doctors*, 5 January 1990).

There is no doubt that limited stereotypical images of nurses are maintained in what has become an intrinsic part of afternoon television.

CASUALTY

This hospital drama set in an Accident and Emergency Department of a General Hospital was first screened in September 1986. It deals not only with the work of casualty nurses but also with their private lives. Interestingly, this soap drama has received much comment and scrutiny from government and doctors as well as nurses (Cole 1986).

The aspect which these three groups have picked up on is the question of whether *Casualty* represents reality. The notion of reality is a problem not only in terms of the diverse occupational roles undertaken by the nurse, but also in terms of the media being more than a mere reflection of reality. Thus, nurses' actual day-to-day work would not make good soap drama. In contrast, the perceived hi-tech, emergency drama of an Accident and Emergency Department has this potential. As Cole (1986) notes of *Casualty*, the mundane aspects of work are omitted while the excitement, drama and danger aspects are emphasized.

Cole (1986) points out that many real-life casualty nurses he interviewed felt that the emphasis in *Casualty* on the nurses' life styles – for example, drinking alcohol, smoking and 'sleeping around' – was unrealistic.

With respect to the issue of stereotypes, however, it has been argued that *Casualty* has made attempts to overcome conventional stereotypes by utilizing role reversal. This is seen in the situation of a male charge nurse and a female doctor, but, as Cole (1986: 19) notes in his survey of what Accident and Emergency nurses thought of *Casualty*, one nurse comented that it has 'Simply swapped one set of stereotypes for another. The terrifying Sister and the effeminate male nurse have gone, and they've put in a token coloured bloke, a female doctor and an alcoholic'.

Despite these criticisms, a consideration of the representation of nurses in *Casualty* reveals some important developments from their representation in *Young Doctors*. The nurses in *Casualty* are portrayed as playing an important part in patient care in the Accident and Emergency Department. The care given ranges from physical to psychological care. Thus, with regards to psychological care, the Sister is portrayed as giving important explanation and reassurance to a patient involved in a road traffic accident (*Casualty*, 23 September 1989).

With regards to doctor/nurse relationships, Cole's survey (1986: 20) revealed a change in the way that doctor/nurse relations are represented: 'It was felt that the working relationship between doctors and nurses – showing them as partners rather than master and servants – provided a welcome change to the usual media stereotype'.

The change in representation in *Casualty* is thus important in terms of highlighting the fact that representations of the nurse can change and are changing.

Changing the image of nursing

The fact that *Casualty* is felt to provide a more 'progressive' representation of nursing as compared with other programmes may be symbolic with regards to change. Developments such as these may be accompanied by notable changes within media representations as a whole. Examples are given in the *Nursing Times* for the year 1988. In *Nursing Times* (24 February 1988) comment was passed on the BBC Radio 4 programme *Medicine Now* (10 February) highlighting the important role of nurses in primary health care, particularly with respect to screening and preventative health. It was also noted by *Nursing Times* that nurses were more vocal, and were being interviewed more often on the news. So, as *Nursing Times* (10 August 1988) commented, the media are just as likely to approach Trevor Clay (the then general secretary of the Royal College of Nursing) for a comment on the NHS as the British Medical Association.

Such examples highlight two important points. First, they reveal the direction of change in which nursing seems to be aiming, that is, a recognition of its role in health care. Secondly, they show that this change is being legitimized by the media. However, this development could be viewed as rather limited change, for, as has been indicated, certain representations, such as *Young Doctors*, are still prevalent within the popular media and the image of the nurse in *Carry On Nurse* is now most certainly a permanent part of the history of popular culture. Nevertheless, while concerns remain, it is also important to note finally that the changes have come about through the determination of nursing to re-evaluate its own image and reassess its future.

Gallagher (1987) argues that the concern with the image of the nurse in the media is based on the fact that nursing is concerned with its general public image. Thus as Gallagher (1987: 674) notes: 'in just a few years the nursing profession has become aware that its image must satisfy those who work in the profession and inspire confidence among the general public'.

One of the criticisms aimed at the pioneering work of the Kalisches by both Gallagher (1987) and Aydelotte (1987) is that *the media* are seen as the main problem in the perpetuation of a detrimental public image of the nurse. Thus, there is assumed to be a direct relationship between media representation and nursing status. In contrast, it has been argued that the media form just part of a wider discourse within society which creates a complex framework through which a particular ideology maintains nursing status by the passage of various meanings and messages. Consequently, Aydelotte (1987: 214) notes:

Nowhere among the strategies do the Kalisches propose that nursing looks seriously at what it is, what nurses themselves do in practice or what characteristics nurses themselves possess, the very basis upon which public image and self image rest.

This perspective is useful. In brief, Aydelotte advocates the importance of change *within* nursing to facilitate change in the media representation of the nurse. This involves a consideration of the way in which the practice of nursing directly feeds into an ideology which ultimately inhibits change in nursing. The meanings of the ideology are not fixed but can 'shift' according to need. Thus, the fact that nursing is demanding changes in its public image, and has recently been vocalizing that need in terms of, for example, changes in pay structure, has corresponded with changes in the way that nurses are represented in the media. This is not to suggest a direct correlation between the two, nor is it to suggest that all change in the media representation of the nurse will necessarily be deemed progressive.

There will now be a consideration of the ways in which nursing is striving to make changes in its public image. First, there will be a consideration in terms of a general attempt to change, to move away from the attributes associated with a secondary job status towards a position of control, i.e. through professionalization. Within this shift the media are potentially implicated in terms of their contribution in perpetuating the attributes associated with this secondary job status. The second way relates to a specific case study of recruitment. This example is important because it indicates the degree to which nursing has supported the ideologies which perpetuate the status quo and also highlights how nursing has utilized the media to portray a particular representation of itself.

The case of professionalization

The need for nursing to reassess and revalue itself is constantly an issue within nursing. Thus, Project 2000 is the result of the assessment of the way in which nurses are trained, and, similarly, the clinical grading (though problematic in terms of its implementation) is an attempt to re-evaluate nurses' skills and experiences. These re-evaluations are part of the process of nursing trying to gain public recognition of its skills and also of its contribution to health care. In other words, nursing is asserting changes in its public image. These changes can be seen as attempts to undermine the attributes associated with nursing being of secondary job status to, and of making a less valuable contribution to, health care than medicine. These are the very factors which have been traditionally associated with the meaning and ideology incorporated within the media representation of the nurse.

The way in which nursing is instigating change must be considered. Progress within nursing tends to be seen in terms of increased status, control and autonomy. Interestingly, as Salvage (1985) indicates, these are factors which are most associated with the medical profession. This has all led to much discussion within nursing of the idea of professionalism. Salvage makes an important distinction between being 'a profession' and professionalism. Thus, although nursing may not be recognized as a profession in the strictest sense (because, for example, of the diversity of the people covered by the title 'nurse'), it can still aspire to professionalism. This notion of professionalism is seen by Salvage (1985: 93) as meaning 'better standards of practice achieved through improving training, raising entry requirements and changing attitudes'.

The goal of professionalism although problematic highlights the way in which nursing is changing. However, the notion of professionalism is not just about the striving for occupational change, but is ultimately about the concern within nursing for the need of a change in public image.

The case of recruitment

A useful example to consider in order to gain an understanding of how nursing wants to portray itself publicly is within the area of recruitment. The importance of such commercials has recently been highlighted by Vousden (1989a: 26): '[they] will probably do as much to shape people's opinions of nursing as anything, other than perhaps their portrayal in popular television programmes, so the advertisements have to get it right.'

Recruitment is currently an area of much importance for several reasons: first, the falling numbers of appropriately qualified school leavers; secondly, the high turnover rate (particularly among newly qualified nurses); and, thirdly, the problems relating to the image of nursing, particularly relating to status, pay and conditions. It is interesting, then, to consider the images which nurses themselves validate through recruitment advertisements.

Vousden (1989b) stresses the fact that the earliest campaigns always used an attractive female nurse to encourage people to train, and gave little information about what nursing was about. Hence, whatever the accepted view within society about nursing at this time, a white, female, young, attractive nurse was at that time a face acceptable to nursing. Vousden (1989b: 52) highlights the use in the 1970s of the advertisement of a young girl in a nurse's outfit with a bandaged teddy bear. The caption was 'The best nurses have the essential qualifications before they go to school.' In this representation can be perceived elements of girlishness, so undermining the importance of nurse training and education just as well as any of the sex-symbol or angel stereotypes could. Further, the meaning behind such an image and caption seems to imply a certain innate quality which can be compared to the meaning behind the 'angel' image emphasizing the 'naturalness' of nursing skills and so again devaluing the role of nurse education. Finally, the utilization of the image of the child suggests a certain quality of dependency, which associates well with the handmaiden stereotype in which the nurse is dependent on the doctor.

In the 1980s the DHSS ran a campaign to recruit more men into nursing. This campaign was run under the heading 'Are You Man Enough to do Women's Work?' with the hope that recruiting more men into nursing would raise the status of nursing and counteract the effects of the 'demographic timebomb' (Cottingham 1987). In terms of trying to resolve the perceived problem of the association of 'femaleness' with nursing work, the campaign may actually have had the effect of aggravating the problem.

The recent Department of Health campaign for recruitment (which has been endorsed by the nursing establishment) is interesting to consider. It was produced in an attempt to make nursing attractive to potential recruits and was again in response to the so-called 'demographic timebomb'. Two television advertisements, depicting 'real-life' nurses, were shown in 1988 and 1989. They were aimed at the southeast region of the country to appeal to 17–25 years olds (Millar 1988). This campaign particularly attempted to recognize criticisms of earlier recruitment advertisements. In the event, criticisms of this recent campaign by the nursing unions among others have largely been in terms of the money spent on the campaign, arguing that it would have been better targeted at improving conditions to retain existing staff (Millar 1988). However, this latest set of advertisements are particularly important as signposts to the focus on change.

Millar notes that the latest advertisements glamorize the role of nursing. This glamorization particularly relates to the concentration on emergency situations (a cardiac arrest, for example) and the reality of nursing is ignored. Thus Mackenzie, General Secretary of COHSE, argues: 'The reality of a nurse's life is struggling to make ends meet and a daily workload which leaves nurses weeping with despair' (cited in Millar 1988: 906).

Such criticisms are important but ignore that these adverts *are* attempting to recruit, not deter (and so a certain bias in presentation will almost inevitably result). Further, one must recognize that these representations have developed and changed, revealing a progression from the notion of 'nurse' being totally encapsulated within the notion of 'woman' to the current representations which emphasize more fully nurses as workers.

The future

The way in which the nurse has been represented within the media has been revealed to be subject to some change, while elements of the traditional stereotypes still remain. It is important that nursing continues to recognize the relevance of campaigning about media images, stereotypes and representations, and yet moves beyond simply campaigning around what are regarded as detrimental images. These particular concerns are, of course, important, but it is also crucial that nursing takes account of the contribution it has itself made over the years to the perpetuation of the ideology behind these images.

The changes that nursing is making to alter its public image and consequently its status have been shown to be an attempt to move away from the meanings which are incorporated within the traditional stereotypes. The striving towards professionalism and all its connotations is understandable when nursing is associating the attributes of professionalism with the privileges that doctors enjoy. However, the notions of professionalism may be seen as problematic, leading to the concern of whether the notion of professionalism per se is the way in which nursing should be developing as an occupation. This had led to the idea in some quarters that any notion of change must involve a rethinking of what exactly nursing as an occupation involves. Nursing must consider and revalue the diversity and range of precisely 'who the nurse is'. This re-evaluation involves a consideration of nurses' role in health care. This must involve an acknowledgement of the special role of the nurse in terms of the close contact that nurses have with patients, for, as Salvage (1986: 170) warns:

This contact is something we have now and could develop more strongly, but we risk losing it in the blind pursuit of professionalism along medical lines, which – as doctors demonstrate – tends to create divisions between people rather than bring them together.

The re-evaluation of nursing also involves a recognition of the fact that nursing *is* an occupation constituted mainly of women. Again, as Salvage urges: 'stop trying to professionalise nursing to take it away from women's work and acknowledge "that this is the single most important issue in nursing"' ('Women's issues', 1989). This reassertion is probably one of the most difficult to accomplish in light of the fact that the issue of 'women's work' is actually used to undermine nursing, just as women's work in general is undermined in society. Traditionally, the message that nurses are women has run consistently through the representations of the nurse in the media. More recently, nursing has tried to distance itself from this image by advocating professionalization and trying to recruit more men into nursing. However, there is still a major problem for women in nursing, symbolized by the number of men who achieve promotion in nursing relative to women.

A variety of issues need to be considered here, including, for example, the facilities offered to nurses at their place of work in terms of child-care provisions and flexibility of shift patterns. A career structure which allows men to achieve a higher representation in the upper echelons of what is still a female-dominated occupation has little to do with how the recruitment campaigns are presented and much more to do with fundamental structural issues within nursing.

By re-evalauting its role and by utilizing the unique position of contact that nursing has with patients, nursing must demand its right to comment on and be taken seriously on not only health care issues, but also changes within its own occupation. While there has been progress in this area, the rights of nursing to demand equality with medicine and a voice in issues of health care at a local and national level must involve an increased political awareness (Gott 1985). The prerequisite to gaining power and influence in participating in important decision-making processes is noted by Gott (1985: 276) in nurses needing 'to believe in the validity of their own case. Until they do so, corporately they will be neither political [nor professional]'.

These points are not being stressed in order to devalue the attempts of nurses to campaign against detrimental images, nor is it an attempt to undermine the anger that is felt within nursing about the way in which nursing is represented in the media. Indeed, it is important that nursing not only recognizes the influence of the media on the formation of perceptions about nursing, but also vocalizes these feelings of concern. It is important though that nursing 'takes stock' and reconsiders not only why the way nursing is represented in the media is of such concern, but also the extent to which nursing can identify its own contribution to the perpetuation of such representations. These issues are crucial with regard to change and the development of nursing. Change in nursing and consequently change in media representations will not occur unless fundamental issues are tackled. These issues must not be ignored in favour of what are superficially perceived as obvious routes to status acquisition which in themselves place little value on the day-to-day experience of the nurse's role in health care.

References

Austin, J., Champion, V. and Tzeng, O. 1985. Cross-cultural comparison on nursing image. *International Journal of Nursing Studies* 22(3): 231–9.

Aydelotte, M. 1987. The changing image of the nurse. *Image*, Winter 19(4): 213–14.

Betterton, R. 1987. *Looking On.* London: Pandora.

Bologh, R. 1979. Alienation in the patient role: source of ambivalence and humour in comic get well cards. *Sociology of Health and Illness* 1(2): 137–57.

Cole, A. 1986. Making a drama out of a crisis. *Nursing Times*, 10 December, 82(50): 19–20.

Cottingham, M. 1987. Putting men in the picture. *Nursing Times*, 20 May, 83(20): 28–9.

Ehrenreich, B. and English, D. 1973. *Witches, Midwives and Nurses: A History of Women Healers.* New York: Feminist Press.

Fagin, C. 1983. Nursing as metaphor. *American Journal of Nursing*, September, 1362.

Gallagher, P. 1987. Media image of nursing. *Nursing*, June, 3(18): 674–6.

Gott, M. 1985. Politics and professionalism in nursing. *Nurse Education Today* 5:274–6.

Hall, S. 1981. The whites of their eyes. In G. Bridges and R. Brunt (eds), *Silver Linings.* London: Lawrence & Wishart.

Kaler, S., Levy, D. and Schall, M. 1989. Stereotypes of professional roles. *Image*, Summer, 21(2): 85–9.

Kalisch, P. and Kalisch, B. 1986. A comparative analysis of nurse and physician characters in the entertainment media. *Journal of Advanced Nursing* 11: 179–95.

Kalisch, P. and Kalisch, B. 1987. *The Changing Image of the Nurse*. California: Addison-Wesley.

Kalisch, P., Kalisch, B. and Scobey, M. 1983. *Images of Nurses on Television*. New York: Springer.

Kappeler, S. 1986. *The Pornography of Representation*. Cambridge: Polity Press.

Karpf, A. 1988a. Broken images. *Nursing Times*, 18 May, 84(20): 16–17.

Karpf, A. 1988b. *Doctoring the Media: The Reporting of Health and Medicine*. London: Routledge.

Kuhn, A. 1982. *Women's Pictures*. London: Routledge & Kegan Paul.

Millar, B. 1988. The TV gloss that masks despair. *The Health Service Journal*, 11 August: 905–6.

Muff, J. (ed.) 1982. *Socialization, Sexism and Stereotyping: Women's Issues in Nursing*. St Louis: Mosby.

Salvage, J. 1985. *The Politics of Nursing*. London: Heinemann.

Salvage, J. 1988. Professionalisation – or struggle for survival? A consideration of the current proposals for the reform of nursing in the UK. *Journal of Advanced Nursing* 13(4): 515–19.

Salvage, J. 1989. Shifting boundaries. *Nursing Times*, 8 March, 85(100): 24.

Salvage, J. 1989b. Support your CNO. *Nursing Times*, 21 June, 85(25): 26.

Vousden, M. 1988. What the papers said. *Nursing Times*, 17 February, 84(7): 18.

Vousden, M. 1989a. Selling nursing. *Nursing Times*, 23 August, 85(34): 25–9.

Vousden, M. 1989b. This year's model. *Nursing Times*, 6 September, 85(36): 50–2.

'Women's Issues'. 1989. *Lampada*, (RCN newspaper), April/May, Issue no. 19,3.

CHAPTER THREE

Nursing, advertising and sponsorship: some ethical issues

Ruth Chadwick

Introduction

Clause 14 of the second edition of the UKCC Code of Professional Conduct for the Nurse, Midwife and Health Visitor states that every registered nurse, midwife and health visitor shall '[a]void the use of professional qualifications in the promotion of commercial products in order not to compromise the independence of professional judgement on which patients/clients rely' (UKCC 1984). In 1985 the UKCC issued an elaboration of this particular clause of the Code of Professional Conduct. The current trend in health care provision towards a market-based system, however, has produced some problems for nurses in this area, and the UKCC has recently circulated a further document on advertising and commercial sponsorship in response to the 'variety of innovative schemes and proposals ... being devised and considered to generate income to supplement resources allocated to health authorities and boards from Government sources' (UKCC 1990: 1).

It is the purpose of this chapter to look at the ethical issues involved in advertising by nurses, with special reference to the matters covered by the recent UKCC statement: the wearing of logos on uniforms, advertising in the health care environment, and commercial sponsorship. In the context of a society which has embraced publicity, and in which the General Medical Council has recently relaxed its rules on advertising, what are the ethical arguments for the position taken by the UKCC, and how, if at all, can it be defended against objections? Is there something about health care in general, or about nursing in particular, which is incompatible with advertising?

First, it is necessary to be clear about what advertising is.

Advertising

According to the Oxford English Dictionary, an advertisement is a public notice or announcement; a statement calling attention to anything (OED 1971). As Don Evans (1990) has noted, however, ethical questions arise when such an announcement becomes promotional. We may understand a promotional advertisement to be one that attempts to further the success of a particular organization or product by, for example, boosting sales.

Advertising – is it an ethical issue?

It has been suggested (Carroll and Humphrey 1979) that the question of whether advertising is appropriate for nurses is a matter of etiquette rather than of ethics. In the context of nursing ethics, 'etiquette' can be interpreted in the following way: 'the unwritten code of honour by which members of certain professions (esp. the medical and legal) are prohibited from doing certain things deemed likely to . . . lower the dignity of the profession' (OED 1971).

Those who see advertising as an ethical issue for nurses, however, look beyond the notion that advertising might be considered undignified, and stress its capacity for 'undue influence' on patients who are vulnerable (Miles et al. 1989). The claim is that the interests of patients may be adversely affected by the promotion of the interests of particular advertisers. If this is so, we have an ethical issue. Ethics is, after all, concerned with finding principles to resolve conflicts of interests.

Truth-telling and misleading advertisements

There is a view that there is nothing wrong with advertising as such, even when it is promotional; that moral problems arise only in relation to misleading advertisements – ones that make claims for products or organizations which are untrue.

Certainly, if the advertisement is making claims that are false, this introduces the question of harm to those misled, the harm not only of being deceived, but also of being injured by useless or even dangerous products. In the health care setting this is particularly worrying, as the controversy over misleading advertising by pharmaceutical companies illustrates (see Melrose 1982).

But what is misleading is a matter of degree. John Berger, who was instrumental in defining the terms in which recent debates on advertising have been conducted, argued that it is in the nature of advertising to mislead and suggested that: 'Publicity speaks in the future tense and yet the achievement of this future is endlessly deferred' (Berger 1972: 146). In other words, advertising perpetuates itself by promising more than it can deliver. Nevertheless, even if we accept that it is in the nature of advertising to mislead, there will be differences of degree according to the amount of harm that may be brought about by a particular deception. Thus we might consider an advertisement which promotes, in the Third World, a drug which has been banned elsewhere worse than an advertisement in the West for the health-giving properties of some harmless but ineffective food supplement. And again, in some advertisements which draw attention to services offered, it may be difficult to find any false claims: in so far as the advertisement misleads it is because it participates in the system.

The extent to which an advertisement is misleading, however, is not the only factor to be taken into consideration. First, there is the question of the relevance of the beliefs of the person involved in advertising. This will be taken up in the discussion of the wearing of logos on nurses' uniforms.

Secondly, we have to address the issue of whether the appropriateness of advertising is context dependent. In particular, is the health care environment one from which advertising should be excluded, and if so why? This takes us to one of the three aspects of advertising considered in the UKCC circular.

The health care environment will be taken to include not only the physical spaces in which health care is provided (e.g. hospitals and GPs' surgeries), but also advertising which relates to the provision of health services generally (e.g. advertisements which might attract potential clients to those physical spaces). The issues will be approached by looking at justifications of advertising and the extent to which they apply in the health care context. As indicated above, we have as our focus of concern specific types of advertising that might involve nurses, and it is in relation to these that we primarily need to think about moral arguments. But first it is appropriate to reflect a little on advertising in general, and possible lines of argument that might be used to support permitting its use in the health care setting.

Advertising and the health care environment

Berger (1972: 130–1) sets out the standard justification of what he calls 'publicity':

> Publicity is usually explained and justified as a competitive medium which ultimately benefits the public (the consumer) and the most efficient manufacturers – and thus the national economy. It is closely related to certain ideas about freedom: freedom of choice for the purchaser; freedom of enterprise for the manufacturer. The great hoardings and the publicity neons of the cities of capitalism are the immediate visible signs of 'The Free World'.

There are in fact two arguments here. The first is that advertising produces good results by promoting the interests of all, especially the consumer; the second is that advertising should be permitted in the name of freedom.

The interests of consumers

Let us look more closely at the argument that advertising promotes the interests of consumers. The benefit is said to lie in the information they receive about competing products, which enhances their power of choice. The objection to this view is that advertising is essentially not about providing information which enables consumers to choose. Berger's point remains valid, that, while choices may be offered between one type of car and another, 'publicity as a system only makes a single proposal. It proposes to each of us that we transform ourselves, by buying something more' (Berger 1972: 131). Advertising, then, is not about providing information which enables us to choose; it is about making us buy more.

It might be argued that this does not apply to all types of advertising. Don Evans (1990: 23), in discussing advertising by doctors, seems to be supporting a version of the consumer interest argument when he refers to the 'general gain in public awareness of doctors' services produced by advertising' and says that 'the relaxation of restrictions on advertising ... constitutes an important advance on what can be regarded as the provision of good health care'.

Evans seems to be assuming that the Berger point does not apply in the health care setting: that, where what is under consideration is advertising by doctors, it is simply a question of the public being informed about what services are offered by different practices and practitioners, so that potential patients can choose which to consult. There is no suggestion that the purpose of advertising might be to boost consumption of the services offered. The picture given is of people who have particular needs but who realize that not every professional will be equally competent to meet those needs. Advertising will help them to find out who is competent.

It might be argued that in the context of health care these are reasonable assumptions to make. Surely, apart from one or two people who are obsessive about their health (with or without advertising), people consult medical practitioners when they are ill, and so need to know where they can obtain the best care.

First, however, it seems fairly clear that the most effective advertisers are not necessarily the best providers of care. Secondly, we are operating in the context of a political ideology which advocates not only greater consumer choice in health care but also the other side of that coin, which is personal responsibility for health. In such a setting, advertising by doctors may indeed lead people to perceive themselves as having a larger set of health care needs than they would otherwise have done. As Berger pointed out, 'all publicity works upon anxiety' (Berger 1972: 143). An 'unworried well' person might be transformed into a 'worried well' person by the advertising of preventive medicine and screening services, for example.

It is not the purpose of this chapter to downgrade the

importance of preventive medicine and screening. The value and effectiveness of such programmes must be assessed on a case-by-case basis. What *is* being argued is that it is not possible to support advertising, in the health care setting or in any other, simply by claiming that it is in the general interest in that it increases the information available to consumers and leads to an improved service by stimulating competition. The social and political context also has to be borne in mind. We have to ask, for example, whether there are incentives for practitioners to target certain groups in the population, and, if so, what kind of incentives these are, and which groups. These are the sort of questions that have frequently been raised in connection with the recently proposed changes in the NHS.

The interests of advertisers, and the interests of all

Advertisers, however, have interests as well as consumers, and it has to be admitted that advertising makes them a great deal of money, which they argue ultimately benefits the economy and thus the interests of all. It is so profitable to large companies to advertise that they are willing to pay handsomely for space in which to do it, to those with space available to sell.

An argument about the interests of advertisers is unlikely, however, to carry weight with the nursing profession. As the Code of Professional Conduct indicates, it is the duty of every nurse to act to promote the well-being and interests of patients/clients (UKCC 1984). The argument therefore needs to be extended beyond the interests of advertisers to the interests of all. In the health care context it is fairly clear how this would go. The health care environment has space that could be used for advertising; the Health Service needs money; advertisers will pay the Health Service money for the use of their space; everyone will benefit, including the patients who can be provided with improved facilities out of the income so generated.

This is a difficult argument to counter. If it really can be shown that it is to the ultimate benefit of patients to allow advertising in the Health Service, then how can it be argued against? In order to answer this we need to look first at Berger's freedom argument and the related issues of autonomy and paternalism.

Freedom

As regards the freedom argument, this is a theme about which we have heard much in the recent past as the barriers between East and West have fallen. But Berger's point that publicity is related to 'certain ideas' about freedom draws our attention to the fact that there are other ideas which are being denied in this form of argument. Freedom is an 'essentially contested' concept (see Gallie 1955–6): there are opposing, irreconcilable political philosophies, in which 'freedom' takes on different meanings. The freedom to compete, which capitalism promotes, is opposed to the notion of freedom from poverty and want, conditions which are to a certain extent effects of the implementation of the first notion of freedom.

From its beginning, the National Health Service incorporated into its aims the second notion of freedom, that of freedom from, not poverty and want, but avoidable ill health and disease. There is now under way a deliberate attempt to replace this 'freedom from' concept by the 'freedom to' concept, interpreted as freedom to market, and freedom to choose. This again is linked with the (at least partial) replacement of the idea that the state has a responsibility for health by the view that individuals should take personal responsibility for their own health.

As the meaning of freedom is contested, then, the freedom argument is problematic.

Autonomy and paternalism

There has been a related longstanding conflict between two models of health care: the autonomy model and the beneficence model. The autonomy model, resting on the principle of autonomy, suggests that, because adults of sound mind have a capacity to think, decide and act on the basis of such thought and decision (Gillon 1985), we should respect the decisions they make and so facilitate, for example, informed consent. The beneficence model, on the other hand, adopts the view that people who are ill may not be in the best position to make decisions about their own welfare; illness diminishes the capacity for autonomy, and it is thus up to health care professionals (primarily doctors) to make decisions about what is in the best interests of their patients.

In the context of this debate, to try to prohibit advertising in the health care setting on the grounds that patients are vulnerable may seem to be a paternalistic siding with the beneficence model. Don Evans (1990: 24) argues against too strict a control on advertising by doctors on these grounds: 'Too tight a control by the GMC will harm the interests of the consumer and will represent an unwelcome paternalism. We do not want to see every doctor's advertisement qualified by a GMC warning "Danger: this advertisement may damage your health".'

There does seem to be a potential problem here for anyone who wants to oppose paternalism in health care and yet prohibit advertising on the grounds that patients are in a vulnerable condition. If we think that, despite their vulnerability, they are perfectly capable of making autonomous decisions about their treatment, why are they not, despite their vulnerability, equally capable of responding to advertising in an autonomous way?

There are three points to be made here. The first two relate to the situation of those in the physical spaces of the health care environment, the third to advertising in health care generally.

Berger has something to say about the relation between the advertisement and the recipient:

> Usually it is we who pass the image – walking, travelling, turning a page; on the tv screen it is somewhat different but even then we are theoretically the active agent – we can look away, turn down the sound, make some coffee. Yet despite this, one has the impression that publicity images are continually passing us .. We are static; they are dynamic . . . (Berger 1972: 130)

It is fairly clear that in the health care setting people waiting for appointments will be 'static' in the literal sense. Thus in a letter to *The Times*, Malcolm Miles and others wrote:

> Most people enter a hospital in fear of a disease they or a relative may have. When they wait for an appointment they are stressed – a fact which the cunning psychology of advertising could exploit. Amidst the notices dislayed, an advertisement may take on an authority, as if from the caring professions, to which it has no claim; yet its vulnerable recipients may make no such distinction (Miles *et al.* 1989: 13).

The second point is made by the UKCC in its recent circular, and that is that the physical surroundings can in themselves contribute to, or detract from, the therapeutic process. So it is suggested that the physical environment 'should be conducive to healing, recovery, care and calm' (UKCC 1990: 2). The description given by Berger, of being continually passed by a plethora of advertising images, hardly meets this requirement.

The third and final point under this heading is the most important. It disputes the validity of the analogy between advertising and the 'informing' part of informed consent, and so holds that the prohibition of advertising is not unjustifiably paternalistic.

The importance of patient autonomy has been increasingly emphasized, at least since the mid-twentieth century, to the extent that the autonomy model is the dominant model of health care, especially in the USA, but also in the United Kingdom. It implies that health care professionals should avoid using their authority to influence patients unduly, but should try to facilitate the expression of informed choices by them.

Advertising, on the other hand, as we have seen, is not primarily about facilitating informed choice. if it is the case that it feeds on anxiety in order to produce a particular result, it is not autonomy enhancing. So it is quite consistent for one who supports the autonomy model of health care to oppose advertising to those who are ill.

Without being unduly paternalistic, then, the above arguments suggest that a concern for patients' interests will lead to the opposing of advertising in the health care environment. It is still arguable, however, that patients have other interests, in improved facilities, which could outweigh these considerations. This will be considered further in the context of examining the arguments for and against logos on nurses' uniforms.

Logos on uniforms

Logos have become a pervasive feature of our culture. We buy clothing and carry bags with brand names prominently displayed. The fact that it is found not only acceptable but desirable to adorn our own persons with advertising that is designed for the promotional benefit of others is particularly significant: it shows how deep the uncritical acceptance of publicity is.

Given this background, why should it be thought impermissible for this feature of our society to spread into the Health Service, particularly if it is done in a discreet way?

The position of the UKCC on logos is as follows:

> The use of professional uniforms, or the use of the clothing worn by professional staff who do not wear uniform, to carry advertising through the use of emblems or other embellishments used for commercial promotion is not acceptable as this implies the endorsement of the product or service so advertised by the individual practitioner. (UKCC 1990: 1).

Since the wearing of logos implies endorsement, then, it constitutes a violation of Clause 14, which prohibits the use of professional qualifications to promote commercial products.

Means and ends

But why should this be so? What if nurses really do think that the products of a certain company are worthy of promotion, as being the best? This recalls the truth-telling argument outlined above, where the relevance of the agent's beliefs was mentioned.

There are two possible scenarios to consider. The first is where an individual nurse wishes to endorse a particular product or company and uses his or her professional qualifications to give backing to it. The problem with this is that if he or she uses professional qualifications to do so it can be seen as endorsement, not by an individual, but by the profession, and in this sense it is a misleading advertisement.

The second type of case concerns a group of nurses in, for example, a hospital setting who are instructed by management to wear uniforms carrying logos, because to do so will bring the hospital a considerable sum of money. We have talked about the selling of space in health care settings to advertisers, but what is now being suggested is, in effect, the selling or hiring out of the persons of nurses. Now it is conceivable, though statistically unlikely, that every single nurse will agree that this product should be endorsed, but it is probable that at least some will disagree, or not have given thought to the matter. In that case they as individuals are being asked to join in the endorsement of a product to which they do not give their wholehearted support. And not only may they not support the product, they may also of course be opposed to this form of advertising. In such a case an appropriate way of describing what is going on may be to use a Kantian argument to the effect that nurses are being illegitimately used as means to ends they do not agree with, rather than as ends in themselves.

One possible reply to this would be that nurses are in very many aspects of their work used as means. In the first place, they are used as a means to the end of promoting patient welfare. This, however, is an end with which they presumably agree if they are to enter the profession in the first place. Advertising is not such an end. In several other types of situation, of course, they may have to do things with which they personally do not agree, but they have an obligation to cooperate with other members of the health care team in order to promote the interests of patients.

There are limits to which nurses are expected to accept things, however. It is part of the point of the UKCC Code of Professional Conduct to encourage nurses to be people who challenge (Pyne 1988). The ultimate test is whether or not they believe that a particular course of action is in the interests of patients.

This brings us once more to the crux of the matter. Is it in the interests of patients to raise money by such methods as wearing logos on uniforms?

The answer to this does not only depend on a crude analysis of the amounts of money that can be made available by different methods, e.g. public funding versus commercial sponsorship. There are wider questions about the ethos of the service, public expectations and the nature of nursing as a profession.

Nursing as a profession: two kinds of power relationship

The notion of publicly provided health care has its origins in the ethics of charity on the one hand, and in public responsibility for welfare, on the other. Of those who work in the Health Service, nurses in particular have been associated with notions of altruism and an ethic of care. The image of the medical profession has been associated to a greater extent with career advancement and social position than has that of nurses.

The image of nurses has changed from that of doctors'

handmaidens to that of professionals in their own right. But the realities of the power relationships in the health care context are still of interest and of particular relevance in thinking about logos for nurses' uniforms.

First, nurses still have less power than doctors, in that doctors have ultimate authority in determining how patients should be treated. Their power, however, does not stop at this, but spreads in other directions. While doctors may perhaps be seen using pens emblazoned with the name of a pharmaceutical company, it is difficult to imagine them wearing logo-bearing uniforms, however much money it might raise for their patients. But if it were acceptable for nurses, why not for doctors? This may say something about the relative status of the two professions. (An additional point, however, is that the advertising of pharmaceutical companies to doctors is largely aimed at persuading doctors to prescribe certain drugs, rather than encouraging patients to buy.)

The point about the relative power of doctors and nurses is one that has frequently been made. Also significant is the difference in power between the nurse and the patient. Here it is the practitioner who has the power. As has already been suggested, patients who are ill are vulnerable. In this situation they want to put their trust in somebody, and it is nurses in whom it is commonly placed. The advertisers, of course, will be well aware of this. Not only are there more nurses than there are doctors, but they spend more time with patients, in which they can develop a relationship of trust. The potential for influencing patients is thus enormous.

An argument against the use of nurses for advertising through logos, then, might be that this is an illegitimate exploitation of differences in power that already exist – first, of nurse vis-à-vis other professional groups, and secondly of patients, who are in a vulnerable position with regard to health professionals generally, including nurses.

The professional and the patient

Beyond this, however, there is a point about the ways in which nurses and patients are viewed. We have already said something about the way in which the image of nurses generally has changed. Reg Pyne has argued that the UKCC Code of Professional Code of Conduct presents an image of what a nurse is (Pyne 1988). This image, according to the UKCC, is one that is incompatible with the nurse as advertiser. The nurse's primary duty is to act at all times to promote the welfare of patients. While it has been suggested that the strongest argument in favour of advertising is that it can contribute towards this end by raising money for new or improved facilities, the reply to this can be put in the following way: using nurses to advertise to patients alters, not only the image of the nurse, but also that of the patients. To see patients as customers marks a radical change in how they are regarded, a change which patients themselves might resent, and which might lead to a weakening of that very trust which advertisers would like to exploit.

In another context Ronald Green makes this point in relation to fee-splitting (the practice of paying a percentage to doctors who refer patients to clinics). He notes 'a fear that fee-splitting encourages a "trafficking" in sick people and a view of patients as financial resources rather than persons. A further assumption is that even the appearance of such practices might seriously undermine patients' trust' (Green 1990: 24). The point being made here is that, if patients suspect tht someone has something to gain financially out of certain advice they are given, they are likely to distrust both that advice and the professionals who give it to them.

In addition to this argument about the possible undesirable consequences for trust in the professional–client relationship, there is a problem about the implications for respect for the person.

Those who uphold a principle of respect for persons may vary in how they interpret it, and it is beyond the scope of this chapter to examine the principle in detail. There has been, however, a move towards calling the recipients of care 'clients' rather than 'patients'. This is supposed to reflect more respect for them as persons in the sense that 'patient' implies a passive role, when we should rather be thinking of the recipients of care in accordance with the principle of autonomy, as actively involved in decisions about their treatment. So far, so good. What is suspect about such moves is the suggestion that in order to show respect for recipients of a service it is necessary to regard them as customers, the implication being that it is people who pay for a service who command respect. As Bernard Williams has pointed out, the relevant factor about people who want to receive health care is whether or not they are ill, not whether or not they have money (Williams 1969).

Commercial sponsorship

On commercial sponsorship the UKCC has this to say:

> The same principles set out . . . in relation to advertising, that is independence of professional judgement based on the needs of patients and clients, unfettered by undue commercial influence, should equally apply to any commercial sponsorship arrangements. (UKCC 1990: 2).

What is envisaged here is the kind of situation where a nurse's salary is paid for by a commercial company. It has become much more common recently for persons in all kinds of occupations to seek funding for their posts in such ways.

For the UKCC the important consideration is that such sponsorship should not compromise the independence of the nurse's judgement. Whether it does will depend on the degree of distance between the sponsor and the nurse's work. For example, if the sponsorship also entailed the wearing of a particular logo then it would be ruled out in accordance with the argument in the preceding section. Similarly, if the sponsorship involved recommending one and only one particular brand of products not patients, the nurse's independence would be undermined.

In some cases, however, sponsorship of particular posts is compatible with there being no particular promotional message passed on to patients and clients. In such cases perhaps the argument that it promotes the interests of all can be made out. A nurse is provided with employment; patients are provided with care; the public purse is relieved of some pressure.

The argument against this is that, despite the apparent harmlessness of such arrangements, their increasing number reinforces the idea that health is not a public responsibility; that it is up to private concerns to finance it. In the long term it is difficult to see this as being in the interests of all, for a large concession is being made to the culture of publicity, which has been argued in this chapter to be an inappropriate one for the health service.

Conclusion

Our consideration of the debates surrounding advertising, then, has highlighted arguments, from a moral point of view, that support the stance taken by the UKCC, and casts doubt on the applicability, in the health care context, of the standard justifications of advertising.

References

Berger, J. 1972. *Ways of Seeing*. Harmondsworth: Penguin.

Carroll, M. A. and Humphrey, R. A. 1979. *Moral Problems in Nursing: Case Studies*. Washington DC: University Press of America.

Evans, D. 1990. Ethics and advertising. *Bulletin of Medical Ethics* 59: 21–4.

Gallie, W. B. 1955–6. Essentially contested concepts. *Proceedings of the Aristotelian Society* 56: 167–98.

Gillon, R. 1985. Autonomy and consent. In M. Lockwood (ed.), *Moral Dilemmas in Modern Medicine*, pp. 111–25. Oxford: Oxford University Press.

Green, R. M. 1990. Medical joint-venturing: an ethical perspective. *Hastings Center Report* 20(4): 22–6.

Melrose, D. 1982. *Bitter Pills: Medicines and the Third World Poor*. Oxford: Oxfam.

Miles, M., Morrison, V., Weeks, J., Crimmin, M. and Shand, W. 1989. Letter to *The Times*, 11 November.

Oxford English Dictionary. 1971. Oxford: Oxford University Press.

Pyne, R. 1988. On being accountable. *Health Visitor* 61: 173–5.

UKCC. 1984. *Code of Professional Conduct for the Nurse, Midwife and Health Visitor*, 2nd edn. London: United Kingdom Central Council for Nursing, Midwifery and Health Visiting.

UKCC. 1985. *Advertising by Registered Nurses, Midwives and Health Visitors: an Elaboration of Clause 14 of the Code of Professional Conduct*. London: United Kingdom Central Council for Nursing, Midwifery and Health Visiting.

UKCC. 1990. *Statement on Advertising and Commercial Sponsorship and the Position of Nurses, Midwives and Health Visitors and the Health Care Environment*. London: United Kingdom Central Council for Nursing, Midwifery and Health Visiting.

Williams, B. 1969. The idea of equality. In J. Feinberg (ed.), *Moral Concepts*, pp. 153–71. Oxford: Oxford University Press.

CHAPTER FOUR

NHS nursing:
vocation, career or just a job?

Brian Francis, Moira Peelo and Keith Soothill

Introduction

There has been intense recent interest in attitudes of nurses to conditions of work within the National Health Service, and much speculation as to why nurses are leaving the National Health Service. Much of the latter discussion has concentrated on the issue of pay. Many may believe that the recent pay award for nurses will resolve the problems currently being experienced within the nursing profession. However, while most nurses, prior to the pay award, regarded pay as the most important issue (Soothill and Mackay 1988), there are a range of other concerns troubling a substantial number of nurses which we may neglect at our peril. It is to these other issues and attitudes that we principally turn in this analysis.

The crucial point to recognize is that nurses are not a homogeneous group. This fact is often overlooked by politicians, managers, unions and the media, for whom the demand for higher pay for nurses has provided a narrow focus for widely expressed concern about the NHS. Politicians are suddenly introduced to the problems of nursing without knowledge or interest in the subtleties of the issues; managers are trying to introduce working practices which encourage conformity rather than diversity; unions are seeking the common interests which bind their members together; and the media want a straightforward message which appeals to the sensibilities of their readers. For the rest, however, the picture is much more complex: even among nurses, what are seen as issues for some nurses are not mentioned by others and vice versa. Until we begin to understand the varying demands, interests and needs within the nursing profession and the complex patterns of nurses' concern, we cannot understand why nurses continue to leave the profession.

Concern about nurses' conditions, pay, status and duties is not new: nineteenth-century reformers wished to attract trained personnel into hospitals but some, like Mrs Bedford Fenwick, were concerned that high pay might attract the wrong sort of recruit (Leeson and Gray 1978). The move away from untrained, lower-class nurses to more genteel recruits highlighted tension between, on the one hand, nursing as an extension of a domestic role, with emphasis on hygiene as well as motherly care; and, on the other, a desire for professional status which made problematic the carrying out of duties usually performed by lower domestic servants (Gamarnikow 1978). Florence Nightingale, we are told, saw these non-nursing duties as character-building; however, not all shared her view in a period which saw attempts to get nurses registered, and hence officially recognized (Leeson and Gray 1978). In spite of the flourishing of other work roles in the health sector (ward auxiliaries, dieticians, etc.), the use and misuse of nursing staff remains an issue today. Similarly, tension remains between the view of nursing as a truly caring 'vocation', and notions of professionalism; concern for the emotional as well as physical well-being of patients has traditionally been a part of a nursing vocation, whatever other skills and knowledge are required. Downe (1990) has written that the pursuit of skills-based professional status for nurses is dangerous if it does not also ensure better care for clients, since this unmeasurable element reflects a state of 'being' a nurse which is an essential ingredient rather than a sign of weakness.

What was not in doubt in the nineteenth-century nursing reforms, however, was the subsidiary role of nursing to medicine: Witz (1985), in describing the struggle for registration of midwives, illustrated how such changes in nursing coincided with the striving of doctors for professional dominance of medicine. Game and Pringle (1983: 94) have called the division of labour in the health sector 'a sexual division in its most blatant form' both in the nursing/female, medicine/male model and in its actual work ethos and practices. Gamarnikow (1978: 121) described the sexual division of labour as 'a patriarchal ideological structure in that it reproduces patriarchal relations in extra-familial labour processes', and nursing illustrates this with its emphasis on 'the interconnections between femininity, motherhood, housekeeping'. Yet, in spite of the equation of nursing with these values and attributes, recruitment into nursing is seen as an issue concerning young women, and a caption to a press photo of two nurses tells all – 'Crisis in care . . . up to half of all girl school leavers will have to become nurses to meet the demands of the 21st Century' (*Guardian*, 30 July 1988). While adolescent girls do, according to Martin and Roberts (1984: 60), see their futures as dominated by family and domestic commitments, they often 'expect to return after having a family' to paid employment. At the very least, one might expect this sector to have most experience in accommodating the needs of its older female employees. However, Game and Pringle described how, in spite of evidence that, in Australia, large percentages of nurses are married women with children, hours of work are particularly difficult to combine with family life.

At a time when the emphasis was on bad pay, Mackay (1988a) attempted to widen the terms of the debate by indicating that the lack of career prospect also plays a significant part in why nurses leave the NHS. Mackay (1988b) has shown that nurses were extremely dissatisfied: nurses reported that they were very frustrated, for they simply did not have the time to look after their patients properly. They recognized they were failing to meeting their own standards of care. These were the nurses' perceptions and they felt that it should be to staffing levels above all else that local managers – who were not in a position to offer extra pay – should first turn their attention. Mackay (1988c) also focused on the misuse of nurses and reminded that the Briggs Report on Nursing (1972) found fairly high levels of misuse of nurses regarding 'non nursing chores'. While the situation has probably worsened in the last decade and a half, it cannot continue if the predicted shortfall in learner recruits (the 'demographic explosion') takes place in the 1990s. Many are now beginning to recognize that nurses will have to be used more carefully and their talents nurtured if there are not enough to go around. In brief, we must now attend to their concerns. We maintain that a more sophisticated statistical approach enables us to recognize the range of differing expectations held by nurses, and the variety of demands they make of nursing – issues which need to be addressed if the predicted shortfall in nursing recruitment is to be avoided.

Data collection and initial analysis

A random sample of one in three nurses in post in a district health authority in the north of England was taken in July 1986 and a questionnaire was posted to their home address. We surveyed a wide range of posts: from students and pupil nurses up to and including sisters and charge nurses. After one follow-up letter, a total of over 60 per cent of nurses responded to the questionnaire, providing a group of 435 'stayers'.

Standard questionnaire items on age, sex, post, marital history and residence were included as well as a section on life events and a bank of attitudinal questions on nursing and the NHS (Bagguley 1988). Following Mercer (1979), we asked nurses to rate the importance (on a five-point scale later collapsed to a four-point scale for subsequent analysis) of each of 11 improvements which would encourage trained nurses to stay in the National Health Service. We also asked the sample to identify reasons (from a checklist of ten reasons) which might cause them to leave nursing, and followed up with additional questions in which we asked the nurses for their attitudes to matters of salary (much too high, too high, about right, too low or much too low), promotion prospects (very good, quite good, not very good or poor), career opportunities (sufficient or not sufficient), community care (strongly approve, approve, indifferent, disapprove or strongly disapprove) and whether absenteeism was thought to be a problem (yes, no or sometimes). In total, there were 26 attitudinal items.

Searching for one major factor which causes nurses to leave would provide an inaccurate and simplistic picture, for, as respondents came to sort out the reasons which might affect their decision to leave, the picture was diverse. In fact, none of the ten reasons attracted more than 35 per cent as a likely reason, while, conversely, none attracted less than 5 per cent. When one comes to personal motivation for possible leaving, it is the diversity of reasons which merits attention.

When analysing frequencies, the temptation to look for one causal factor can be great: for example, in our series of questions both replicating the work of other studies and introducing new areas of interest, the topic of pay emerged in various guises: 76 per cent thought the present level of salary for nurses 'too low' or 'much too low'; over 94 per cent regarded increased salaries as 'important or very important' as an improvement necessary to encourage trained nurses to stay (with 62 per cent of these answering 'very important'). Indeed, 'increased salaries' was the reason given as 'important' or 'very important' most often from among the list provided. But when the respondents were asked what might cause them to leave nursing, 'dislike of nursing pay' was no longer the dominant reason given.

However, as Table 4.1 shows, while no single item constitutes a main cause for leaving, the responses are by no means totally random. Table 4.1 summarizes the responses of our stayers' sample to the various attitudinal items, cross-classified by current age. Here some patterns begin to emerge. Of those under 25 years, having a baby, a dislike of nursing pay or a possible preference for nursing outside the NHS emerged as the three most predominant reasons given as possibly causing them to leave nursing. The likelihood of these reasons being offered declined markedly with age. A new set of possibilities for leaving rose to prominence among those aged 40 or over: nearly one-third saw looking after dependants as a possible reason most frequently stated. However, closer attention to Table 4.1 shows that the possibility of having a baby as a reason decreases markedly with age and looking after dependants increases markedly with age; looking after children, however, as a possible source for leaving is fairly constant at all age groups apart from the oldest. So, taking these examples in turn, suitable maternity leave arrangements might interest younger nurses, day centres for elderly dependants may be helpful to older nurses, while creche/nursing facilities may well appeal to nurses of all age groups (this is, of course, reflected in the responses on creche/nursing facilities in Table 4.1 – row 2(k)).

Attitudes apparently related to age are fascinating but hazardous, and cross-sectional data can be misleading. It is dangerous to interpret this effect as a change of attitude as a nurse proceeds through a career path. For example, while one can accept on biological grounds that the chances of a nurse being likely to leave to have a baby will decrease markedly when she is over 40, one cannot have similar confidence that the 35 per cent who were under 25 and said they might leave nursing owing to a possible preference for nursing outside the NHS will change their attitude towards nursing outside the NHS as they grow older. In other words, it seems unlikely that when they are aged 40 years or over only 11 per cent will be attracted by the possibility of nursing

Table 4.1 Attitudes to nursing and current age

Attitude	Age group				
	Under 25 (%)	25–29 (%)	30–39 (%)	Over 40 (%)	All nurses (weighted %)
1 *What might cause you to leave nursing?*					
1(a) Marriage	7.1	4.1	5.7	3.9	5.3
1(b) Baby	61.9	47.4	24.4	7.8	35.4
1(c) Partner moving jobs	24.8	28.9	24.4	11.8	22.5
1(d) Looking after children	31.0	34.0	22.0	7.8	23.7
1(e) Looking after dependants	15.0	23.7	20.3	28.4	21.6
1(f) Wanting a rest from paid work	2.7	9.3	9.8	9.8	7.8
1(g) Dislike of nursing work	9.7	9.3	7.3	2.9	7.4
1(h) Dislike of nursing pay	37.2	32.0	27.6	10.8	27.1
1(i) Wanting to get out of nursing	18.6	24.7	23.6	7.8	18.9
1(j) Prefer nursing outside NHS	34.5	16.5	16.3	10.8	19.8
2 *What improvements are necessary to encourage trained nurses to stay?* (Response: *'very important'*)					
2(a) Relaxation of discipline	8.0	3.1	4.9	2.0	4.6
2(b) Better promotion possibilities	37.2	47.4	32.5	28.4	36.1
2(c) Increased salaries	71.7	69.1	61.0	46.1	62.1
2(d) Regular training opportunities	46.9	48.5	52.8	52.9	50.3
2(e) More auxiliary help	19.5	20.6	15.4	25.5	20.0
2(f) More flexible hours	11.5	21.6	30.9	36.3	25.1
2(g) Special responsibility pay	35.4	43.3	48.0	43.1	42.5
2(h) Shorter working week	6.2	6.2	16.3	16.7	11.5
2(i) Split time between hospital and community	5.3	6.2	7.3	13.7	8.0
2(j) More nursing accommodation	11.5	17.5	8.1	22.8	14.5
2(k) Creche/nursing facilities	34.8	46.9	46.3	35.6	41.0
3 *Additional attitudinal questions*					
3(a) Present level of salary? (Too low or much too low)	95.5	80.4	72.4	58.0	76.8
3(b) Does nursing offer sufficient career opportunities? (Yes)	50.0	36.5	36.4	41.2	41.1
3(c) Do you consider the promotion prospects for someone like yourself? (Quite good or very good)	38.4	25.8	32.0	22.0	29.9
3(d) Do you see absenteeism among nurses as being a problem?	57.7	62.9	59.3	55.9	58.9
3(e) How do you feel about the present moves to community care? (Disapprove or strongly disapprove)	7.2	15.5	11.4	22.6	13.8
Sample size	113	97	123	102	435

outside the NHS. (Of course, when it comes to that point in time with this cohort, many more may have exercised their option of working outside the NHS before reaching 40, and the percentage in the group that remain may be similar to 11 per cent.)

The current cohort of those aged under 25 will have spent all their years in nursing since the Conservative government came to power in 1979 and in an era when the growth of private medical care has been actively encouraged and the concept made more generally acceptable. In short, the social and political context when the attitudes of our young nurses in the study were being formed was very different from that of the older nurses in the study. Hence, one can see the dramatic shift in the attitude of those aged under 25 when 35 per cent say they may prefer nursing outside the NHS and those aged 25 and over when only 13 per cent take a similar attitude. So while Table 4.1 tends to suggest that attitudes to the NHS seem to be associated with age reached, we feel that caution should be exercised in making such a ready connection that attitudes may change with age.

One way of examining these possibilities is to assume that there are groups of nurses with differing attitudes to the NHS and nursing, and that the proportion of these groups differs in each age. We investigate this possibility by looking for clusters of nurses with relatively similar responses to the attitude items.

The classification and its results

Various authors over the last 20 years have suggested a wide variety of algorithms for determining patterns in data. Gordon (1981) is one of many to suggest that many methods currently in use have no strong statistical basis, making it difficult to determine the number of groups. Latent class analysis provides solutions to a number of difficulties of standard cluster analysis. First, the number of different groups or types of activity may be assessed by examining the 'goodness of fit' of the various solutions (two group, three group, etc.) to the data – this is formally measured by the 'deviance', which is based on the likelihood function. Secondly, the analysis gives a set of probabilities (referred to here as response probabilities) which provide information on the importance of each response in each question in distinguishing between the groups. Formally stated, each response probability is:

the probability of an individual in a particular group giving a particular response to a particular item. Finally, latent class analysis does not give a rigid assignment of individuals to groups but instead provides a set of 'posterior probabilities' for each individual, giving the individual probability of assignment to or membership of each group. Thus an individual has a probability of belonging to a number of groups, and this is often a more realistic assumption to make.

Latent class analysis has been used extensively in sociological applications (Clogg 1979), one example being the classification of a survey population into groups based on their responses to a questionnaire designed to measure prejudice among blacks (Tuch 1981). The algorithmic approach used here follows Aitkin et al. (1981a), who re-analysed data from the Teaching Styles and Pupil Progress study of Bennett (1976), which produced a classification of teachers into a number of teaching styles. The algorithm used by Aitkin et al. was extended by Hinde to deal with multinomial responses and with missing data, and was subsequently used in a study on the Welsh language background of children (Baker and Hinde 1984). We used the same computer algorithm, which is written in the statistical programming language GENSTAT. No attempt is made here to describe latent class analysis in detail, as other authors (Lazarsfeld and Henry 1968; Aitkin et al. 1981b; Everitt 1984) have produced detailed treatments.

Four groups of nursing attitudes were identified by the analysis (the appendix provides the statistical information). An advantage with probabilistic clustering procedures is that the technique does not attempt to shoehorn nurses into groups, but allows for the possibility that some nurses will be difficult to assign to the groups found, and may have equal probabilities of belonging to a number of groups. The analysis instead gives us probabilities for each nurse to belong to each of the four groups, and we can therefore attempt to classify our sample of nurses into the four groups by looking for high probabilities of individual nurses belonging to a particular group. We adopted a criterion of assigning a nurse to a group if the nurse's probability of belonging to that group is greater than 0.75. On that assumption, the four-group solution produces the assignment of nurses in the sample to the groups shown in Table 4.2.

We now examine the four-group solution in greater detail. Table 4.3 shows the response probabilities for this classification.

Table 4.2 The four-group solution: assignment of nurses to groups

	Group				
	1	2	3	4	Unclassified
Number of nurses	79	77	82	123	74

Major differences between the probabilities can be identified. For example, there is a probability of 0.60 that Group 4 nurses will give 'baby' as a reason for leaving nursing, compared with a probability of 0.13 of Group 1 nurses giving the same reason. Group 2 nurses have a probability of 0.70 of giving 'dislike of nursing pay' as a reason for leaving nursing, compared with substantially lower probabilities in the other three groups. Group 3 nurses have a high probability (0.74) of seeing 'more flexible hours' as very important to encourage trained nurses to stay, compared with low probabilities for the other three groups.

We can continue this process, and attempt to produce a description of each of the four groups produced by the clustering procedure. Although the groups are defined in terms of probabilities of giving answers to certain questions, we can think of these probabilities in terms of expected proportions of nurses giving a particular answer if a hypothetical sample of nurses of the group under examination had been taken. We can therefore adopt a straightforward approach and treat high probabilities as being indicative of concerns specifically raised by each of the groups.

Group 1: Nursing come what may

Curiously, there are no matters which specifically concern nurses classified as Group 1 more than any of the other three groups. Of the total body of nurses in the sample, these are the ones who see the least problems in nursing at present; furthermore, they are also nurses who see less in their own situation, such as having a baby, partner moving jobs, looking after children and so on, which is likely to cause them to leave nursing. Whatever may happen, they seem to be saying that they will be staying in nursing. Nursing pay is not likely to drive them away into other work; indeed, while the probability of giving the answers 'too low' or 'much too low' for the level of salary being paid to nurses at that time is still high (0.73), they have a low probability (0.34) of answering 'very

Table 4.3 Response probabilities for each group – four-group solution

Attitude	Group 1	2	3	4
1. What might cause you to leave nursing?				
1(a) Marriage	0.02	0.08	0.02	0.08
1(b) Baby	0.14	0.43	0.14	0.60
1(c) Partner moving jobs	0.09	0.38	0.16	0.26
1(d) Looking after children	0.02	0.30	0.08	0.45
1(e) Looking after dependants	0.14	0.22	0.15	0.31
1(f) Wanting a rest from paid work	0.10	0.12	0.07	0.04
1(g) Dislike of nursing work	0.00	0.21	0.15	0.31
1(h) Dislike of nursing pay	0.12	0.70	0.16	0.16
1(i) Wanting to get out of nursing	0.15	0.46	0.16	0.05
1(j) Prefer nursing outside NHS	0.19	0.34	0.13	0.15
2. What improvements are necessary to encourage trained nurses to stay? *(Response: 'very important')*				
2(a) Relaxation of discipline	0.00	0.09	0.08	0.04
2(b) Better promotion possibilities	0.16	0.58	0.60	0.26
2(c) Increased salaries	0.34	0.84	0.84	0.58
2(d) Regular training opportunities	0.29	0.59	0.84	0.44
2(e) More auxiliary help	0.11	0.24	0.50	0.10
2(f) More flexible hours	0.10	0.20	0.74	0.12
2(g) Special responsibility pay	0.12	0.60	0.85	0.32
2(h) Shorter working week	0.04	0.14	0.35	0.04
2(i) Split time between hospital and community	0.04	0.05	0.28	0.03
2(j) More nursing accommodation	0.09	0.22	0.30	0.07
2(k) Creche/nursing facilities	0.19	0.46	0.63	0.43
3. Additional attitudinal questions				
3(a) Present level of salary? (Too low or much too low)	0.73	0.96	0.70	0.70
3(b) Does nursing offer sufficient career opportunities? (Yes)	0.37	0.19	0.38	0.82
3(c) Do you consider the promotion prospects for someone like yourself? (Quite good or very good)	0.12	0.06	0.29	0.65
3(d) Do you see absenteeism among nurses as being a problem?	0.58	0.71	0.68	0.53
3(e) how do you feel about the present moves to community care? (Disapprove or strongly disapprove)	0.26	0.24	0.22	0.05

important' when salary is considered as an improvement to encourage nurses to stay. It seems little will deter them from continuing in nursing and, further, they make few new demands upon the system. Compared with other nurses they do not bemoan the pay, poor promotion possibilities, lack of training opportunities etc. Quite simply, nursing is their life whatever the trials and tribulations.

Group 2: Nursing, but for how much longer?

These nurses disproportionately feel they are more likely to leave nursing for a wide variety of reasons. The strongest differences can be seen on the responses of disliking nursing work and pay, or just simply wanting to get out of nursing. The likelihood of preferring nursing outside the NHS is also higher than for the other groups. However, they also seem likely to leave for other external factors, such as having a baby, looking after children or looking after dependants. They feel that improvements are necessary in promotion, salaries and training, but are less likely than Group 3 to rate other improvements as being 'very important'. If this group has a single source of disillusionment, it is pay, with the highest probability among the groups of rating their own salary as inadequate. Hence, these can be identified as nurses seeking a well-paid occupation, and perhaps rapidly coming to the conclusion that NHS nursing is not for them.

Group 3: Nursing: battling it out

This group is characterized by its low probabilities of giving reasons for wanting to leave nursing, and in this respect are somewhat similar to Group 1 nurses. However, their attitude to the improvements questions tell a different story. This group has extremely high probabilities of seeing a wide range of improvements as 'very important', from increased salaries to issues such as a shorter working week and increased responsibility pay. Their responses indicate they are particularly concerned about the level of nursing pay and all the trappings which transform a mundane job into a career (e.g. training opportunities, promotion possibilities, special responsibility pay, more auxiliary help). Group 3 nurses are also unlikely to leave because of family reasons. This does not mean that they would not have children, but they do not wish to leave paid employment to look after them. Hence they, more than any of the other three groups, feel that creche/nursing facilities are among the improvements which are necessary to encourage trained nurses to stay. They now find themselves in nursing and like it, and they want it to be uninterrupted and rewarding. They seem on the whole likely to be stayers, but, unlike Group 1, remain extremely concerned about the pay and conditions of the nursing profession.

Group 4: Nursing: 'just a job'

This is another quite distinct grouping in which there is a much more ready response to factors and demands external to nursing. These are the nurses who it seems are more likely to leave as a result of marriage, having a baby, partner moving jobs, looking after children, looking after dependants. For them nursing largely seems to offer sufficient opportunities and there is a much greater satisfaction about 'the promotion prospects for someone like yourself'. They do not express concern about flexible hours, nursing accommodation, and so on as a way of encouraging trained nurses to stay. Creche facilities have less interest for them than for Group 3, for many probably intend to give up work to care for their children. It should be noted that they also express serious concern about the pay and so, if it is 'just a job', it needs to be paid satisfactorily. Certainly they are very much less concerned about the problem of career opportunities and probably have thought much less about alternative kinds of work. However, one suspects that, if the private health sector outside the NHS was thought to pay well, then this group of nurses would be among those attracted to move. In brief, these nurses are interested in well-paid nursing jobs but recognize that they may leave nursing because of family commitments.

Discussion

As Everitt (1980) has said, cluster analysis techniques provide methods of breaking complex data sets into manageable groups. We have seen that latent class analysis provides a model-based approach for investigating the number of groups, and provides a picture of the attitudinal response of such groups. Our evidence indicates that nurses are not a homogeneous group, but hold very different expectations from nursing. This outcome has serious implications for recruitment policy, as it implies the futility of a one-solution strategy as an approach to staffing problems.

Our statistical analysis of a random sample of nurses from one district health authority suggested that four groups may be the most appropriate way of understanding their responses to a set of attitudinal items. The most frequent constellation of attitudes (28 per cent) resulted in seeing primarily 'nursing as a job' (Group 4). The remaining groups split evenly, with just under one-fifth of the sample in each group. Hence, it is obviously misleading to consider the nursing profession as a homogeneous group or even as having one major group with a dominant set of attitudes. Once these groups have been established we are then able to build up group profiles by examining the characteristics of nurses who have been assigned to a particular group. Analysed this way, one is able to retain the complexity inherent in the sample, rather than making assumptions about the sample and any subsets. It is possible, for example, to cross-classify the group variable by a number of descriptive variables (such as age, marital status, number of children at home, specialty, etc.) and by further attitudinal variables not included in the original analysis. These variables help to provide background information, but this kind of analysis in no way validates the groups; so, for example, it is perfectly possible for people of similar profiles in relation to age and marital status to be assigned to different groups by virtue of their attitudes.

Building up group profiles makes clear that this method of analysis reveals levels of complexity which should not be ignored. Age, for example, emerged as an important difference between the groups. So Group 1 nurses ('nursing come what may') were more likely to be aged 30–39 or 40+ than to be aged 25–29; Group 2 ('nursing, but for how much longer?') nurses were more likely to be aged 30–39 or younger, but were unlikely to be 40+; Group 3 ('battling it out') also included many aged 30–39 plus those of 40+; over 40 per cent of Group 4 nurses ('just a job') were under 25, with a further 20 per cent under 30. In what ways these age differences between groups matter is more complex and lends itself to more interpretations than might, at first, be imagined. These under 25, as we have seen earlier, have grown up and trained in a period in which opportunities outside the NHS have grown for nurses, and must seem to be realistic options. The job market has, in this respect, altered. Also, the expectation of marriage and childrearing breaks, in this predominantly female profession, echoes the hairdressers in Attwood and Hatton's study (1983), whose expected 'life' as a hairdresser was five years before taking the anticipated break. These 'lifecycle' events, however, did not exclude a return to hairdressing, but were a prelude to working in the less glamorous salons. As such, the hairdressing industry perceived these young women as failures in not following a specific and expected route; their nursing counterparts may also return to non-NHS jobs, nursing homes or other private work rather than disappear completely from the nursing scene.

Dex (1988: 148) has illustrated that 'there are considerable variations between women, not just by age and lifecycle, but according to their experience, education and prospects' which influence the attitudes of women to work. Brown (1976: 39, 40) has also argued for a need to understand 'the ways in which the labour market operates', and the constraints set upon the worker, to further our understanding of the 'relationship between "structure" and "consciousness", rather than looking at workers' perceptions alone. In nursing, Firth and Britton (1989) have highlighted some situational elements in professional 'burnout', notably that supportive action by managers could reduce absenteeism. The complex relationships between daily experience of working life and longer-term expectations of nursing are illustrated by Clifton (1990), who has written of the ways in which management styles and goals can cut across a nurse's commitment to caring for the whole patient rather than mechanistically carrying out tasks.

In this study, in addition to generational and cyclical aspects of age, it became apparent that there are situational aspects which need to be borne in mind. Group 4 nurses, containing a high proportion of students, were the least qualified, and perceive nursing as offering sufficient training opportunities. By comparison, Groups 2 and 3 contained high proportions of midwives and mental health nurses, and their responses indicate levels of discontent over the ways in which their qualifications and experience are used; we have already seen that both groups are likely to view 'special responsibility pay' as a necessary incentive to retain trained staff (see Table 4.3). Group 1 nurses, who were more content than Groups 2 and 3, contained a high proportion of the sample's community nurses. Another aspect of the relationship between situation and age was highlighted by group 3: they were highly likely to be combining childrearing with an occupation to which they were committed, yet apparently found the conditions of work difficult and unrewarding. Perhaps not surprisingly, they saw creche and nursery facilities as important provisions which might encourage trained nurses to stay. This particular set of concerns is at odds with the traditional picture of a nurse as young and single; a picture, incidentally, which Vicinus (1985: 118) shows us to be inappropriate even a century ago when nurses faced the expectation of early retirement and so took the option of private nursing, which provided 'better pay and longer working life'.

We have indicated that there are currently considerable divergencies in attitudes towards nursing among nurses, and there is little chance of a longitudinal study clarifying what is actually happening. These attitudes are complex, and appear to reflect interaction between conditions of work and an individual's personal circumstances, expectations and experience. As these nurses clearly differ in their situations, ages and workplaces it becomes harder to talk of 'nurses' as one group. Whittaker and Olesen (1964) point to how the legend of Florence Nightingale, widely accepted as the culture-heroine of the nursing profession, has many faces and many functions. The differing faces of this legend reflect prevailing ideologies in nursing, and each generation claims something specific from the Florence Nightingale legend as its own: 'to those asked to accept and incorporate change [the legend] shows a face which reflects the very change desired. To some women it projects the face of traditional womanhood, to others it shows how traditional femininity could be combined with a career' (Whittaker and Olesen 1964: 130). From this analysis, we would argue that it is unwise to attempt to delineate one model of nursing in the NHS. In order to recruit the necessary workforce we must recognize that there are different attitudes within nursing, and come to terms with the different needs they reflect.

Appendix

Examination of the deviances for various numbers of groups from one to five provides us with evidence to determine the number of groups of attitudes present. If the observed deviance reductions shown in Table 4.4

Table 4.4 Deviances for the classification problem

Number of groups	Deviance	Deviance difference	Largest of 19 simulated differences
1	17957		
		396	118.4
2	17563		
		270	123.0
3	17293		
		201	123.2
4	17092		
		125	124.7
5	16967		

are greater than the largest of 19 simulated deviance reductions, then there is evidence that these reductions in deviance are unlikely to have occurred by chance, and thus evidence for the higher number of groups. Table 4.4 shows that there are large reductions in deviance from the one- to the two-group solutions, from the two- to the three-group solutions and from the three-group to the four-group solutions. Monte Carlo testing procedures allow us to determine the importance of these deviance reductions by generating random data with the characteristics of the sample assuming a certain number of groups, then carrying out a latent class analysis on these data assuming that there is a further group present. In this way, we can simulate deviance reductions for comparing three groups over two groups, four groups over three groups, etc. We can see from the table that there is strong evidence for the existence of two groups over one group, for three groups over two groups, and for four groups over three groups. The evidence for five groups is less strong, as the deviance reduction is close to the simulated test value, and we do not consider the five-group solution further.

Glossary

algorithms a set of mathematical calculations to carry out a statistical or mathematical technique.

attitudinal questions a set of questions on a questionnaire which ask the respondent for their opinions on various issues.

clustering methods a set of statistical techniques which attempt to classify individuals into groups, and where the individuals within a group are more similar in some respect than individuals from different groups.

cross-sectional data information which is collected on one occasion at the same date or in the same time period for a number of individuals. This is usually contrasted with longitudinal data, where information on the same individual is collected over time, on more than one occasion.

deviance a number which measures the 'goodness of fit' of a statistical model to the data. In our example, the statistical model is the assumption of a certain number of groups. The deviance decreases as the number of groups increases, until a perfect fit is obtained when every individual belongs to his or her own individual group.

fit to estimate mathematically a set of numbers based on a set of assumptions about the structure of the data. In our example, the set of numbers are **probabilities,** and the assumptions are the number of differing groups which are present in the sample.

five-point scale in response to an **attitudinal question,** the respondent will have a choice of one of five categories in which to record their view on the question topic. The categories often measure agreement or disagreement with a statement, and, if so, will usually be ordered, with category 1 representing the most extreme category of disagreement and category 5 the most extreme category of agreement. Other scales are also used.

frequencies counts of numbers of individuals (i.e. not proportions, percentages, or measurements).

GENSTAT a statistical computer package or program.

homogeneous group a group with similar opinions and behaviour patterns.

latent class analysis a statistical technique for carrying out **probabilistic clustering.** Literally, classes or groups which are not observed but which are latent or hidden in the data.

likelihood function a mathematical formula which represents the **probability** of observing the data which were actually observed under a set of assumptions (on the number of groups).

Monte Carlo testing often referred to also as simulation, the techique uses random numbers to generate sets of data assuming a particular hypothesis (for example, 'there are three groups present in the data'), then uses those sets of data to examine the effect of assuming different assumptions (for example, 'there are four groups present in the data').

multinomial responses responses to a single question which are categorized into more than two groups.

probabilistic clustering a method of clustering which, rather than giving an absolute assignment of individuals to groups, instead provides **probabilities** for an individual to belong to each of the groups.

probability a probability is a measure of how likely an event is to occur. Probabilities always lie between zero and one inclusive.

Acknowledgement

We are grateful to the Leverhulme Trust for providing financial support for the above research.

References

Aitkin, M. A., Bennett, S. N. and Hesketh, J. 1981a. Teaching styles and pupil progress: a reanalysis. *British Journal of Educational Psychology* 51: 170–86.

Aitkin, M. A., Anderson, D. A. and Hinde, J. P. 1981b. Statistical modelling of data on teaching styles. *Journal of the Royal Statistical Society* A, 144: 419–61.

Attwood, M. and Hatton, F. 1983. 'Getting on', Gender differences in career development: a case study in the hairdressing industry. In E. Gamarnikow, D. H. J. Morgan, J. Purvis and D. E. Taylorson (eds), *Gender, Class and Work*, London: Heinemann.

Bagguley, P. 1988. *A Report of a Study of Turnover and Work Dissatisfaction amongst UK Professional Nurses.* University of Lancaster.

Baker, C. and Hinde, J. 1984. Language background classification. *Journal of Multilingual and Multicultural Development* 5: 43–56.

Bennett, S. N. 1976. *Teaching Styles and Pupil Progress.* London: Open Books.

Briggs, A. 1972. *Report of the Committee on Nursing*, Cmnd 5115. London: HMSO.

Brown, R. 1976. Women as employees: some comments on research in industrial sociology. In D. L. Barker and S. Allen (eds), *Dependence and Exploitation in Work and Marriage*, London: Longman.

Clifton, B. 1990. Who's helping who . . . *Health Matters*, June, Issue 4: 18.

Clogg, C. 1979. Some latent structure models for the analysis of Likert type data. *Social Science Research* 8: 287–301.

Dex, S. 1988. *Women's Attitudes towards Work.* London: Macmillan.

Downe, S. 1990. A noble vocation. *Nursing Times*, 3 October, 86 (40): 24.

Everitt, B. 1980. *Cluster Analysis.* London: Heinemann.

Everitt, B. 1984. *An Introduction to Latent Variable Models.* London: Chapman & Hall.

Firth, H. and Britton, P. 1989. 'Burnout', absence and turnover amongst British nursing staff. *Journal of Occupational Psychology* 62: 55–9.

Gamarnikow, E. 1978. Sexual division of labour: the case of nursing. In A. Kuhn and A. Wolpe (eds), *Feminism and Materialism.* London: Routledge & Kegan Paul.

Game, A. and Pringle, R. 1983. *Gender at Work.* London: Pluto Press.

Gordon, A. D. 1981. *Classification.* London: Chapman & Hall.

Lazarsfeld, P. F. and Henry, N. W. 1968. *Latent Structure Analysis.* Boston, Mass.: Houghton Mifflin.

Leeson, J. and Gray, J. 1978. *Women and Medicine.* London: Tavistock.

Mackay, L. 1988a. Career woman. *Nursing Times*, 9 March, 84(10).

Mackay, L. 1988b. The nurses nearest the door. *Guardian*, 13 January.

Mackay, L. 1988c. No time to care. *Nursing Times*, 16 March, 84(11).

Mackay, L. 1989. *Nursing a Problem.* Milton Keynes: Open University Press.

Martin, J. and Roberts, C. 1984. *Women and Employment: A Lifetime Perspective*. London: HMSO.

Mercer, G. M. 1979. *The Employment of Nurses*. London: Croom Helm.

Soothill, K. and Mackay, L. 1988. Submission to Pay Review Board.

Tuch, S. A. 1981. Analysing recent trends in prejudice towards blacks: insights from latent class models. *American Journal of Sociology* 87: 130–42.

Vicinus, M. 1985. *Independent Women: Work and Community for Single Women 1850–1920*. London: Virago Press.

Whittaker, E. and Olesen, V. 1964. The faces of Florence Nightingale: functions of the heroine legend in an occupational sub-culture. *Human Organisation* 23(2): 123–30.

Witz, A. 1985. *Midwifery and Medicine*. Lancaster Regionalism Group, Working Paper 13.

CHAPTER FIVE

Conceptions of the nature of persons by doctors, nurses and teachers

Christine Henry

This chapter focuses upon part of a major research project and discusses a small qualitative study of doctors', nurses' and teachers' conceptions of the nature of persons. It concentrates upon moral, formal and commonsense conceptions of persons, showing how past experience and professional education influence the acquisition of the conceptions of persons held by these professionals.

The chapter concludes by examining the ethical and educational implications of these various conceptions and how particular conceptions may have implications for the way we treat and care for patients, and consequently offers recommendations for the education of doctors, nurses and teachers.

Conceptions of the nature of persons

First it is essential to seek some understanding of what is meant by the concept of the person and who legitimately can be counted as a person before emphasizing the idea that a better comprehension is necessarily central for good health care.

The concept of the person with some of its uses stands for what humans essentially are, and more than one answer to the question of what constitutes a person can be given. Nevertheless, it may be helpful to identify three possible models that are useful in understanding the concept of a person. The three models are only tentative conceptual schemes and must not be viewed as definitions of the person. However, each model will allow for diversity in perspectives, with the underpinning assumption that each model is insufficient in itself. The concept of the person defies definition in the formal and descriptive sense. Further, it is claimed by some philosophers to be a primitive concept and difficult to analyse.

The morallevaluative model of the person

A moral conception of the person is put forward by Abelson (1977), who claims that the term 'person' is normative and evaluative like the term 'good'. Abelson also remarks that we do not have any established criteria for applying person status. In other words, it is open to us whether we ascribe person status or not, and neither logic nor language can give the answer to who should and who should not be given the title 'person'. Even when we observe the behaviour of others, although we may find grounds for person ascription it is not logically conclusive because behaviour does not entail such status. Further, Abelson states that the ascription of personhood does not rest entirely on respect for human beings. It is possible that the mental defective and the very small infant can be given semi-person status and this does happen within the healthcare field. Similarly, recent history reflects the reality of a whole race of people being deprived of full person status – for example, the treatment of the Jewish people in Nazi Germany. Abelson argues that the term 'person' is an open-ended evaluative term and therefore empirically unanalysable. However, he claims that the individual person is a subject of psychological and moral predicates and therefore independent of biological classification. If this is the case then it is possible from this moral and evaluative model to ascribe person status to non-humans. The term 'person' is therefore not a natural concept and defies biological classification.

Not only is the term difficult to define in formal ways but it is a term that is viewed as species neutral. Abelson remarks that in everyday language there may be some confusion between the two terms 'person' and 'human'. The term 'person' is viewed as purely normative whereas the term 'human' is semi-normative and descriptive. The term 'human' will convey a limited reference to the species and at the same time refer to characteristics of humans.

The latter semi-normative elements involve the characteristics that are valued. The term 'human' can be used interchangeably with the term 'person' in everyday commonsense ways (for example, 'Well, she's only human after all'). This indicates that being human is valued in that we are not machine-like, or perfect in a formal or descriptive sense. Abelson suggests that in our everyday use we often imply that the terms 'human' and 'person' are the same or have the same meaning.

This model emphasizes value and a moral sense of the term 'person'. Harris (1985) remarks that a person will be any being capable of valuing its own existence. Although it is not as simple as Harris claims, it implies that there does not appear to be any sort of necessary truth that all persons are human beings. Midgley (1983) also remarks that other animals besides ourselves may value their own existence and from this point of view are capable of being a person. This serves to support Abelson's claim that the concept of the person is open-ended and evaluative like the term 'good'. Shoemaker and Swinburne (1984) support the idea that the animal is the form in which the person is physically realized at a given time. Locke (1632–1704) remarks that human beings in one sense are animals and he distinguishes between the identity of a person and that of a man, holding that the former does not involve the identity of an animal (Henry, 1986).

The formal traditional model of persons

Why is it that some human beings are identified as having only semi-person status? This may relate to a more formal model of the person influenced by a number of Western traditional philosophers. One of the criticisms levelled at Midgley's statement that other animals may value their own existence is its attribution of the features of a special kind of consciousness and features of rationality to other animals. These special features are particularly attributed to the human mind and have been viewed as person features and what differentiates ourselves as human beings from other sentient beings. Further, it may be one of the reasons why in commonsense terms the severely mentally handicapped, the very young infant, the confused elderly and the patient on a life support machine are not viewed as persons in the full sense of the term. Not only do traditional philosophical views influence the conceptions of the nature of persons, but also the type of education that is given can reflect traditional values and the need for attributing defining features in order to categorize, recognize or make sense of individuals and their situation.

Hampshire (1959) claims that persons are distinguishable from other sentient beings because they are capable of putting their thoughts into words (Singer 1979). A person must be able to communicate in general but also let his or her intentions be known. Strawson (1959) supports this by claiming that we do not ascribe psychological concepts such as memory, motivation or intention to other animals. However, Midgley disagrees and claims that we have no right to diminish the inner lives of the rest of creation. Further, in commonsense everyday terms we often do attribute psychological features to other animals who share our lives and with whom we have special relationships (for example our family dog). In this sense Midgley supports and advocates a value perspective which is more open-ended and links to a commonsense view rather than the formal traditional or ideal model.

Dennett (1979) presents some possible themes or features that have been identified as necessary but not sufficient conditions of personhood and may summarize an ideal/formal model of the person. He claims that we require an intelligent conscious feeling agent to coincide with a moral notion of a person who is accountable, having rights and responsibilities. He claims that the notion of a conscious feeling agent is a necessary if not sufficient condition of moral personhood. Dennett outlines a further six themes identifying other necessary but not sufficient conditions of personhood. Dennett's six familiar themes are useful for seeing different ways in which an individual might identify person features. Further, the themes may be used as distinguishing features between persons and non-persons. However, the danger arises when only one model of the conception of the nature of persons is used. It is therefore essential to remember that even the formal model must remain an open-ended list of features and be taken as an ideal model only, that we can only approximate to the idea anyhow, and that there must be caution in attempts at defining persons by attributing identifiable features.

Dennett suggests that the first and most obvious condition is that persons are seen as rational beings. This theme indicates that reason involves higher-order notions of knowledge, language and intelligence. Secondly, states of consciousness are attributed and psychological features such as intentions are predicated to these states. The third theme depends upon whether something counting as a person rests upon a particular stance being adopted towards it. In other words, individuals are treated in a certain way and to some extent this is part of being a person. This theme involves a social element. A reminder of how Nazi Germany treated a whole group of people as non-persons reflects how it is possible to influence the treatment and care of people in the health care field simply by taking a particular stance towards individuals; i.e. treating them as persons or treating them as things or non-persons. Dennett remarks that the first three themes are mutually dependent – i.e. the person is rational, intentional and a subject (not object) of a particular stance. These three themes are a necessary but not sufficient proviso for the fourth theme of reciprocity, which implies that a being who has a personal stance taken towards it must be capable of reciprocating in some way. This fourth theme in turn is a necessary but not sufficient condition of communication. This fifth theme of communication is a necessary condition of Dennett's sixth and final theme. Persons are distinguishable from other sentient beings by being conscious in a special way. Self-consciousness is a condition for persons being moral agents.

These themes of Dennett's can be identified as a common cluster of person features. However, Dennett's themes may be viewed as an ideal feature list for the nature of persons, which would be difficult or impossible to apply in certain cases.

The social commonsense model of persons

An alternative way of understanding the concept of the person links closely with a commonsense view. Teichman (1972) states that in commonsense terms we treat humanity as the deciding mark for the ascription of person status. Teichman, like Abelson, suggests that in ordinary use the word 'person' and the extension of the term 'human being' give the impression of being identical. She observes that the only natural persons we actually meet in real life are human beings, although she acknowledges that it is logically possible for another variety of natural persons to exist on other planets, i.e. non-human persons.

An extension of this viewpoint could be the inclusion of other animals on this planet that are strikingly like us (i.e. like us psychologically, with intentions and so on). What is important from Teichman's point of view is that the intension (meaning and application) of the word 'person' allows for this possibility. Teichman's view is not only social but involves the idea of the term being meaningfully applicable. Further, any meaningfully socially constructed view is not decriptive but involves values and an element of open-endedness. Teichman emphasizes that the conceptions of the nature of persons involve the idea of a social fellowship or relationship within the social context. However, Teichman points out that the notion of having a particular kind of body, whether misshapen or unusual but recognizably human, rules out parrots, dolphins and chimpanzees, although the latter in some ways are similar to human beings. She emphasizes an alternative view of a social and human commonsense model of the person. This perspective is restricted to the human social world and therefore fits with the idea that as human persons we use the term 'human being' as a starting point. Further, there may be a self-creating element with the term that arises from out of our own interpretive world (phenomenological world). This latter point links to the idea of what is meaningful to ourselves when ascribing person status.

Teichman's view relates to Wittgenstein's approach in that language (in the human context) is essentially social. The meaning of the word is to be found not in logical analysis but in its use within a particular language game to which it belongs. These language games are not just a matter of words and use but also include feelings, gestures, attitudes and skills. These complex related elements compose a particular 'form of life'. A form of life is part of our interpretive world. For example, Wittgenstein claimed that other animals have different forms of life and if a lion could speak we would not understand him. The language used in each game overlaps, sharing the same words but having different meanings. Application of Wittgenstein's view can be illustrated crudely in the use of the word 'human'. For example, in a particular language game between medical biologists it may be specifically used to mean biological membership of a species, whereas a group of nurses or general practitioners may use the term 'human' to mean the same as 'person' when talking about the patient or client. The same word is used in each language game but has a different meaning (Henry 1986). The two terms 'human' and 'person' can also come together in some language games but act differently in others. The major focus of this model concerns everyday functions of language, the use of which can be associated with a human commonsense view of the world, which in broad terms considers the social context to be important. Once again this model like the previous models cannot offer a definition of the nature of persons and is not sufficient on its own.

The three models offer different viewpoints but hopefully can coexist with other more varied perceptions and help to push back the boundaries of understanding and show how confusions can arise with the conceptions of the nature of persons that are held by health professionals. The conceptions that we have will, in turn, influence the way we treat and care for individuals within the health care system.

The next section focuses upon a small research study of doctors', nurses' and teachers' conceptions of the nature of persons.

The research approach and results

The major research project from which this small study is taken was concerned with commonsense conceptions of the nature of persons amongst children, adolescents and adults. Whilst the main study focused upon social cognitive developmental psychology, a rich source of data emerged concerning ethical and professional issues, particularly with the doctors, nurses and teachers who formed the sample of adults in the study. Whilst the number of adult respondents was small (24 adults), it is important to point out that not only were the adult group part of a main study but also that the research was qualitative by nature of its originality, with its emphasis upon exploratory procedures rather than formulation of generalizations. Further, the author takes a philosophical stance in that research of this nature not only allows for further exploratory research to be carried out at a future date and therefore lays down a foundational framework in which to proceed, but also contributes to the body of knowledge that will expand levels of understanding of perceptions of ourselves as professionals.

Specific attention was paid to two aspects: (a) the criteria for person/non-person distinctions, including temporal phases in personhood – namely the nature of origins (i.e. birth) and cessation (i.e. death), and (b) the content of persons and the meaning of person predicates – for example, features of the mind (i.e. consciousness, rationality, self-reflection and, to some extent, emotion).

The major form of collecting data was the semi-structured interview, although other methods such as a semantic differential rating scale were used as support. The transcribed interviews were subjected to a detailed content analysis from which categories were devised and ordered into frequency response tables. This was to give an overview of the similarities and differences in responses to the conceptions of the nature of persons held within and between groups. A clustan computer format yielded a cluster analysis on the two areas of person/non-person distinctions and content and features applied to persons.

Given the framework of both philosophical aspects inherent in the conceptualization of the nature of persons and the initial lack of previous research, it was thought desirable that the investigation should explore aspects of person conceptions initially from a cognitive developmental point of view, particularly with the children and adolescents, and from an ethical and educational point of view with the adult group. The latter exploratory study will be the focus of this final section. The author felt that expressing views on the conceptions of the nature of persons demanded a more personal approach and the semi-structured interview was seen as appropriate. Whilst it was recognized that there were several disadvantages relating to interviews (such as the limit on the number of respondents, sources of error relating to the interviewer, the instrument itself and overall reliability and validity), these factors can be and were partially overcome by minimizing subjectivity and bias from the interviewer, respondent and the substantive content of the questions. As Valentine (1982) remarks, the problems raised by taking introspective reports are no more serious than the problems raised by other methods. In fact, no one method of collecting data guarantees certainty.

Doctors', nurses' and teachers' conceptions of the nature of persons

Generally, from a philosophical standpoint younger children in the main study did not differentiate between the two terms 'human' and 'person'. The term 'human', as Teichman suggested, was therefore used as a starting point for the acquisition of a concept of the person. However, the older groups including the adults showed a more qualitative distinction between persons and non-persons utilizing more rational constructs in their conceptions and variations in the conceptions were evident.

PERSONS AND NON-PERSON DISTINCTIONS

The general hypotheses from the main study concerned cognitive developmental psychology. Nevertheless, certain important areas implicit within the hypotheses relate closely to concerns for doctors, nurses and teachers. The research involved representations or images of the person and attempted to tease out construals in this conceptual field that are often taken for granted within the health care domains.

Through the process of growing older the individual may have more variable experience, be influenced by the learning environment and therefore become less bound by context. The adult group's conceptions of persons, particularly in the distinctions between persons and non-persons, not only use more abstract and inferential constructs but also approximate towards a more ideal/formal model of the person.

The doctors, nurses and teachers highlighted the fact that abstract features should be attributed to persons. This sort of concept acquisiton can be dependent upon their own experiences, which are more variable, and therefore influenced by the learning environment. It was apparent that the adult group used more psychological attributes to distinguish between persons and non-persons.

The doctors, nurses and teachers emphasized that the beginnings of persons (i.e. origins) were variable, although an innate potentiality for persons (before birth) had a preference overall. This could cause some confusion in relation to abortion and embryonic research. There was also a divided preference for views of the ending of persons in constructs for finite and infinite life spans relating to the conceptions of death of persons.

There is obvious variation in response in the adults for divided preferences, like birth and pre-birth categories, which may reflect aspects of variation in interpretation and individual experiences.

FEATURES AND CONTENT OF PERSONS

The doctors, nurses and teachers show variation in their conceptions of the nature of mind. The variations indicate experience and individual preferences, although overall they show a preference for dualistic conceptions (mind being non-material and body being material). However, the doctors in particular show a preference for the mind conceived as brain, mind as aspects of the brain and mind as sum of parts. These constructs may be influenced by their education and training and indicate a sophisticated monistic and materialistic viewpoint.

The adult group particularly reflected Dennett's ideal type of model in that there was a high response to features of rationality, consciousness and self-awareness, treated as a person and symbolic language.

Teichman (1985) remarks that an attempted analysis of the concept of the person cannot be taken for granted in that it will to some extent be guided by ordinary use. However, particularly in relation to content, the doctors, nurses and teachers did not necessarily adhere to this view. The group had a tendency to approximate towards an ideal/formal model for features and content attributed to persons. Teichman suggests that it is usually only philosophy students who add features such as self-consciousness and rationality to persons. The highly selected sample of adults were chosen from the professional fields of medicine, nursing and teaching. Therefore to some extent their conceptions may have been influenced by their education and training. This in turn may highlight the Western traditional philosophy that influences formal higher education.

There was little use of the ethical or moral model of the conceptions of the nature of persons within the adult group. The moral view not only relates to viewing the person as a non-biological term but also demands some thinking in ethical terms. Further, in professional life the doctors, nurses and teachers must utilize this rather abstract and moral viewpoint. This emphasizes the importance of an ethical curriculum for the professionals.

More knowledge is explored in thinking about the self and others, utilizing as a starting point the discussion of the three tentative models within a new curriculum. In doing this more direction is given to how we may behave and treat others. Underpinning this is also the basic tenet of Wittgenstein in that meaning is within use. In other words, how we use a particular term like 'person' will reflect the meaning we give to it. There is a need to consolidate some of our thinking regarding the nature of persons because of the moral and social issues involved in the practice of health care and the essential central concern for respect for persons.

Ethical and educational issues

Obviously the conceptions of the nature of persons have more than one interpretation. For instance, on the one hand it may mean that each person is rational and self-conscious, or on the other hand each individual can be ascribed person status on the understanding that neither logic nor language will solve the problem for us as to who should or should not be counted as a person. The first interpretation relates to attributing features to each individual, and the doctors, nurses and teachers had a tendency to do this. In some ways it is restrictive and not useful for moral or social issues. The moral and social aspects are involved in how we view others in the world and in decisions and actions we take. The second interpretation is more open and can be linked to the commonsense model, and also will involve as a consequence respect for persons. What is important through education is to sort out some of the confusions that arise in ascribing person status to ourselves and others who we care for and the moral issues involved in treatment of non-persons as well as persons who share our world. It seems that there are no clear natural dividing lines between some non-persons and persons – for example the six-month-old fetus. Whilst it would be silly to give votes to oysters, just as it would be silly to call them persons, it is the borderline cases that cause us problems (Russell 1974). Perhaps it is worth noting that the commonsense model gets out of the tricky position of distinguishing between ourselves and other animals by referring to a human identifiable shape or differences in forms of life (e.g. if a lion could speak we would not understand him). The formal or ideal feature list could exclude other animals by not attributing major person features to them such as intentions or self-consciousness. However, this is rather a dangerous form of application because the feature list is open-ended and ought not to be applied in absolute terms. The moral/evaluative model makes it possible to ascribe the term 'person' to non-humans, perhaps including other animals that share our world. If it is meaningful then it is possible to have non-human persons. However, there are contradictions within and between these selective models.

In examining the conceptions of the nature of persons for this particular group of doctors, nurses and teachers several questions arise in relation to the ethics of care. Does the distinction between persons and non-persons depend upon whether the term 'person' is meaningfully applicable or not? The fetus is human and a potential member of a rational species, a potential person, but is it a person? (Rational species is different from biological membership – see Teichman 1985.) Can it be inferred that the severely defective infant, the madly insane, the confused elderly individual and the individual on a life support system are in some way exempt from some very important elements of personhood? These are important questions to ask when considering the perspectives which nurses have regarding individuals in their care. Let us consider the situation within an intensive care unit where a young person has an intact brain stem but the upper parts of the brain have been irrevocably traumatized. This presents a position were the major physical functions of heartbeat, breathing and excretion can be maintained because the brain stem has remained viable. However, because the upper part of the brain is severely damaged it means that cognitive processes such as thoughts, feelings and emotions may no longer be expressed. This situation can cause a great deal of anxiety not just for nurses but also for the relatives.

Historically, death was signified by the stopping of the heart and the eventual putrefaction of the body. This is not such a definitive process today. Consider the position of the relatives who can see monitors which record heartbeat and breathing. Further, the body is still warm to touch and the individual's cheeks may have colour in them. All of these traits illustrate the presence of life. Despite this fact, the relatives will never again experience those special elements expressed by their loved one which made him or her unique as a person. They will never hear laughter, share a joke or experience the joy or pain of a relationship which has been such an important part of living.

This is not an abstract scenario; it is something which nurses may have to face often. It is therefore important that we examine the various threads involved in understanding personhood. Is the young patient with brain damage still a person despite losing the facility to express important cognitive elements so central to personhood? There can be no doubt that an intact brain stem will maintain bodily functions, but we have to ask whether or not there is more to being a person than merely having a biological realm? Respect ought to be attributed to the young person by the nurses and therefore a moral definition of personhood is maintained. Further, the relatives may clearly attribute person-hood to their loved one simply because it is meaningful to do so, in that they have known and experienced a relationship with him or her. All of these issues graphically illustrate the importance of examining our understanding of personhood in the light of everyday nursing practice. This is why ethical and philosophical analysis needs to play a central role in the education process for health professionals.

Part of the ethical curriculum for doctors, nurses and teachers should include exploration and discussion of the conceptions of the nature of persons. Downie and Telfer (1980) point out that natural science explanations of the world are based upon conceptions of things. However, within the health care domains it is essential to explore forms of knowledge more appropriately matched to conceptions of care and subsequently persons. Persons are not things unless we choose to avoid giving them person status (as in Nazi Germany). Reflecting on the new forms of knowledge needed in the professionals' curriculum may encourage a more healthy respect that can enhance care and treatment of persons in the health care system.

Glossary

cognitive relating to the faculty of knowing and perceiving things.

consciousness the mind's capacity to reflect upon itself. It is analogous with the psychological concept of perception.

dualistic in philosophical terms this usually relates to the notion that the mind and the body are to be viewed as two separate entities. The philosopher who is thought to have first developed this theme was René Descartes.

empirical developing and reinforcing knowledge through observation and experiment.

monistic this is the complete opposite of dualism; it holds the basic tenet that minds and bodies do not differ in their intrinsic nature. This ties in with contemporary ideas concerning holism.

person beings who are capable of making choices and then acting upon those decisions. Persons also possess a reflective awareness usually referred to as 'self-consciousness'.

rationality possessing the ability to reason.

semantic differential a research tool which analyses the different meanings and interpretations that language may hold.

sentient the abilty to sense and feel the world around us.

References

Abelson, R. 1977. *Persons: A study in philosophical psychology*. London: Macmillan.

Dennett, D. 1979. *Brainstorms*. Sussex: Harvester Press.

Downie, R. and Telfer, E. 1986. *Caring and Curing*. London: Methuen.

Hampshire, S. 1959. *Thought and Action*. London: Chatto & Windus.

Harris, J. 1985. *The Value of Life*. London: Routledge & Kegan Paul.

Henry, I. C. 1986. The conceptions of the nature of persons amongst children, adolescents and adults. Unpublished PhD thesis, Leeds University.

Midgley, M. 1983. *Animals and Why They Matter: A journey around the species barrier*. Harmondsworth: Penguin.

Russell, B. 1974. *History of Western Philosophy*. London: Allen & Unwin.

Shoemaker, R. and Swinbourne, S. 1984. *Personal Identity*. London: Basil Blackwell.

Singer, P. 1979. *Practical Ethics*. Cambridge: Cambridge University Press.

Strawson, P. F. 1959. *Individuals*. London: Methuen.

Teichman, J. 1972. Wittgenstein on persons and human beings. In *Understanding Wittgenstein*, pp. 133–48. Royal Institute of Philosophy Lectures, London: Macmillan.

Teichman, J. 1985. The definition of person. *Journal of the Royal Institute of Philosophy* 60: 175–85.

Valentine, E. 1982. *Conceptual Issues in Psychology*. London: Allen & Unwin.

PART II

Education

Major changes have occurred and will occur in nursing education, and the content and the nature of the new curriculum will influence the professional's role and the delivery of health care itself.

Understanding the nature of change within nursing education rests upon long-term effects for the professionals themselves and the quality in health care practice. Kevin Kendrick and Anne Simpson (Chapter 6) reveal some fundamental issues surrounding the dynamic challenge for nurse education and highlight concerns that may be viewed as controversial. Kendrick and Simpson underpin their standpoint from a social and philosophical stance and advocate that a positive approach to the changes must be driven forward with a high level of professionalism. Research findings quoted by Kendrick and Simpson clearly support the view that nurse education in the past has failed to meet the needs of a substantial number of students. Further, Kendrick and Simpson and Chapman and Fields (Chapter 7) remark that knowledge underpinning the nursing professional's education programmes must move away from a biomedical focused model.

Tom Chapman and Helen Fields, like Kendrick and Simpson, emphasize the need for a more integrated and flexible knowledge base that enhances and substantiates a 'caring' rather than a 'curing' profession. Chapman and Fields discuss in some detail particular educational strategies and emphasize the interpersonal and therapeutic skills for a Project 2000 curriculum.

The changes in nurse education will obviously influence not only the perceptions of nursing but aspects of professional practice and accountability. Ruth Balogh (Chapter 8) discusses performance indicators and professional accountability relating to nurse education and clinical practice. She remarks that, in the past, schools of nursing have had a rather ambiguous status, hence the need for radical changes in nurse education. The changes ought to clarify the perceptions we have of nursing and what nursing education ought to be in the future. Balogh is concerned with not just measuring the output of qualified practitioners but also the ethical dimension that underpins professional accountability for the future practitioner. She gives an overview of professional accountability which outlines performance and quality.

Part II concludes with Glen Pashley's view (Chapter 9) of psychiatric nurse educators' and practitioners' conceptions of mental illness. Her study emphasizes that nurses utilize a commonsense view and reflects the need to enhance the curriculum further to include more integrated knowledge from psychology, sociology and the law. This leads appropriately into Part III, which focuses upon clinical issues.

CHAPTER SIX

The nurses' reformation: philosophy and pragmatics of Project 2000

Kevin Kendrick and Anne Simpson

Henry and Pashley (1990) remark that one of the major policies for effecting change in nursing practice and education is most certainly Project 2000. The advent of Project 2000 has presented the nursing profession with a stimulating and dynamic challenge. If the major themes suggested by the project are implemented, then the next ten years will see fundamental changes in both nurse education and practice. Despite its relative infancy, debates about the efficacy of the proposals already cause divisions amongst managers, practitioners and educationalists. It is inevitable that the nature and extent of the proposed reforms should be met with a degree of controversy. A rather pessimistic position for the past and present education for nurses is supported by a number of research findings.

(1) Chapman (1988) argues that nurse education is exploitive because students spend 60 per cent of their training period being used as an invaluable but cheap form of labour. Demographic changes have presented a sudden threat to this labour supply as the number of 18 year olds continues to decline.

(2) Hancock (1986) reveals that the NHS continues to invest a great deal of money in training individuals who then go on to enter occupations as diverse as department store assistants and air hostesses.

(3) A study by the United Kingdom Central Council for Nursing,

Midwifery and Health Visiting (UKCC 1982) has revealed
that 21 per cent of nursing students leave during training or in
the period immediately following qualification. Continued
disillusionment and low morale are further reflected in the
finding that 10 per cent of trained staff continue to leave the
profession every year.

These findings clearly suggest that the present system of nurse
education is failing to meet the needs of a substantial number of
learners.

Further, nursing has remained in the shadow of medicine and
the philosophy of biomedicine has strongly influenced the
development of both basic and post-basic courses in nurse
education. The emphasis has been on the cure-oriented basis of
medicine rather than on developing themes which enhance the
concept of care as being central to nursing. The uniqueness of
nursing and its status as an autonomous and accountable
profession have long been explored by North America and parts
of Europe. The lack of impetus to move away from the medical
influence has meant that certain beliefs and values continue to
have an effect upon the way learners perceive care-giving in the
clinical arena.

The new Project 2000 curriculum will not only enhance the
nursing profession's existing qualities, but also provide the
opportunity to use more diverse forms of relevant knowledge. The
out-dated curriculum is viewed often as a watered-down medical
approach. However, nurses and nurse educators have known for
some time that their professional practice involves much more
than a medical-oriented model for care (Henry and Pashley 1989).

The medical model and the practice of nursing

The principles of biomedicine have been used as a model and
knowledge base for Western health care practice for over three
hundred years.

There is no doubt that the biomedical model has enjoyed a great
deal of success. Today we take it for granted that an inflamed
appendix will be removed within the confines of relatively safe
and effective surgery. However, although the medical model may
be considered appropriate for dealing with the physical aspects of

a person, there are many who feel it is of limited use as a basis for delivering nursing care. Birke and Silvertown (1984) argue that the biomedical model reduces the patient to the lowest common denominator in terms of cells, atoms and molecules. They use the phrase 'biological reductionism' to describe this position and claim that it allows very little room for the expression of higher-order concepts such as thoughts, feelings and emotions.

If nursing is ever to reach a position where practitioners are accepted as being of equal parity with their medical colleagues, then a method must be implemented which destroys the power relationships which have been allowed to exist for far too long. The immensity of such a task cannot be overstated and a multifactorial approach must be considered if professional equality is ever to become a reality.

The initiatives which have been proposed by Project 2000 give us a viable framework for developing a professional base which demands autonomy and accountability for all nursing prac-titioners. The Project proposes major changes in nurse education to help achieve these goals. As Henry and Pashley (1990: 45–6) state:

> as nurses' professional confidence grows relationships between them and other health care professions, in particular the medical profession, should also improve. It is essential that there is equality between the nursing and medical professions. No longer will the central role of the nurse be that of the doctor's assistant. Such a major change in direction for the profession can only be achieved through the new education programme.

It is important that we re-evaluate the role which the learner plays in the ward environment. If a student perceives his/her role as being a cheap form of labour then it is little wonder that morale is so low and staff wastage so high. The passage from nursing novice to skilled practitioner should be one of discovery and enlightenment. If this is to be achieved then we must consider the much-debated theory–practice gap. One of the major themes underpinning Project 2000 is that the dichotomy which exists between theory and practice should be confronted. The so-called 'gap' between the two areas, in the final analysis, is something of a misnomer. We often compartmentalize the different professional strands into 'practice', 'management' and 'education'. Perhaps such an approach is merely divisive and further adds to confusion. It may be more constructive to think of all these areas as being part of the 'clinical' equation because each brings a different influence to bear upon the delivery of care. If the educational reforms suggested by the project are to be implemented, then a collective approach must be adopted by the various professional areas.

Moving towards protected learning in the clinical setting

We have already noted that an influencing factor regarding staff wastage and low morale could be the apprenticeship-style of training which has traditionally been preferred. This area has been investigated by the Royal College of Nursing (1985) and various suggestions were put forward as possible avenues for bringing about a more viable learning environment.

It is often the case that students experience a 'culture shock' when exposed to their first clinical experience. There are many covert rules and agendas which the student has to tentatively discover and come to terms with. In addition, students may also find themselves suddenly faced with circumstances which may be completely alien to them. The initial confrontation with concepts such as pain, fear, anguish, emotional trauma and death can leave the student feeling frightened and totally inadequate. If these areas are not met with compassion and sensitivity then it can result in a harrowing experience for the student who will be left with a very negative impression of practice.

The Royal College of Nursing recognizes that students can encounter major difficulties during the early months of training. To try and restrict the possibility of students being exposed to situations which are not commensurate with experience, the first year of training could be undertaken in areas which offer a high degree of protection. The second year of training should see the students having gained in confidence and practical skills. This will enable them to make a greater contribution to the practical side of their placements. During the third year, the students will be expected to operate from a more autonomous base. The central themes will be self-learning and a much greater contribution to service-giving during placements. This staggered introduction to the complexities of the ward would help students to develop a broad knowledge and skills base without the traumatic effects which feeling incompetent can bring.

The RCN has agreed that nursing students should enjoy the same academic standards and conditions as their colleagues undertaking courses in higher education. This would involve an eclectic approach where students could choose from a variety of extracurricular activities ranging from information technology to modern languages. This would equip the student with options to build a varied range of interests which could contribute greatly to both personal and professional development. If this suggestion were to become a reality it would lead traditional nurse training very much into the ethos of an educational process. This is an important point. 'Nurse training' should be replaced with a 'nurse education' if the continued search for professionalization is to be effective. Henry and Pashley (1989: 70) consider this issue and make the following point:

> the term 'education' ought to be emphasised much more forcefully. It is changes in the education curriculum that, in the long term, will have the impact and influence in producing a profession in its own right, running parallel with, but uniquely different to, medicine. However, for many of us who have been conditioned by an archaic but effective system, it sometimes feels safer if we hide those changes under the old title of training.

The curriculum changes which are being discussed and implemented by educationalists strongly reflect the themes of Project 2000. The traditional nurse training has been recognized as inadequate for meeting the needs of both students and patients. The emphasis is being placed upon a more care-oriented approach to practice. This represents a refreshing move away from the medical influence, which places 'cure' at the centre of its objectives. Whilst it is always essential that medicine seeks to improve a patient's prognosis, it is not always possible to achieve a cure. However, the concept of care is central to nursing and this is not always reliant upon the patient regaining a positon of health. It has taken a great deal of time to accept that caring and curing are not mutually exclusive.

By placing the concept of care at the centre of nursing it has
become possible to introduce a greater diversity of subjects. The
biological sciences are still essential if students are to understand
the physical realm. However, it is now more acceptable to apply
the social sciences to illustrate the vast conceptual web which
makes up the patients' background and environment. This takes
us away from the nebulous approach of viewing the patient as
distinct from a social world merely because of hospitalization.
Adopting these ideas gives students the opportunity to develop
rigorous academic theory which can both complement and
underpin their practice.

Student nurses have always been quick to sense an injustice or
problem with patient care. However, it takes a great deal of
confidence to play the role of advocate within a system where
power psychology is so prevalent. The introduction of health care
ethics can play a vital role in helping students to develop
analytical tools which help them deal with moral issues. The area
between patient autonomy and medical paternalism is classically
problematic and very much open to advocacy. Ethics can help the
student to challenge the value systems in which they work as well
as improving their insights and skills of analysis.

This discussion has supported the recommendations of Project
2000 in two key areas. It is essential that students are given a
protected introduction to the demanding complexities of practice.
The suggestions which have been considered here would go a long
way towards achieving this. However, it is also clear that nurse
training has not equipped the student with sufficient support to
cope with all the areas of practice. The curriculum changes will
help to give students the necessary foundation on which to
develop effective theoretical and applied skills. The impact of
these proposals has yet to be seen because of their relative infancy.
Bysshe (1990: 21) discusses what it is hoped will be achieved:
'The UKCC hopes this system will produce a better educated
nurse with better opportunities, academic recognition and professional status. As a consequence, there should be a reduction in
wastage rates both during and after training.'

The changing face of nurse education holds a great deal of
promise for students who are new entrants to the profession. The
changes can provide a stimulating and dynamic programme for
developing a body of knowledge which can be successfully applied
to practice. However, the problems of low morale and wastage are

not restricted to students. Many qualified staff leave the profession every year and we need to consider what Project 2000 has suggested as a means of improving their position.

Trained staff and Project 2000: will it be a qualified success?

We have exmained the major themes and suggestions which Project 2000 hopes will enhance the learning experience of the students. However, it is possible that qualified staff will think that the proposals were concerned just for learners. This is a misconception which must be dealt with through the continued promulgation of the opportunities available to trained staff.

Accountability is a key element for membership of a profession. Another important factor is the regular updating of material which forms the body of knowledge underpinning practice. Continuing education can play a major role in assisting trained staff to build upon existing skills. The partnerships which are being forged between traditional nursing schools and the higher education sector can help to facilitate and develop opportunities for qualified nurses. The idea of the RGN (Registered General Nurse) qualification having some degree of academic weighting is widely accepted by a growing number of institutions. This reflects the themes of Project 2000 because it is a fitting acknowledgement of the study and practical application which the training programme demands.

Many colleges have already made it possible for qualified nurses to enter higher education through the Credit Accumulation Transfer Scheme (CATS). Moreover, the content of RGN training is sufficient to allow exemption from certain modules on a given course of study. The CATS system is very complex because it considers the qualifications and experience of each candidate before exemptions are considered. The guidelines are no longer a rigid and universally applied scenario of 'O' and 'A' level passes. The complexity of this situation can be shown by considering the number of courses the English National Board validates at a post-basic level. Each of these courses has to be viewed in the light of the academic criteria which help decide what credits an individual may take to gain exemption. However, these are administrative difficulties which will become less obstructive as the process becomes more familiar. The scheme should be greeted with enthusiasm because it is designed to meet the student's needs on a very individualized level. The student may choose a subject area, which is usually presented in the form of a module. These modules may be increased at a pace which suits the student. Over time, the number of modules will increase and this gives the student a credit weighting which can lead to an academic award. The starting point may be the award of a certificate; this can be developed to diploma, first degree or onto Master's level. The emphasis is placed upon students progressing as far along the academic process as they need or wish to.

Another advantage with this is that it allows the students freedom of choice in developing a learning programme which fits their own needs. The student may choose a course which is made up of a diverse range of subjects and which combines a variety of academic disciplines. However, if the student wishes to take a clearly defined course of study then this may also be facilitated through the scheme. This is a new and innovatory approach to dealing with the learning demands of a professional group. Nurses have been denied access to higher education because of the lack of credibility which was given to professional qualifications. This has been radically challenged and ultimately changed. Qualified nurses have so much to offer higher education in terms of professional and life experience. The emphasis is placed upon the institutions to ensure that this is a reciprocal arrangement.

The institutions of higher education must operate from a flexible base if they are to accommodate the needs of qualified nurses. The peculiarities of rostering prevent nurses from attending lectures at the usually designated times. This can present a number of problematic issues which must be confronted before a viable solution is found. Perhaps some answers may be discovered through developing part-time courses and introducing distance learning packages.

The task which lies before educators is considerable. The nature of the reforms will demand a change in perspectives and attitudes. There is a certain degree of security in an unaltered state. Project 2000 has presented a force for change which leaves us all with questions and concerns. This is the nature of the dynamic; if professional autonomy is to be achieved then we must embrace the themes which Project 2000 offers. Queries can be answered as the proposals are implemented and ideas exchanged. The following quote from Henry and Pashley (1989: 7) reflects the direction which nurse education is taking:

> logically, the two areas of higher education and nursing education should develop a partnership that offers mutual support and therefore creates a positive force for change. The higher education sector can inform, support and offer a rich source of expertise in research and relevant forms of knowledge, whereas the professioal educators are the creators of applied knowledge and innovators of new philosophies of care. Such a partnership would allow for something good to happen in health care.

Some pragmatic considerations

There are many queries concerning Project 2000 and the answers will only be seen with its practical application and the passage of time. This does not stop us speculating as to what these possible outcomes may be. One of the major concerns is that as qualified nurses become involved with academia they will leave a void of skilled practitioners at the interface of care-giving. The possibility of a graduate profession is viewed, by some nurses, as a development which will put a great deal of emphasis upon the health care assistant or support worker. This would seem to defeat the object of a highly skilled nurse practising at the bedside.

This need not be the obvious scenario; the educational opportunities for qualified staff should help to ensure that a research-based practitioner is starting to emerge onto the wards. A great deal of encouragement is also being given to mature students to enter the profession and most of these wish to remain on the service side. If the opportunities for enrolled nurses to enter conversion courses become more flexible then this will provide another avenue for ensuring that a high standard of care is given at ward level. Moreover, it will also provide the means for enrolled nurses to enter higher education. These points help to illustrate that Project 2000 can actually lead to an increase in the number of highly skilled staff giving care at a 'grassroots' level.

We have tried to discuss Project 2000 with a degree of guarded optimism. The themes and suggestions which the Project has presented only provide a framework for change. If the proposals are to become reality then a great deal of commitment must come from nurses working in all professional areas. This can only be achieved through a working partnership; managerial initiatives, the educational process and excellence in the delivery of care can help to achieve this.

References

Birke, L. and Silvertown, J. 1984. *More Than the Parts: Biology and Politics*. London: Pluto Press.

Bysshe, J. 1990. Strength, status and respect. *Nursing: The Journal of Clinical Practice, Education and Management* 4(1): 20–3.

Chapman, C. 1988. Cousins in crisis. *Nursing Times* 84(8): 32–3.

Hancock, C. 1986. The staffing equation. *Nursing Times* 82(16): 40–1.

Henry, C. and Pashley, G. 1989. Vital links. *Nursing Times* 85(20): 70–1.

Henry, C. and Pashley, G. 1990. Carving out the nursing nineties. *Nursing Times* 86(3): 45–6.

Royal College of Nursing. 1985. *The Education of Nurses: A New Dispensation*. London: RCN.

UKCC. 1982. *The Development of Nurse Education*. London: United Kingdom Central Council for Nursing, Midwifery and Health Visiting.

CHAPTER SEVEN

Interpersonal and therapeutic skills in the 'New Curriculum' for nurse education

Tom Chapman and Helen Fields

The stimulus of nurse curriculum reform

Many initiatives, coming in the wake of Project 2000, have made it plain that the education and professional preparation of nurses is at an important crossroads. A succession of documents emanating from the UKCC make it quite clear that the council envisages a 'total and radical' restructuring of nurse education. In the first of nine Project 2000 papers, the council stated that:

> the aim will be to look at foundation training de novo, with no options foreclosed and with no proposals, however radical, eliminated without proper study. ... This re-look at training will need to take into account societal needs and be based on assumptions and perceptions about the role of those practitioners who undertake the functions of nursing, midwifery and health visiting. (UKCC 1985: 2).

This bold statement of intent opens up the possibility of developing many curricular innovations which presage an exciting, and potentially creative, period for those educators who have the courage to respond positively to the challenge this opportunity provides. The public perception of nursing also seems to have reached something of a watershed. An enhanced status for nursing, essential to the recruitment of high-quality students, in a wider context of serious problems of recruitment and retention, is more than ever dependent on the quality of education and future career prospects. In grasping and developing the opportunity presented by Project 2000, the nursing professional should be mindful of the fact that, apart from Eire, every other country in the English-speaking world educates and prepares its nurses within mainstream higher education.

At the beginning of the 1990s, nurse educators have a considerable measure of autonomy in determining the nature and quality of educative programmes for the foreseeable future. The time is ripe not only to prepare nurses for a more varied and responsible role, but also to attempt to influence the main nature of the role itself, and, hence, its public perception. Creative, dynamic and responsive educational programmes, designed to prepare nurse professionals for future challenges in health care, will, if rooted in a more rigorous academic atmosphere, nourish and strengthen the status of the profession itself. This is surely one of the keys to future recruitment.

As a member of the one of the oldest of the helping professions, the nurse, in both hospital and community settings, is required to respond to clients' needs in a humane, caring and effective manner. With the general exception of mental handicap and mental health nursing, it would appear that those interpersonal skills aimed at enhancing the psychological, emotional and social well-being of clients have, until recently, been largely neglected in that aspect of nurse education which sets the tone for professional socialization – the curriculum. Until the advent of individualized care processes and conceptual nursing frameworks, the focus of professional training had largely been on task performance, with competence measured primarily in terms of practical, psycho-motor and administrative skills, which are observable and relatively easy to assess. Since patients or clients, as the 'consumers' of the health services, carry so much 'emotional baggage' with them, it is becoming increasingly recognized that their problems can only be adequately conceived and managed in a holistic sense – in their physical, psychological, social and spiritual totality.

The increased attention to 'theory' which is facilitated in higher education will provide the opportunity to acquire a greater depth of knowledge and understanding of the complex interactions between the various dimensions encompassed within a holistic perspective. According to De Basio (1989: 4), such a knowledge

base is essential to the practice of nursing because clients
continually make adaptations and adjustments to their internal
and external environments. Nursing is becoming increasingly
recognized as being much more than a problem identification and
solving process (see Faulkner 1985). Individualized care is
predicated on some degree of understanding of the client's
background, personality, feelings, values, beliefs, and so on.
Professional nursing is essentially an interpersonal process requiring the integration of clinical and humanistic skills (see Peplau
1988; Travelbee 1971; De Basio 1989).

One of the major Project 2000 pre-registration learning
outcomes identified by the UKCC (1988) is that of 'using
appropriate interpersonal and communication skills to enable the
development of helpful caring relationships with patients/clients,
and their families/friends, and to initiate and complete therapeutic
relationships with patients'. The Division of Mental Health of the
World Health Organization (1986) has similarly stressed that
nursing care should have as one of its major goals 'imparting
effective interpersonal skills to help people identify their own
psychosocial and physical needs and to use their own resources to
meet them'. Such a goal is entirely consistent with the focus on
health promotion, increasing personal responsibility for healthy
living and extension of the nurse's role to include those
interpersonal skills designed to maximize the 'therapeutic potential' of the nurse–patient relationship (see Peplau 1988; Barber
1991). Additionally, this kind of emphasis can create the
conditions whereby nurses can embrace more readily the concept
of advocacy, in so far as this relates to acting in a way which helps
to give meaningful guidance, counsel and support to patients/clients,
or families, who may be in vulnerable, and potentially threatening,
situations and circumstances.

Whilst it can be argued that some nurses have always
interpreted their role in this way, it is reasonable to argue that, in
general, adequate and systematic preparation and education for
such a role has not existed in nurse education in Britain (see
Aidroos 1985). In an empirical study of the effectiveness and
relevance of student learning in three 'training schools', Gott
(1984: 50) found that 'The development of social (communication) skills was not a stated curricular goal and no form of
training in, or development of, skills was offered'. Paradoxically,
teachers did appear to value communication and interpersonal

skills, and frequently encouraged students to consider 'patients' psychological and emotional needs . . . and emotions (embarrassment, distress, anxiety)'. In none of the schools studied, however, was there any opportunity to put this advice into practice. The few learning opportunities that were realized were theoretical. Gott concluded that such skills were neglected because teachers themselves felt insecure about their knowledge of the skills, and because more 'important' things had to be taught (nursing practices). From her observation of student nurse/patient communication on the wards, Gott discovered that 85 per cent of communications students used with patients were 'inhibitory'. Student nurses controlled the content and length of interchanges, initiating and concluding 90 per cent of all communications with patients. She also found that, despite the fact that patients clearly valued 'social communications' from nurses, they were almost totally provided with 'functional' ones concerned with treatment or care. It would seem that the vital message from this study is that, unless students themselves are provided with the opportunity to learn about and engage in the practice of interpersonal skills, in a systematic fashion in a supportive environment, they are unlikely to practise 'whole task' behaviour commensurate with the tenets of the holistic perspective.

It seems clear that some continued exploration is called for on how interpersonal and communication skills can be facilitated and enhanced in nurse education programmes. Our position is that they are fundamental ingredients of a caring relationship, and should be considered to be central to curriculum development. We would argue that educating future nurses to understand their own feelings makes them better attuned to empathize with others, and that the ability to empathize is the basis for helping (see Tschudin 1987: 33). Plainly, it is not sufficient to leave such fundamental skills to chance, with reliance placed on personality disposition, 'natural caring instincts', or indeed the existence of role models to demonstrate appropriate interpersonal skills in practical settings.

It is the intention of this chapter to make out a case for giving particular consideration to the various interpersonal skills required by nurses in education programmes currently being planned and implemented. It is anticipated that such programmes will provide future nurses with the confidence to engage proactively in extending the scope of their responsibilities in non-clinical settings.

By 'therapeutic' skills, in this context, we mean those skills which calm, comfort, reassure, support, restore confidence and self-belief; in other words, interpersonal skills which are intrinsic to what might be called the 'art of caring'. The objective is to introduce a set of values and a model of interpersonal dynamics intended to improve the quality of interpersonal communication skills, and hence the quality of 'care' and 'therapy' on offer. We have in mind a distinctive type of 'professional socialization' which sets the tone for nurse–client interaction. Indeed, the progressive philosophy which underpins the ethos of Project 2000 directly encourages the elevation of human relationships to the centre of the curriculum, and not their relegation to the periphery, as has so often been the case in the past.

Needless to say, the ultimate success or failure of this type of 'psychological engineering' will depend on the extent to which individual students feel better equipped to cope with the demands and stresses of their chosen career. It seems self-evident that the internalization of any aspect of an educative programme depends on the students' conviction that it actually 'makes a difference' to, or alters, in some constructive and lasting sense, the way they see themselves, and the way they wish to act (practice). Consequently, the self-knowledge necessary before any meaningful personal change can take place in the student will be obtained only by experiential learning (see Chapman 1974).

Philosophical and theoretical bases

It is useful to start from the basic premise that nursing is a 'helping profession', which should have as its main aim the optimum personal development of clients (consumers) of nursing services. Such a stipulation requires attention to bio-psycho-social-spiritual needs, and as such directs us to consider much more than basic 'health needs'. This prompts the question, 'How, then, can we utilize knowledge drawn from the human sciences to promote more effective practice in the helping professions?' To achieve this goal, some study of the dynamics of human behaviour drawn from selected aspects of humanistic psychology will be helpful. This will lead to an appreciation of the value of a humanistic frame of reference in the increasingly wider contexts of nursing.

Within humanistic psychology, the theoretical orientation known as perceptual psychology has special utility since it provides a framework for understanding clients as people who have needs, motives and identities, immediately applicable to the practical problems that health care professionals are faced with.

Accordingly, it is not surprising that perceptual psychology is called the 'practitioners' psychology' (Combs *et al.* 1971, Combs 1989). In America, this particular theoretical orientation has been put to the test in professional practice. As far as we are aware, its potential in the field of nursing in Britain has not been adequately explored.

In a very real sense nursing is an applied profession in which the successful practitioner does something with her/his knowledge. Knowledge alone, however, is no guarantee of effective helping practice, unless it can be channelled into enabling nurses to recognize and respond to specified needs of clients. An examination of recent policy documents reveals a marked shift in formal stipulations relating to conceptions of clients' needs (see UKCC 1985, 1988; Secretary of State for Health 1989; Secretary of State for Health *et al.* 1989). This policy change reveals an increased respect for the rights of the consumers of public services and an increase in the responsibility and accountability of health professionals, and implies radical changes in practice. In summary, this new ethos requires professionals to relate to clients as individuals with unique needs – to be treated with dignity, respect, and consideration; to be fully consulted on all decisions which affect their health status; and to be regarded as being capable, within sensible limits, of acting with self-responsibility.

Countless research studies in the fields of teaching, medicine and psychotherapy have revealed that effective practitioners are not distinguished by the 'methods' they use. It seems that the conception that there is one best method of teaching, in any absolute sense, is a mistaken one. It is almost certain that the same holds true for the practices of all the helping professions. Perceptual psychology provides us with a most plausible explanation. The underlying reason why successful practice is not associated with any particular method is that it is the client's perception of both the method and the professional who is applying it, in combination, which is important. In other words, it is the *meaning* of the intervention of the professional for the client that significantly determines the outcome. This 'meaning', for the client, is interpreted in relation to its relevance and effects on her/his 'self-concept' (see Chapman 1975). As a theoretical orientation within humanistic psychology, perceptual psychology is predicated on the fundamental importance of the concept of self in human interaction. Perceptual psychology is also closely allied with 'counselling psychology', with which it shares a common intellectual heritage.

Because of its essentially practical approach to helping people who present with a problem which is impairing their personal well-being, 'counselling' provides an invaluable frame of reference for the acquisition of those very skills which underpin good nursing practice. In the context of nurse education, we take 'counselling' to be more than a set of skills employed in a limited range of situations. Counselling is represented here in the sense used by Burnard (1989: 4) as an 'often idiosyncratic mixture of personal qualities, practical skills and interpersonal aspect of the health professional's job'. Importantly, since caring for people who are psychologically distressed inevitably places carers them-selves under stress, counselling-based programmes are invaluable in helping them to take care of themselves. Furthermore, since one facet of good practice is to reduce the gap between 'the all-knowing, all-powerful, all-adequate professional and the unin-formed, powerless, student, patient or client' (Nurse 1983: 250), the approach of person-centred counselling, in particular, may be profitably explored and adapted to nursing care.

The humanistic approach to counselling elevates those human values which also underpin the ideals of Project 2000 – empowerment, authenticity and autonomy. It is posited that sensitization to counselling skills and 'person-centredness' would improve interpersonal communication in all organizational and professional contexts in which 'nursing' takes place, and help nurture the relationship which develops between the nurse and client. Person-centredness as a way of relating to other people suggests a set of beliefs, values and attitudes, and not some standardized routine. It is the quality of the therapeutic relation-ship that is intrinsically valuable to the client, and not any particular technique or method (see Merry 1990). The theory and practice of person-centredness, in the context of nurse education, should encourage the internalization of an approach to nursing which enables and facilitates, as students gain trust in the process and, importantly, in their own grasp of it.

The contribution of humanistic psychology

We believe that much may be learned from considering some of the conceptual formulations employed by the American psychologist and psychotherapist, Carl Rogers. When faced with the need to set out the implications of psychotherapy for education, Rogers (1967: 279–96) coined the expression 'significant learning' to describe a process which is more than an accumulation of facts; it is a deeply social process, 'which makes a difference' in a fundamental way to the actions, behaviour and personal growth of those individuals who internalize and are penetrated by such learning, with its therapeutic undertones. To paraphrase Rogers, and at the same time adapting the learning outcomes to the nursing context, one would expect this type of orientation to produce people with an improved capacity to (a) accept themselves and their feelings more fully; (b) become more confident and self-directing; (c) become more flexible and less rigid in their perceptions; (d) become more accepting of others; and (e) become more open to evidence (1967: 280–1). Plainly, the ideals of Project 2000 and the ethos of 'consumerism' are commensurate with the kind of education and professional socialization which is derived from this theoretical perspective.

A nurse education curriculum designed to achieve such outcomes will be one which is rooted in a philosophical and conceptual approach which is sympathetic and dedicated to the concepts of 'helping' and 'caring'. Pre-registration nurse education should, therefore, include interpersonal and therapeutic skills as a core theme underpinning the five basic concepts of the person, society, health, health care, and nursing. These five concepts are those identified by the ENB (1989) in their Guidelines and Criteria for Project 2000 Course Development.

Desired outcomes and curricular orientations

Some of the desired outcomes which are envisaged from the adoption of the precepts and values which derive from counselling psychology are as follows:

● improved communication, in an atmosphere of trust
● a decrease in frustration, uncertainty, anxiety, and other anti-therapeutic states which result from poor communication

- a reduction in the number of clients who feel they are powerless and unable to exercise choice or express their wishes
- a general reduction in iatrogenesis (i.e. a process of dependence created by medical/professional bureaucracy)
- elevation of status of clients as consumers
- improved coping ability on the part of both nurse and client
- the development of a more 'therapeutic' and caring environment
- better undertanding of health problems (in perspective)
- the adoption, by clients, of more positive attitudes towards themselves and their health-related problems
- improved efficiency as a consequence of more effective decision-making
- a greater facilitation of advocacy skills.

Needless to say, all of these outcomes are contingent on the level and extent to which the clients of nursing services are exposed to 'therapeutic' interventions.

From the standpoint of nurses themselves, systematic and thoroughgoing attention to 'interpersonal skills' in the curriculum of nurse education in Britain is likely to lead to an improvement in self-esteem and self-confidence, both during the programme of preparation and after qualification (see Aidroos 1985; Bond 1986; Kagan et al. 1986; Tschudin 1987). In time, as this aspect of the curriculum is developed, it should ensure a greater likelihood of interpersonal support in a profession where vulnerability to stress is widely recognized. Firth et al. (1986), for example, have highlighted the conspicuous lack of psychological and emotional support for both students in training and nursing professionals. Other important outcomes are likely to include improved teamwork and communication; enhanced competence in guiding clients towards accepting greater personal responsibility for their care; and greater confidence in coping with distressed clients and their families.

The interpersonal skills that the new curriculum should address may be enhanced by the inclusion of:

- an orientation to the client's needs
- the ability to listen (active listening, sensitivity to non-verbal cues)
- the ability to offer 'free attention' (noting and accepting − not judging)
- the ability to suspend preconception

- the ability to offer empathy (empathy-demonstrating skills need to be learnt; empathy as a communication skill)
- the ability to feel (and show) acceptance, respect and warmth
- the ability to interact from a standpoint of 'genuineness'
- the ability to help clients (at all ability levels) to develop programmes to adjust to, and cope with, their presenting circumstances. (In some instances, to act on behalf of those who have long- or short-term coping deficits.)

An important motivating factor in the mastery of these skills, maximizing the prospects that they will be internalized, will be that the skills should as far as possible be related to the everyday circumstances of nursing. Needless to say, the supervision of student nurses' learning experiences by competent teachers/ counsellors is essential to the skill-gaining process, whatever the context and application. There is clearly a need for in-service training and adequately funded staff development programmes. For high-quality care to evolve, the personal and professional development of nurse educators, student nurses and qualified practitioners need to be 'dovetailed'. Clinical managers need also to recognize and manage resources for peer support and supervision in a profession where the performance of care is invariably accompanied by distress (Barber 1991). In a very real sense the extent to which employers and managers of health care provider units are prepared to support the pronouncements embraced in Project 2000 philosophy will be evidenced by their willingness, or otherwise, to support staff development initiatives of this kind. The prescriptions which derive from this type of philosophy are instrinsically enabling. In a political climate centred around a consumer-oriented service economy which elevates the virtue of 'self-help', it seems that an important task for nursing will be to facilitate and nurture those personal qualities in clients themselves, in order to encourage them to play a more proactive role in the promotion of their own and their families' health.

Summary

In summary, nursing is a caring and helping profession in which the dynamics of interpersonal interaction have rarely been given systematic attention to the extent that is now afforded by the scope for radical reappraisal of nurse education offered by Project 2000. To this end, a study of the basic tenets of humanistic psychology and, in particular, certain facets of counselling psychology embraced in person-centred approaches will be valuable. Since the nature of interpersonal exchanges will fundamentally affect the quality of care the client receives, attention to the processes of human interaction should be a fundamental concern throughout nurse education. If programmes are to be accessible to students, and of value to future practitioners, they must be based on coherent and consistent philosophical and theoretical frameworks and include substantial experiential learning. After all, as Kurt Lewin once asserted, there is nothing more practical than good theory.

Whilst it is plainly far beyond the scope of pre-registration programmes to incorporate counsellor training in any comprehensive fashion, it is possible to introduce and apply some broad principles and relevant interpersonal skills in order to properly sensitize student nurses to the importance of the human dimension of their practice. In this way, we would argue, standards of care will improve, as will public confidence in nursing, as we adjust to a period of increasing sovereignty for the consumer. Equally, it might well prove to be the case that, by putting a more professional stamp on this special and vital aspect of the role of the 'practitioner-nurse', nursing will be able to distinguish itself from other health-related professions. Unless the profession confidently asserts the principles which underpin good nursing practice, care that makes a difference in people's lives will be swamped by commercialism, cost-benefit ratios, product-planning, outcome evaluation, throughput, and the 'quick fix'.

At a time of philosophical and moral disarray and unprecedented change in the Health Service, the art of 'caring' is in danger of being undermined. Clearly, at this conjuncture, nurse educators have an important, and urgent, role to play. Increasing opportunities to broaden academic and professional horizons should be progressed firmly, and with conviction. To this end, we would like to reiterate the claim of the chairman of the RCN's Commission on Nursing Education, Dr Harry Judge, that, if only the profession would say clearly and unambiguously what it wants, then it stands an excellent chance of achieving it (RCN 1986: 4).

References

Aidroos, N. 1985. Interpersonal skills. In A. T. Altschul (ed.), *Recent Advances in Nursing 12*. Edinburgh: Churchill Livingstone.

Barber, P. 1991. Caring: the nature of a therapeutic relationship. In A. Perry and M. Jolley (eds), *Nursing: A Knowledge Base for Practice*. London: Edward Arnold.

Bond, M. 1986. *Stress and Self-awareness: A Guide for Nurses*. London: Chapman & Hall.

Burnard, P. 1989. *Counselling Skills for Health Professionals*. London: Chapman and Hall.

Chapman, T. 1974. The humanistic tradition in Psychology and its relevance for education, *Self and Society* 2(4).

Chapman, T. 1975. The relationship between children's self-concepts and the expectations of teachers, *Self and Society* 3(8).

Combs, A. W. *et al.* 1971. *Helping Relationships*. Boston, Allyn & Bacon.

Combs, A. W. 1989. *A Theory of Therapy: Guidelines for Counselling Practice*. London: Sage.

De Basio, P. A. 1989. *Mental Health Nursing: A Holistic Approach*, 3rd edn. St Louis: C. V. Mosby.

Department of Health. 1989. *Working for Patients*, Cm 555. London: HMSO.

Department of Health. 1989. *Caring for People*, Cm 849. London: HMSO.

ENB. 1989. *Project 2000: A New Preparation for Practice. Guidelines and Criteria for Course Development and Collaborative Links between Approved NHS Training Institutions and Centres of Higher Education*. January. London: English National Board for Nursing, Midwifery and Health Visiting.

Faulkner, A. 1985. *Nursing: A Creative Approach*. Eastbourne: Baillière Tindall.

Firth, H. *et al.* 1986. Interpersonal support amongst nurses at work. *Journal of Advanced Nursing* 11: 273–82.

Gott, M. 1984. *Learning Nursing*. London: RCN.

Kagan, C. *et al.* 1986. *A Manual of Interpersonal Skills for Nurses*. London: Harper & Row.

Merry, T. 1990. Client-centred therapy: some trends and some troubles. *Counselling* 1(1): 17–18.

Nurse, G. 1980. *Counselling and the Nurse*, 2nd edn. Aylesbury, Bucks: HM&M Publishers.

Nurse, G. 1983. Counselling. In J. Clark and J. Henderson, *Community Health*. Edinburgh: Churchill Livingstone.

Peplau, H. E. 1988. *Interpersonal Relations in Nursing*, 2nd edn. London: Macmillan.

Rogers, C. 1967. *On Becoming a Person*. London: Constable.

Royal College of Nursing 1986. Comments on the UKCC's Project 2000 proposals. London: RCN.

Travelbee, J. 1971. *Interpersonal Aspects of Nursing*, 2nd edn. Philadelphia: F. A. Davies.

Tschudin, V. 1987. *Counselling Skills for Nurses*, 2nd edn. London: Baillière Tindall.

UKCC. 1985. *Project Paper 1: Introducing Project 2000*. London: United Kingdom Central Council for Nursing, Midwifery and Health Visiting.

UKCC. 1988. *Consultation Paper: Proposed Rules for the Standard, Kind and Content of Future of Pre-Registration Nursing Education*. London: United Kingdom Central Council for Nursing, Midwifery and Health Visiting.

WHO. 1986. Division of Mental Health Nursing Unit, *Integration of Mental Health Concepts and Skills in Nursing*. Geneva: World Health Organization.

CHAPTER EIGHT

Performance indicators and changing patterns of accountability in nurse education

Ruth Balogh

Introduction

In this chapter I wish to show some of the ways in which questions of accountability relate to discussions about how to develop performance indicators (PIs) for nurse training institutions. The evidence I draw upon is derived from material gathered over a two-year period of research for the English National Board for Nursing, Midwifery and Health Visiting (ENB), which commissioned Alan Beattie to direct a project on the subject at the University of London Institute of Education. The aim of this research was to explore the feasibility of developing PIs for nurse (and midwife) training institutions. The account I give of this research is intended to show how the initial findings led to further work on implementation issues, and finally to a series of recommendations for the ENB to consider in formulating policy. Accordingly, the views in this section of the chapter are presented as the collective views of the research team and termed as such.

The project itself took place between 1987 and 1989 – a period it would be no exaggeration to describe as one of upheaval in the arrangements for the delivery of nurse and midwife training. Policies and the information required for their implementation are highly interlinked, and therefore it seemed useful first to locate this ENB initiative within a more general background of recent changes in public sector policy, then to focus more particularly on nursing and midwifery education, and to present some of our research findings within this context of wide-ranging policy debates, concluding with a discussion about some of the general issues of accountability which are raised by the systematic and routine collection of this type of information.

The growth of public sector services

The idea of gathering information to assess the performance of public sector services has been, since the development of the welfare state at least, closely linked with the public expenditure process. Pressure to examine costs arose from a general trend throughout the developed world in the twentieth century towards growth in public expenditure, especially on social, environmental and economic services, and there is considerable debate among economists as to why this should be so. Peacock and Wiseman (1967) suggest that periods of social upheaval (such as the Second World War) have been a critical influence through creating an 'imposition effect' whereby the public become more willing to bear a high taxation burden, and at the same time an 'inspection effect' in which additional social problems are identified.

The complexities of these debates aside, this analysis does draw our attention to a central issue in any discussion about how to assess performance in the public services, namely the complex and changing accountability structure of modern society. Individual taxpayers today must be seen as both contributors to and recipients of public services in potentially differential degrees at different points in the life cycle. They may, furthermore, also be accountable as professional service-providers, or as educators of the professionals of tomorrow, or indeed both. The precise nature of these accountabilities is, however, itself a shifting phenomenon, for, as Peacock and Wiseman argue, they exist against a backdrop of changing ideas about how social problems should be defined and changing social priorities in different historical circumstances. Schon, in his influential book *The Reflective Practitioner* (1983), goes so far as to describe 'a crisis of confidence in professional knowledge . . . which seems to be rooted in a growing skepticism about professional effectiveness'. Accountable to whom? – and how? – are questions that may need to be posed more frequently than they can be answered.

The performance of public sector services

Although the introduction of policies requiring performance indicators for the public sector generated a considerable amount of work in the 1980s, the notion of monitoring activity and performance is by no means new. Indeed, the nursing professon can legitimately claim an early advocate in the shape of Florence Nightingale, who wanted regular and systematic recording and publication of hospital in-patient activity 'to enable the work of hospitals to be assessed' (Goldacre and Griffin 1983).

The National Health Service, perhaps of all the public sector services in the postwar period, has inquired most regularly into the costs and effectiveness of its operations. Within four months of the launch of the NHS in 1948, it had become apparent that the original costs for its first year had been underestimated by £49 million, and Bevan noted to his cabinet colleagues – in terms which would be entirely appropriate in the 1980s – that 'the justification of the cost will depend upon how far we get full value for money' (quoted in Klein 1983: 34).

Successive governments, both Labour and Conservative, have pursued this question of value for money in the NHS in their different ways, with Labour administrations trying to reconcile rising costs with the principles of equity and effectiveness, and Conservative administrations attempting to justify the raising of additional revenues by (for instance) the introduction of prescription charges within a general policy of non-intervention. The early questions about the costs of health care in part derived from the very fact that costs had not entered into the initial debates about what form the proposed NHS should take; indeed, it had been assumed that the provision of health care free at the point of delivery would *save* money, and it was a matter of some surprise that from the very beginning annual budgets were constantly having to be revised upwards. A committee chaired by Guillebaud was set up in 1953 to investigate the problem, and found that costs had indeed risen against early estimates, but, if they were taken as a proportion of gross national product, this proportion had actually fallen from 3.75 per cent to 3.25 per cent. The committee drew attention to the need for better information on NHS activity, but though it recommended the appointment of a statistician at the Ministry of Health, it also argued against setting up a framework to relate costs to performance on the grounds that suitable indicators of performance were difficult to identify and even more difficult to measure (Ministry of Health 1956).

The 1960s and 1970s brought with them attempts to introduce rational planning methods into the public sector. A plethora of new techniques emerged, complete with acronyms: Programme Analysis and Review (PAR), Planning Programming and Budgeting Systems (PPBS), Zero-Based Budgeting and Cost-Benefit Analysis (CBA), all of which sought to challenge the existing principle that 'the largest determining factor of the size and content of this year's budget is last year's budget' (Wildavsky, quoted in Likierman 1988: 39), by determining budgets on more rational criteria. The Plowden Committee's reform of the public spending process did not go this far, but it did transform it by introducing annual surveys of departmental spending which were scrutinized by the Public Expenditure Survey Committee (PESC), chaired by the Treasury. For the first time a systematic attempt was being made to discover how funds had been distributed by spending departments and to use this information for future planning.

In the NHS, the reorganization of 1974 made it possible to compare the funding for different health authorities on the basis of the populations for which they were responsible, and wide differences were revealed on expenditure per head. The Resource Allocation Working Party was convened to remedy this in 1976, but, coinciding as it did with a period of recession, much of the redistribution of funding was implemented as cuts.

During the mid-1970s governments began gradually to introduce a change to the basis on which budget plans were calculated from volume to cash. In the early days of PESC, departments calculated the value of the goods and services they planned to buy according to volume, and any unanticipated rises in price were covered by the Treasury. Cash planning, on the other hand, assumes a general rate of inflation through which costs will rise and resources are allocated accordingly.

This change, from volume planning to cash and later cash-limited planning, brought with it a shift in emphasis for managers from service needs (which are more readily translated into volume terms than cash terms) to 'top–down' concerns about resource distribution priorities. But for the Conservative administration of the

1980s, there was still room for change, and in September 1982 the Financial Management Initiative was launched, a top–down initiative whose aim was to hold managers more accountable for the use of resources through cash-limiting budgets, setting targets and monitoring performance. It was through this initiative that the accounting concepts of *Economy, Efficiency* and *Effectiveness* (the 'three Es') became a statutory element in public life, initially for local government services via the 1982 Local Government Finance Act (HMSO 1982) which empowered auditors to look beyond their traditional concerns of accuracy and propriety to 'satisfy himself . . . that the authority has made proper arrangements to secure economy, efficiency and effectiveness' (Audit Commission 1983: para. 40).

Thus the trend throughout the public sector in the 1980s to gather information on performance in order to argue more closely on resource allocation priorities was clearly associated with tighter, top–down mechanisms of accountability. In the NHS, PIs were introduced along with new mechanisms of ministerial review in early 1982, 'as a measure to improve accountability'. Likewise in the universities, new, more streamlined management structures were recommended to accompany the development of PIs in the Jarratt Report (1985) on efficiency in universities.

The case of nursing and midwifery education

Nurse and midwife education has in recent years occupied a position in the public sector which can best be described as not entirely within the NHS yet only tenuously linked with higher and further education, and one of the key items of evidence which has dominated discussions about policy in this area – student wastage rates – would today be called a performance indicator. As far back as 1947, the Wood Report (Ministry of Health 1947: para. 149) recommended full student status for nurses, so that 'the dissociation of training from staffing needs . . . will place the student under the control of the training authority . . . and not under that of the hospital', and it was high wastage rates among student nurses (nationally running at 54 per cent at the time) which in the committee's view indicated the need for such a radical review of training programmes. To further encourage independence from the hospitals, the committee also recommended that training should be funded separately.

Though the Wood Report met with hostility from many senior members of the nursing profession, these policy issues – of where nurse education should be located, how it should be funded, and what should be the contractual status of the student – have remained a central focus for debate in the succeeding 40 years, underlined again in the Briggs Report (1972) which looked more closely at wastage rates by comparing them with other types of predominantly female student and employee, and culminating in the Project 2000 proposals put forward by the United Kingdom Central Council for Nursing, Midwifery and Health Visiting (UKCC) in 1985.

The ambiguous status of nurse training schools during the 1980s – partly funded by the new national boards and partly funded by the health authorities, and with variations in Scotland and Northern Ireland – perhaps protected them from the more robust features of the Financial Management Initiative which were encouraging some of their colleagues in further and general education to develop PIs for training programmes and institutions. But by 1985 the national boards had come under the wing of the annual ministerial review process via the Department of Health and Social Security, and the ENB – by far the biggest of the boards, dispensing £90 million annually (in 1988) for teaching costs to 14 regional education advisory groups (EAGs) – agreed to develop PIs for training institutions to assist in its own annual reviews of the EAGs. The Board adopted a dual strategy, first by encouraging EAGs to start work at local level to develop PIs and secondly by commissioning research from the University of London Institute of Education – the PI project.

During the course of this research, the pace of change in nursing and midwifery education accelerated rapidly. Policy dilemmas which had simmered away for years suddenly became subjects no longer for debate but for resolution. But most important for the PI project was the almost universal call in policy documents that the introduction and ongoing implementation of these new policies depended upon developing more uniform and routine systems to collect information about what goes on in training institutions – in other words, PIs. The various policy initiatives are outlined below, illustrating the central and linking role which PIs are set to play in the future management of nurse and midwife education.

Project 2000

The radical proposals known as Project 2000 were agreed by the UKCC in 1985, but it took until spring 1988 for the Minister of Health to announce, at the annual RCN conference, that the government was prepared to support them. Eventually, they will change the way nurse education is structured from a labour market model, in which schools supply manpower directly to hospitals, to an educational investment model where students are supernumerary, where qualifications to register are approved within higher education, and for which training for the different branches of the profession is more flexible, with a greater contribution from placements in community settings.

Throughout its discussions with the nursing and midwifery professions, the government has been keen to estimate the costs of the Project 2000 proposals. Price Waterhouse, in a cost appraisal undertaken for the UKCC (UKCC and Price Waterhouse 1987), acknowledged that the benefits of reducing the clinical responsibilities of students were very difficult to quantify and therefore weigh against the more easily estimated costs of employing qualified substitutes in their places. However, the first 'demonstration districts', in submitting proposals to the Department of Health, were required to supply basic information which could be turned into ratios of the type used in routine cost-based performance assessment – for instance, proposed student–staff ratios, and cost per student. This exercise, which took place in early 1989, revealed some important discrepancies, not only between the estimated costs of Project 2000 in different districts, but also differences between costing methods and, perhaps most important of all, major problems concerning the quality of financial and other information available to education managers. Such discrepancies, it was argued, clearly pointed to a need for generating performance-type information on a routine basis.

Clinical career structure

Recommended by the Pay Review Body early in 1988, this initiative has sought to determine responsibilities and therefore grades through job appraisal using an information base which is similar to and indeed, for teachers, overlaps with training institution PIs. The criteria used for allocating grades have differed between districts and regions, and the process has been strongly contended, with appeals against grades still, in 1990, taking up a major proportion of senior nurse and midwife managers' time.

The criteria for educational gradings are establishing new relationships between the quantity and range of activities undertaken at training institution level and the numbers of teaching staff at particular grades needed to carry out these activities. The routine availability of PI-type information is, therefore, an essential prerequisite for the operation of the new grading system in training institutions.

ENB internal review

In 1988 the ENB commissioned outside consultants Deloitte Haskins and Sells to carry out a review of the 'interface between the ENB and the training institutions' which reported in early 1989 (ENB 1989a). It recommends ways in which the Board might tighten up its arrangements to secure more direct lines of accountability in the resource allocation process, including the abolition of education advisory groups and their replacement by local training committees, permitted in the 1979 Act which established the boards. The essential difference between the 14 EAGs and the LTCs would be that there would be only four LTCs based in the ENB's existing local premises; they would function as comittees of the Board, but with greater executive input at local office level. Deloittes take the view that this new structure could not function effectively without extending the ENB's information system to permit the quarterly calculation of cost-based PIs to monitor resource allocation to training institutions.

Regional education and training strategies

It has been through these strategies, developed at RHA level, that the amalgamation of schools of nursing into larger units has been implemented. These amalgamations also require all training institutions to establish links with higher education and to provide courses normally in at least three specialisms. Across the country, strategies were still, during the research time-scale, at varying stages of consultation, and new arrangements were still in some places far from certain. Some Regions commissioned option appraisal studies from management consultants to help them decide the best way to organise local consortia of schools, and the information gathered in these studies was very similar to local PI pilot studies. The ENB's own internal review (see above) identifies these strategies, along with educational PIs, as a key element in taking forward the proposed new arrangements for resource allocation.

Department review of the statutory bodies

As non-governmental public bodies, the statutory bodies which regulate nursing (the ENB, the Welsh National Board, the National Board for Scotland, the National Board for Northern Ireland, and the United Kingdom Central Council) are subject to periodic reviews. The first review since this set of bodies was set up under the 1979 Act was conducted during 1988 by outside consultants Peat Marwick McLintock, whose brief included the possibility of changes to statute. While the consultants sought to avoid such changes, their investigation – made public in September 1989 – found that relationships between the statutory bodies were too cumbersome, and argued for a new framework which would require the assent of Parliament (ENB 1989b: para. 6). Central to the argument are the concepts of efficiency, effectiveness and accountability, as the first of the principal findings shows: 'We have identified a number of factors concerned with organisational arrangements which we believe inhibit the efficiency and effectiveness with which the statutory bodies are able to discharge their responsibilities.'

The review proposes that the boards cease to be elected bodies and become an executive with direct ownership of training institutions, thus severing their financial links with the NHS. In contrast, the UKCC's role as the professional body would be clarified: Council would be both funded and elected by the practitioners and would take responsibility for standards-setting.

This, the consultants argue, will enable education managers to use resource-based PIs which will more accurately reflect the true financial situations of training institutions than is possible under present arrangements where not only is funding split between the boards and the local health authorities, but considerable local variation exists over the division of budgetary responsibilities. In particular, the use of student–staff ratios (SSRs) is recommended 'as an aid to improved resource allocation rather than as a measure of achievement'. However, this cannot proceed until definitions of SSRs are not only based on some rationale, but above all harmonized; currently there are variations in definitions over what counts as a teacher, for instance whether unqualified teachers should be included in the calculations. Further research is required, it is argued, to 'establish appropriate values of SSRs in different circumstances'. It is further recommended that the boards develop a 'small set of resource based PIs to be used in monitoring resource usage at institutional level'.

The White Paper: Working for Patients

The publication of the NHS review on 31 January 1989 (Department of Health 1989a) brought all these other initiatives into sharp focus. The idea of introducing 'internal markets' backed up by computerized resource management and clinical budgeting will require the use of cost-related indicators in particular. Project 2000 has necessitated the calculation of some of the 'grey areas' of district health authority resource input into nurse education, the clinical grading structure has established new relationships between labour costs and outputs, and the streamlining of accountabilities proposed in the reviews of the national bodies would result in cost-based PI-type information flowing more directly to the Department of Health.

While the White Paper itself takes no particular stand on the question of how training institutions should be managed, *Working Paper 10* (published in November 1989 and dealing with arrangements for England only) sets out in more detail various options, including strong arguments for schools remaining, for the time being at least, within the NHS and managed through the regions. The Working Paper also explores the way in which the new 'contracting culture' would work for nurse education, and some of the essential elements of contracts will clearly be linked to performance issues, for instance: 'ideally, the contract should be expressed in terms of the output of successful students' (Department of Health 1989b: para. 7).

The restructuring of higher education and community care

The picture of current policy debates in nurse and midwife education and their relationship to performance monitoring would not be complete without some reference to changes in higher education and for care in the community, for both of these areas are required by the recommendations of Project 2000 to play a greater role in nurse education. Radical changes in the funding arrangements for the polytechnics and colleges were introduced on 1 April 1989 when they ceased to be administered through local education authorities (LEAs) and attained their own 'corporate status'. Resources are now distributed through the Polytechnics and Colleges Funding Council and, though consultation and debate continue about the principles on which resources should be distributed, performance-type information is certain to be the basis of new contractual relationships.

Likewise, the White Paper on community-based care, *Caring for People* (Department of Health 1989c), sets out proposals where local authorities, like district health authorities in *Working for Patients*, would become purchasers of 'packages' of care from outside providers, requiring contracts to be drawn up and agreed, and information systems to be developed which would support these contracts.

Government response to the reviews

Taken together, these policy reviews have described and analysed a range of possible options for the future management of nurse and midwife education, with an explicit emphasis on improving accountability. After more than a year's deliberation, the government announced in February 1991 that it approved the Peat Marwick McLintock proposal for the UKCC to become the single elected body, and endorsed the necessity for the national boards to continue to validate training courses.

However, on the question of who should manage nurse and midwife training institutions, there seems to be no preferred model – indeed, each of the four countries is to embark upon implementing rather different arrangements. In Northern Ireland, the national board will continue to manage the colleges of nursing and midwifery, though this model is explicitly rejected for the other three countries. The English colleges will be managed by the regional health authorities as proposed in Working Paper 10, though self-governing status will not be permitted. In Scotland, however, 'The Government would certainly be prepared to consider applications . . . for NHS Trust status' (Secretary of State for Scotland 1991). The Welsh training institutions, meanwhile, are to form consortia which will enable them to be managed from within Welsh institutions of higher education.

The proposals for each of the countries contain, however, recommendations for close liaison with national labour force planning bodies, in the hope that the financing of institutions will be tied to some accurate forecast of future labour force requirements within the NHS. It remains to be seen whether labour force planners are able to devise sufficiently sophisticated models to fulfil this purpose. But the training institutions of the future will certainly need to produce performance indicators which will answer questions about the employment of their leavers.

PIs for the ENB

The project to investigate the feasibility of developing and implementing performance indicators (PIs) for nursing and midwifery training institutions was conducted in two phases over a period of two years. The first phase consisted of a study of the feasibility of developing PIs for training institutions, together with an exploration of the concept of 'qualitative indicators'.

We decided upon an action research approach for the project as the most appropriate way of exploring the problems of how best to develop PIs. This type of approach enabled us to take up the associated sensitive issues concerning evaluation and judgement directly with staff of training institutions by creating a series of discussion forums through which research material could be gathered. To accomplish this, we reviewed the literature from a wide range of sources, and devised techniques of structured consultation through developmental workshops which were held in all the English regions with the help of the regional education advisory groups. The results of these exercises and associated fieldwork are reported upon in *Performance Indicators in Nursing Education: Final Report on a Feasibility Study* (Balogh and Beattie 1988b).

Towards a definition of PIs

Our findings led us to propose a critique of some of the concepts currently used in connection with PIs, and to propose some defining characteristics. In particular, we found an overextension of the qualitative/quantitative dichotomy which had become over-identified with the related, but by no means identical issues of quality and quantity. This overextension found expression in notions such as 'quality cannot be quantified' and that performance indicators could take a qualitative form. While there do exist, beyond the realms of health care and education issues, indicators which express scales of measurement in qualitative terms (the Beaufort wind scale is perhaps the best example), we found no evidence in the literature, or from other ongoing regional pilot PI studies, to support the idea that there are stable and common features concerning the performance of a training institution which could only be expressed in a qualitative way. Conversely, we did find evidence to suggest that quality could sometimes be described, though not encapsulated, numerically. We took PIs to refer to those aspects of a system which are basic to its functioning, and we suggested three minimum properties.

(1) *They are guides rather than absolute measures*
PIs can do no more than, as their name suggests, *indicate*. That they can measure is often assumed, but in practice, even though numerical values may be assigned, they generally fail to show the most basic requirements of measuring instruments – for example, that differences between scores at adjacent points on the scale are equal in weight. The fact that they are guides also points to the need for further information to be sought to elucidate their meaning.

(2) *They have numerical values which describe aspects of a system, most strictly in terms of inputs, activity and outputs*
For educational institutions, this means that PIs are figures about:
student flow – intake sizes, wastage rates, completion rates
teacher inputs and turnover – the range of teacher qualifications and experience
cost inputs – the total costs of teaching, teaching resources, support staff and building maintenance
output of qualified practitioners – employment destinations of successful students.

(3) *Movement in indicators should be subject to unambiguous interpretation* (Best 1986)
This third criterion is in practice difficult to fulfil. It means that there should be no debate about the meaning of, for

example, high scores, and that still higher scores should be consistent with what less high scores denote. However, the student–staff ratio is an example of a commonly used performance indicator whose desirability is usually low both at very low (e.g. 1:1) and very high levels (e.g. 200:1), and which therefore lacks one of the fundamental properties of a measurement scale.

Elsewhere (Balogh and Beattie 1988a), we proposed a further, crucial, consideration:

(4) *The 'three Es' should incorporate a fourth E, which stands for an ethical dimension*
By including this dimension, our aim was to underline the issues of values and accountability which arise every time a decision is taken. The simplest of data sets draws attention to the figures themselves in a way that obscures the fact that its form of presentation has been selected, and that other ways of presenting the figures have *de facto* been rejected. This phenomenon has been called 'the diverted gaze' (Young 1979) – that is, away from debates about the appropriateness of a given concept or variable.

We sought to analyse the conflicts which seemed to lie behind some of the confusions we encountered, and this led us to propose a second phase of research to examine the benefits of implementing a common, nationally agreed data set for performance review, along with the difficulties encountered and prospects for resolving them.

We continued to use an action research strategy, this time by examining implementation issues via a 'vertical' case study, taking the viewpoints of all relevant levels at which planning takes place, from Department of Health, to the ENB, through to the EAG and training institutions in a single region, including the schools of midwifery and the views of health visiting and district nursing course leaders. Some of the workshop-based techniques we used for exploring these issues were further developed and tested and made available nationally in a 'resource guide' containing a sample data set for discussion, along with exercises and suggestions – all derived from the research process – for conducting internal reviews of the quality of educational provision and developing quality strategies. The guide, entitled *Figuring Out Performance* (Balogh, Beattie and Beckerleg 1989) was published by the ENB in July 1989 as a companion to their second Management of Change open learning pack (ENB 1989c). The research findings were reported separately in *Monitoring Performance and Quality in Training Institutions* (Balogh and Beattie 1989).

The implications for accountability of some of the project findings

Throughout our discussions with nurse and midwife teachers, we were impressed by some very simple but key quetions which were an almost universal focus for concern: where do standards and quality fit in? and, how will PIs be used? We sought to analyse in more depth the issues which lay behind these apparently simple questions, and found a rather more complex picture.

Standards and quality

In the first phase of the project, we examined existing PI pilot projects which had been initiated by several regional EAGs. Most of them adopted a dual strategy of gathering 'manpower' figures on wastage and completion rates for students, supplemented by what was often called a 'qualitative review' of the training institution as a whole. Though information on costs was not collected in these exercises, EAGs would have been in a position to draw up crude cost-based PIs (excluding the contribution from local health authorities) by virtue of their own function in distributing funds from the ENB to the training institutions for initial preparation.

It was clear from the difficulties encountered by these local PI projects in subsequently trying to collate the information they had gathered from their 'qualitative reviews' that, though the principle of PIs raising the need for further information was sound, further work was required on what form such information might take and what might be suitable techniques for gathering it. In *Figuring Out Performance* we advised schools about how to embark on an overall 'Quality Strategy' which could incorporate a variety of different techniques including standards-setting exercises, and which could draw upon existing evaluative activities such as the information assembled in the course approval process. The place of PIs in such a strategy would be one of 'core data' – that is, they would provide some basic details about the scale and range of educational provision, ideally over a number of years, though in practice changes in institutional arrangements and course structures will preclude much stability in the definitions of data for some years to come, thus making comparisons over time potentially difficult.

The role of educational standards in developing PIs was much discussed at the developmental workshops, and we found differing viewpoints: some people thought that PIs themselves could be used to specify standards, while others felt that policy statements expressed as standards (e.g. 'learning materials should be easily accessible in the clinical areas') could be called PIs (see, for instance, RCN 1990, where the idea of 'arising PIs' is proposed). The evidence from the case-study workshop activities suggested that neither of these positions was tenable because it is policies themselves which define what constitutes success in their achievement, and local variations over policy are so great that no uniform set of standards could apply to all schools, let alone have any stability over time. We concluded that the guarantee of standards was indeed a basic requirement for performance assessment, but that they should be developed and agreed by parallel processes coming under the umbrella of quality strategies.

The role of PIs in planning and decision-making

We also found a range of views expressed in answer to the question 'How should PIs be used?', not just among senior nurse and midwife teachers in training institutions, but also among Board members and officers, and DoH officials. Moreover, current arrangements had apparently not been conducive to the use of PI-type information for planning and decision-making at either local or national level. The picture of existing information-gathering at training institution level we found to be highly complex, with, for instance, half a day typically set aside for new students to fill in forms, most of which in some sense duplicated each other. Moreover, the ambiguous position occupied by nurse training schools also meant that their financial information was often restricted to those activities funded by the ENB, with precise levels of funding from DHAs frequently unknown.

The situation of EAGs was similarly complex. Though the groups' remit was restricted to initial nurse preparation, the case study EAG made a very strong case for their having access to information about areas outside their responsibility, in particular for post-basic and continuing education, where levels of provision within different DHAs have a considerable impact on the quality of teaching inputs for student nurses.

At the higher levels of ENB and DoH we found a high level of agreement on the necessity for developing PIs, but views varied on how they might be used, ranging from the 'robust' approach that they could be used to specify precise expected levels, for instance on wastage and completion rates, to the view that levels might be specified within a given range of values, to the principle that PIs are merely guides, to be consulted in order to raise questions about possible problem areas. There was some support for the view that PIs ought to form the basis for resource allocation, some of the implications of which are discussed in the next section.

PIs and resource allocation

The question of using PIs for allocating funds was widely debated in all our workshop discussions and interviews. The chief problem which arises can perhaps best be described as one of how to construct an equitable system of incentives, which itself implies the use of rewards and penalties. Furthermore, any system so devised would have to be grafted on to current allocation procedures, which vary between regions, and whose rationale largely flows from the principle observed by Wildavsky that this year's budget is largely determined by last year's budget (quoted in Likierman 1988). Education managers were very concerned that 'if you reward the successful then the unsuccessful have no prospects, it's counterproductive' (EAG financial agent, quoted in Balogh and Beattie 1989).

An important argument against allocating resources on performance criteria derives from the finding that the directors of training institutions felt they had little control over the values which PIs would show. Quite apart from the many local and geographical factors affecting recruitment and availability of qualified staff, our attention was also drawn on many occasions to the influence of local health authority policies on training provision – in particular via the quality of learning environments in practical areas. This is perhaps best illustrated when considering student–staff ratios, where the health authority currently specifies the numbers of students through the provision of placements (the numerator in the ratio) and the school, in consultation both with the EAG and directly with the ENB through course approval, specifies the number of teachers (the denominator). Thus any attempt to change the SSR immediately confronts the problem of 'split accountability' – on the one hand to the health authority and on the other to the ENB.

Further complexities to this question arise because of the transitional state of nursing education, which will persist for some time, especially with regard to the implementation of Project 2000. The old methods of resource allocation, perhaps best described as a 'begging bowl' approach in which the onus fell to training institutions, along up the line to the EAG and the ENB, to present a case of need for further funds, were clearly being questioned by central government policies, especially through the Financial Management Initiative. But though most of our respondents saw the future as being more dominated by rational criteria, it was far from clear what these criteria would be and how they would operate.The chief danger during such periods of transition comes from the difficulty in moving from one model of funding to another without penalizing institutions which have been performing well and with due regard to the need to raise standards in others. In such a climate it is essential for policies to be made explicit and for this reason we recommended the ENB to gather PIs for information only in the first year, and to open the debate on the pros and cons of different methods of allocating funds.

Future patterns of accountability

In this chapter I have tried to trace the roots of the current concern for more streamlined accountability, to argue that they originated in government policies which aimed to tighten the financial accountability of public service managers, and to show how these concerns have manifested in the various new policy initiatives for nurse and midwife education. It is clear that the future management of nurse and midwife education will be planned with greater reference to the monitoring of performance and quality. What is perhaps not so clear is how the role of professional judgement will evolve in this process. With questions of funding increasingly pressing and lines of accountability more clearly defined with regard to resource allocation, there is a danger that these concerns will become the dominant ones. As Donabedian argues (1978: 1), the differing focuses of professional and programme evaluation have 'raised serious ethical problems for the practitioner who is now caught between the two millstones of responsibility towards the individual patient and the collectivity'.

There are some who would argue that financial and professional accountability are not compatible with each other. Elliott (1984) makes this case for general education on the grounds that Value for Money theories are based on a manufacturing model where outputs can be clearly defined, where methods are quantitive rather than qualitative, where evaluation is summative rather than formative, and where the 'audience' is the education authority and the parents or local community.

I would not disagree that all of these distinctions apply. The dominant metaphor of financial management, however, is not so much industrial as blatantly commercial, for even manufacturing companies have problems in defining the appropriateness of their output. However, commercial enterprises assess their performance by crude output measures alone at their peril. They must also guarantee the quality of goods or services on offer *as part of the performance monitoring process*. Operating in a market does theoretically introduce the element of consumer choice as one means of guaranteeing quality, but in many cases product quality may also be bound by legislation or overseen by independent standards-setting bodies, which usually incorporate a professional voice.

My concern would be more about the dangers of the metaphor taking over, and here we might perhaps turn to the literature which derives from the sociology of knowledge for guidance. Schon (1983), for example, in his discourse on *The Reflective Practitioner* argues that such practitioners – indeed the prac- titioners envisaged in Project 2000 – must be aware of different and perhaps competing ways of framing a problem:

When a practitioner becomes aware of his frames, he also

becomes aware of the possibility of alternative ways of framing the reality of his practice. He takes note of the values and norms to which he has given priority, and those he has given less importance, or left out of account altogether.

But, he adds, 'Frame awareness tends to entrain awareness of dilemmas'. The industrial metaphor certainly extends into the vocabulary of performance monitoring, especially with the notion of efficiency ratios which come directly from engineering. An ethical dimension must be incorporated within the three Es for public sector services in order to indicate the essential uncertainties about how, for example, efficiency is to be defined.

We have already taken a brief look at Elliott's second distinction, between quantitative and qualitative methods, and found that they do not necessarily separate so neatly. Behind every statistic some choice, a 'qualitative' one, has been made about what to measure and what to exclude. Certainly an awareness of those qualitative issues is entirely consistent with the professional concerns about how to describe the nuances, details and 'exceptions-to-the-rule' which are the everyday experience of practitioner–client interactions. But this does not mean these nuances cannot be described in a rigorous fashion which is open to debate, and nor does it necessarily exclude the more quantitative features of professional life which may provide a kind of background about the size and range of work undertaken. The principles of peer review have often in the past been conducted using qualitative methods, through the use of independent judgement to protect against possible bias, and more rigorous attention may be needed to these methods in the developing role of professional input to performance monitoring.

Elliott's third distinction, between summative and formative evaluation, may provide us with some important insights. The use of performance monitoring in a summative way implies a focus on a specified 'sum', or short-term end, perhaps without reference to longer-term strategic planning – thereby contradicting the ongoing 'monitoring' aspect of the evaluation. It seems therefore essential to stress this aspect for implementation purposes and, for the ENB at least, we have recommended that PIs be implemented 'within a framework of coherent strategic planning' and that the type of data which are gathered should be continually reviewed (Balogh and Beattie 1989). Embedding PIs within a continuous review process should ensure that the focus will indeed be formative rather than summative.

Lastly, Elliott distinguishes the different audiences to which different kinds of evaluation are addressed. This raises the question of incorporating client satisfaction into the process of performance monitoring – also raised in *Working for Patients* by the creation of market-like conditions which, it is claimed, allow patients greater choice. However, it must be noted that there has been some debate about whether the arrangements envisaged in the White Paper would indeed have this effect (for an analysis of the proposals, see Mullen 1990). Certainly what is being proposed is very far from any image we might have of an open marketplace dealing in goods, and, as I have argued above, the mere existence of some kind of market does not itself guarantee quality. This must be done by other means.

One major problem for the incorporation of consumer or client satisfaction into performance monitoring arises from the fact that services to individual recipients are not delivered by members of one profession alone; the client's perspective in this regard is a multidisciplinary one. There is therefore a need to consider issues like what are the legitimate boundaries of interest of one profession in the activities and policy-setting agendas of another. Donabedian (1978) refers to this issue as one of the defining differences between professional and programme evaluation, and Hepworth (in Levitt 1987) argues that the Financial Management Initiative has raised the question of how far an auditor might legitimately comment on the effectiveness of policy, and whether new relationships between auditors, inspectors and management might be called for. The implications of greater 'consumer' accountability stretch far beyond the boundaries of individual client–practitioner relationships.

Conclusion

I have tried to give a brief overview of some of the issues of professional accountability which are raised by the introduction of new approaches to monitoring performance and quality in nursing and midwifery education. While it is clear that the future management of education will rely much more heavily on these processes, it is also clear that the profession will need to engage in much further work and debate about how the professional voice ought to be expressed within new structures. Taking this debate forward will require at the very least an appreciation of the complex and multiple nature of accountability, where teachers are accountable in many respects:

- to individual patients and to populations of potential patients
- to students in particular and to the students of the future
- to professional peers, whether clinical practitioners or teachers
- to line managers and superiors
- to professional statutory bodies
- to government
- and with regard to the concerns of other professionals with whom they work.

This version of accountability is by no means simple, and, as Schon argues, the entertaining of multiple perspectives brings dilemmas in its wake. But, unless these dilemmas are recognized, there is a real danger of falling into the trap of the 'diverted gaze', and failing to give proper attention to the rich, complex and indeed frequently contested nature of professional practice and management which lies behind the sets of numerical data that new technology allows us to generate and use.

Acknowledgement

The author would like to acknowledge financial support from the ENB for the research on which this chapter is based, and academic support from Alan Beattie, the project director, whose ideas helped in developing many of the lines of argument.

References

Audit Commission. 1983. *Code of Local Government Audit Practice for England and Wales*. London: Audit Commission.
Balogh, R. and Beattie, A. 1988a. Performance review. *Nursing Times*, 4 May, 84(18).
Balogh, R. and Beattie, A. 1988b. *Performance Indicators in Nursing*

Education – Final Report on a Feasibility Study. University of London Institute of Education.

Balogh, R. and Beattie, A. 1989. *Monitoring Performance and Quality in Training Institutions.* University of London Institute of Education.

Balogh, R., Beattie, A. and Beckerleg, S. 1989. *Figuring Out Performance.* Sheffield: English National Board for Nursing, Midwifery and Health Visiting.

Best, G. A. 1986. Performance indicators – a precautionary tale for unit managers. In H. I. Wickings (ed.), *Effective Unit General Management.* London: Kings Fund.

Briggs, A. 1972. *Report of the Committee on Nursing.* Cmnd 5115. London: HMSO.

Department of Health. 1989a. *Working for Patients.* Cmd 555. London: HMSO.

Department of Health. 1989b. *Working for Patients – Education and Training,* Working Paper 10. London: HMSO.

Department of Health. 1989c. *Caring for People.* CM 849. London: HMSO.

Donabedian, A. 1978. *Needed Research in the Assessment and Monitoring of the Quality of Medical Care.* Washington DC: US Department of Health Education and Welfare, National Centre for Health Service Research.

Elliott, I. 1984. The case for school self-evaluation. *Forum,* Autumn, 1.

ENB. 1989a. *Study of the Interface between the ENB and Approved Training Institutions* (Deloittes Report). London: English National Board for Nursing, Midwifery and Health Visiting.

ENB. 1989b. *Review of the United Kingdom Central Council and the Four National Boards for Nursing Midwifery and Health Visiting* (Peat Marwick McLintock Report). London: English National Board for Nursing, Midwifery and Health Visiting.

ENB. 1989c. *Managing Change in Nursing Education.* Sheffield. English National Board for Nursing, Midwifery and Health Visiting.

Goldacre, M. and Griffin, K. 1983. *Performance Indicators – A Commentary on the Literature.* Unit of Clinical Epidemiology, Oxford University.

HMSO. 1982. *Local Government Finance Act.* London.

Jarratt Report. 1985. *Report of the Steering Committee for Efficiency Studies in Universities.* London: Committee of Vice-Chancellors and Principals.

Klein, R. 1983. *The Politics of the National Health Service.* London and New York: Longman.

Levitt, M. S. (ed.) 1987. *New Priorities in Public Spending.* London: Gower House.

Likierman, A. 1988. *Public Expenditure.* Harmondsworth: Penguin Books.

Ministry of Health *et al.* 1947. *Report of the Working Party on Recruitment and Training of Nurses* (Wood Report). London: HMSO.

Ministry of Health. 1956. *Report of the Committee of Enquiry into the Cost of the National Health Service* (Guillebaud Report). Cmnd. 663. London: HMSO.

Mullen, P. M. 1990. Which internal market? The NHS White Paper and internal markets. *Financial Accountability and Management* 6(1): 33–50.

Peacock, A. and Wiseman, J. 1967. *The Growth of Public Expenditure in the United Kingdom*, revised edn. London: Allen & Unwin.

Royal College of Nursing Association of Nursing Education. 1990. *Performance Indicators for the Clinical Learning Environment.* London: RCN.

Schon, D. 1983. *The Reflective Practitioner: How professionals think in action.* New York: Basic Books.

Secretary of State for Scotland. 1991. *Statement by Secretary of State for Scotland on Policy Review of the Statutory Nursing Bodies and the Future Funding and Management of Nursing Midwifery and Health Visiting Education.* Scottish Home and Health Department.

UKCC. 1985. *Project 2000 – a New Preparation for Practice.* London: United Kingdom Central Council for Nursing, Midwifery and Health Visiting.

UKCC and Price Waterhouse. 1987. *Project 2000 – Report on Costs, Benefits and Manpower Implications.* London: United Kingdom Central Council for Nursing, Midwifery and Health Visiting.

Young, R. 1979. Why are figures so significant? The role and critique of quantification. In J. Irvine, I. Miles and J. Evans (eds), *Demystifying Social Statistics.* London: Pluto Press.

CHAPTER NINE

Professional conceptions of mental illness and related issues

Glen Pashley

Psychiatric health professionals are generally in the position of having to treat and care for persons who have been labelled as mentally ill. For this reason it was thought useful to examine just how such professionals conceive of the term 'mental illness'. The term is difficult to define, perhaps even unanalysable. The boundaries of mental illness are a persistent point of debate: it is seen as a myth, as being analogous to physical illness or disease, as maladaptive behaviour, as the result of incongruent thoughts and beliefs or conflicting unconscious desires, as a divided self-concept or as a complex social product that has ultimately formed the basis for psychiatry. Underlying such criteria there seems to be a preconception of what the person is. Indeed, different theories make different assumptions about the person which, in turn, lead to different perspectives of mental illness.

The knowledge base underpinning and supporting the concept of mental illness is not one of a single image but a range of complex, ambiguous and often incommensurable fragments of knowledge drawn from history, philosophy, science, psychiatry, psychology, sociology and the law. It is not surprising then that confusion and disagreement reign regarding what is to count as mental illness and that the boundaries of mental illness are inexact. In order to arrive at a clearer understanding of the term 'mental illness', a multidisciplinary perspective is demanded which takes into account not only the fragmented, formal and descriptive knowledge base, but also the idiosyncratic and shared common-sense knowledge that individual psychiatric health professionals bring to their role. Central to this commonsense aspect will be the person's beliefs, attitudes, and values, the influence of the social context, meaning and use of language and experience in a social world which necessarily contributes to the person's individual ways of perceiving and understanding.

To explore how a number of psychiatric health professionals conceived of mental illness, 25 psychiatric nurses and 10 psychiatric nurse tutors completed a Semantic Differential Scaling Booklet and an open-ended interview.

The semantic differential

The Semantic Differential (S/D) consisted of 11 bipolar adjectives which respondents had to apply to three different types of individuals. The bipolar adjectives focused upon the following terms: personhood status, bad, feelings, intelligent, punishment, responsible, good, treatment, rational, sane and therapy. The types of individuals were: a mentally ill individual, a schizophrenic individual, and an individual with a destructive personality. The S/D was constructed on the basis of a five-point scale. The raw score of 1 was taken to mean that respondents thought, say, the mentally ill individual was rational, a score of 2 would indicate that such an individual was probably rational, a score of 4 was taken to suggest that a mentally ill individual was probably not rational and a score of 5 was taken to mean that such an individual was thought to be definitely not rational. Where respondents had a raw score of 3 this was interpreted that he/she was unsure, simply did not know or wanted to say it would depend upon other influencing factors. The respondents were separated, for discussion purposes, into four groups: male nurses (12), female nurses (13), male tutors (7) and female tutors (3). The findings from the S/D could have been quantitatively and statistically analysed but it was thought, given the abstract and complex nature of the concepts and terms involved, that a more meaningful understanding would be gained through a qualitative and interpretive approach. Therefore, a rather broad, global and generalized interpretation of the response was made.

The mentally ill individual

The mentally ill individual was attributed with full personhood status and was seen as definitely having feelings. He/she was generally perceived to be good rather than bad. It is important to note however that these terms presented a degree of difficulty for some respondents; for example, 12 respondents could not decide whether this type of individual was bad or not, and 27 respondents could not judge whether he/she was good or not. It is likely that these respondents who were more cautious with their judgements and generalizations wanted to say it would depend upon other factors and circumstances. These other influential factors may relate to the professional's own experience, in the sense that they have found mentally ill individuals to be bad at times and good at other times. An interesting point which emphasizes the ambiguity in meaning and use of language is that the term 'bad' is not always seen as the opposite of 'good'; for example, 19 respondents conceived of the mentally ill individual as being definitely not bad, but only 4 respondents thought this type of individual to be definitely good. Interestingly, it was the male and female nurses rather than the tutors who were the most reluctant and cautious in judging the terms 'good' and 'bad'. This relates, perhaps, to the fact that these professionals have the most direct contact with mentally ill individuals and are, therefore, in a position of constantly interacting with individuals who may behave in a good and/or bad manner. However, the meaning and use of language here is important; what one nurse or tutor may mean by the terms 'good' and 'bad' behaviour may not have the same meaning for another nurse or tutor. Further, the meaning that individual respondents attach to such terms will be influenced by beliefs, attitudes, values, the social context in which the behaviour occurs and experience. The S/D does not specify the meaning or use for respondents; it rests with each individual to create his/her own meaning and use given the context which the S/D provides. It is likely that such attributed meaning and use will change in the new context of the interview situation where respondents can discuss their ideas in more depth and introduce their own influential circumstances.

The feature of intelligence as applied to the mentally ill individual reflected another problem area for respondents. Although 20 respondents viewed this type of individual to be intelligent or probably intelligent, 15 felt unable to judge and recorded a raw score of 3. This level of indecision may be a consequence of the concept of intelligence itself being controversial and dependent upon several other cognitive processes for a clearer understanding – for example, thought, memory and problem solving. The female nurses were particularly cautious in attributing this feature to the mentally ill individual.

The features of rationality and sanity were difficult for respondents to judge. No respondents conceived of this type of individual to be completely rational and sane, or completely not rational and not sane; the majority recorded a raw score of 3. The concepts of rationality and sanity are complex, not only in terms of their meaning and interpretation but also in the sense that recognition rests upon subjective inferences, values, beliefs, attitudes, common sense and more formal knowledge and experience. The *Concise Oxford Dictionary* (1987) defines rational as being 'Endowed with reason, reasoning; sensible, sane, moderate, not foolish or absurd or extreme'. However, Berenson (1981) remarks that a misguided dichotomy exists between what is to count as rational and irrational, and that the dichotomy has its roots in a belief that what is rational involves logical thought and what is irrational entails illogical emotion. It is likely that respondents judging the features of rationality and sanity as they understand them applying to the mentally ill individual have in mind the notion of thought disorder. What is important to keep in mind is that thought processes are unobservable and can only be inferred from an individual's actual behaviour. The question arises, is thought accurately reflected in behaviour? and are the observers of that behaviour correct in their interpretation? This is where the centrality of the meaning and use of language, experience and commonsense knowledge can influence our judgements about others.

The attribution of responsibility to the mentally ill individual, like the features of being rational and sane or not, was a difficult area for respondents to assess. Generally speaking, the majority of respondents recorded a raw score of 3, suggesting that they could not decide because it was seen to be dependent upon other fators. The mentally ill individual was thought of as not deserving to be punished; rather he/she should be medically treated or receive some form of psychological therapy. There was a preference by all groups in favour of therapy over and above any type of medically oriented treatment.

The schizophrenic individual

The schizophrenic individual was attributed with full personhood status by all individual respondents, except 1 male nurse. It is difficult to offer any explanation for this viewpoint; perhaps at best it can be assumed that his experience of individuals who have been labelled schizophrenic has left some lasting impressions and doubts as to the nature of their being. The schizophrenic individual, like the mentally ill individual, was definitely thought to have feelings. Similarly, the schizophrenic individual generated problems for respondents when faced with attributing the feature of intelligence. Although 22 respondents viewed this type of individual as intelligent or probably intelligent, 13 were unable to decide and, therefore, recorded a raw score of 3. The schizophrenic individual, like the mentally ill individual, was generally seen to be good rather than bad. However, there was a broad agreement amongst all groups of respondents that the schizophrenic individual is slightly less bad and slightly more good than the mentally ill individual.

The schizophrenic individual was generally conceived to be less rational and less sane than the mentally ill individual. Indeed, 3 respondents viewed the schizophrenic individual as being totally not rational, whereas no respondents had seen the mentally ill individual to be completely not rational. The assumption can be made that respondents may have seen the schizophrenic individual to be less rational and sane because of their professional knowledge of the characteristics often held to be typical of schizophrenia – for example, thought disorder, delusions, hallucinations and withdrawal from reality. These characteristics can all, to some extent, be associated with the terms 'rationality' and 'sanity'. However, these terms presented a problem for respondents to attribute to the schizophrenic individual; the majority were unsure or felt it would be dependent upon other factors.

The feature of responsibility as attributed to the schizophrenic individual was virtually identical to the degree of responsibility levied at the mentally ill individual; in fact, for both types of individuals 21 respondents recorded a raw score of 3, thus reflecting their difficulty in attributing this feature generally. On a commonsense level this seems consistent, since within the meaning of the terms 'schizophrenia' and 'mental illness' there is much room for overlap. However, given that respondents had claimed the schizophrenic individual to be slightly less rational and sane than the mentally ill individual, then it could have been anticipated that the schizophrenic individual would be thought to be relatively less responsible, assuming of course that respondents hold individuals to be responsible on the basis of how rational and sane they are. This was not the case. The majority of respondents did not judge the schizophrenic individual to be less responsible; in fact, the male tutors perceived this type of individual to be more responsible than the mentally ill individual. It is difficult to explain this conception on the basis of the completed S/D, which leaves respondents no room for self-explanation – hence the need for the interview, which allowed respondents to discuss these issues in more depth.

Punishment was generally seen to be slightly less appropriate for the schizophrenic individual than for the mentally ill individual, if indeed it was thought appropriate at all. Just as therapy was deemed to be slightly more suitable for the mentally ill individual, treatment was thought to be slightly more suitable for the schizophrenic individual. This fits with the theoretical belief that schizophrenia is a physical illness or dysfunction which can be treated by physical means. The female nurses were the one group who readily reflected this view, whilst the male nurses and male and female tutors appeared to see more value in both treatment and therapy.

Individual with a personality disorder

The individual with a personality disorder, like the schizophrenic individual, was attributed with full personhood status by all of the respondents except for one female tutor who found she could not judge this feature. The feature of feelings did, to a limited extent, differentiate the individual with a personality disorder from the other two types of individuals. Generally speaking, this type of individual was seen to have fewer feelings than either the mentally ill or the schizophrenic individual.

However, given that individuals with a personality disorder are usually thought to display more heightened and intense feelings than, say, a mentally ill individual, there seems to be an element of inconsistency. Perhaps one possible but tentative explanation for this may relate to the way in which respondents interpret the term feelings. The feelings often associated with personality disorders are: disturbed, violent, self-destructive, impulsive and restless. The feelings often associated with mental illness are: depression, void of emotion and an inability to express emotions. This could be seen to reflect a 'hard' and 'soft' categorization of feelings; the implication being that the individual with a personality disorder is thought by the respondents to have less soft feelings, rather than less feelings *per se*.

The concept of intelligence appeared to be another feature that differentiated the individual with a personality disorder from the mentally ill and the schizophrenic individual. Respondents generally viewed this type of individual to be less intelligent, or found it more difficult to attribute any degree of intelligence than they did for either of the other two types of individuals. Respondents found great difficulty also in attributing the features of bad and/or good to the individual with a personality disorder, although the general tendency was to perceive this individual as bad rather than not bad, and as not good rather than good. In effect, this type of individual was thought to be more bad and less good than either the mentally ill or the schizophrenic individual.

The features of rationality and sanity as they were applied to the individual with a personality disorder presented respondents with some difficulty. The general opinion however was that this type of individual was more rational and sane than either the mentally ill or the schiozophrenic individual. Given this broad trend it follows that respondents might see this type of individual as being more responsible than either of the other two types of individuals. This viewpoint was supported by the respondents in the sense that the majority perceived this type of individual to be responsible or probably responsible for their behaviour. Most respondents were in some doubt as to whether the individual with a personality disorder should be punished, although punishment was generally thought to be more appropriate for this type of individual than it was for either the mentally ill or the schizophrenic individual.

Medical treatment for the individual with a personality disorder was seen to be far less suitable than it was for the mentally ill or the schizophrenic individual. However, the range of scores was diverse, reflecting that respondents had mixed feelings about this issue. Conversely, psychological therapy was seen to be far more suitable for this type of individual than medical treatment. Both the male and the female nurses strongly supported this view, unlike the male and female tutors who thought it to be less appropriate. One possible explanation here is that the nurses, who are constantly using therapy in their everyday work experience, may appreciate its value for a range of different types of individuals far more than do the tutors, who do not have the same and current level of practice and experiential knowledge.

Much of the meaning that respondents had in mind when completing the S/D remains untaped because of the way in which respondents are limited by the research tool itelf; it is somewhat mechanistic in the sense that respondents simply tick a box representing the numbers 1 to 5 in order to indicate their viewpoint. This allows the respondents no room for explaining why they put their tick where they did. However, as an introductory research methodology it has proved most useful and identified several important factors regarding conceptions of mental illness. It expects respondents to make value judgements regarding the attribution of features or properties to different types of individuals. Some respondents appeared to do this with relative ease whereas other respondents were more cautious with their judgements. How easy or cautious respondents are is likely to be influenced by professional knowledge and experience, social, cultural and personal beliefs, attitudes and opinions. The attribution of features to the different types of individuals very much relies upon experience; for example, a psychiatric nurse working in a regional secure unit is likely to have experienced 'bad' behaviour by mentally ill individuals or individuals with a personality disorder to a greater extent than psychiatric nurses working on a ward where patients are being rehabilitated for transition into the community. The notion of experience also involves commonsense knowledge; for example, some respondents may not have had direct contact with or have any formal knowledge regarding personality disorders, but still have a conception of what for them represents an individual with a personality disorder. On the basis of this commonsense knowledge respondents make value judgements and attribute features. However, respondents who scored 3 on the S/D may well not have been prepared to make such value judgements because there are so many unknown influential factors.

A final and important point to note is that the attribution of particular features to the different types of individuals reflects that a sliding scale appeared to be in operation. For example, the individual with a personality disorder was seen to be more bad, to have fewer feelings, to be less intelligent, and to be more rational, sane and responsible than either the mentally ill or the schizophrenic individual. However, it is worth reiterating that many respondents were unsure about several of these features, essentially because of the complexity of such terms.

The S/D was used as a research tool for simply introducing respondents to the broad and particular concepts perceived by the researcher as being relevant to the term 'mental illness'. It was seen as a means of eliciting the subjective and initial responses to such ideas, as a way of discovering in broad and general terms any possible areas of uncertainty, confusion, similarity and difference, and where more in-depth discussion was required. The open-ended interview certainly enhanced this in-depth discussion and also allowed the respondents to introduce their own ideas and concepts and the issues which they felt were central to the term 'mental illness'. The amount and richness of information generated by the interview was extensive, and it is only possible within this chapter to focus selectively on particular terms, concepts and issues that complement some of the broad generalizations derived from the S/D.

The interview

All 35 respondents participated in an in-depth interview which was tape-recorded and later transcribed. A post-coded classification system was developed in order to enhance the qualitative interpretation and understanding of conceptions of mental illness and related issues. As James (1977) remarks, a qualitative interpretation provides 'perspective, insight and understandable decription'. The information which emerged from the respondents' statements was interpreted on the basis of four themes incorporating 27 categories and sub-categories.

Theme 1, Broad Conceptions of Mental Illness, was concerned with how respondents viewed three major aspects of the concept of mental illness, namely, the causes of mental illness, the social influences upon becoming mentally ill and the broad loosely defined features that generally distinguish a mentally ill individual. The following eight 'A' categories comprise this first theme:

A1 Physical causes
A2 Multiplicity of causes
A3 Defined by society/culture
A4 Involves the labelling process
A5 Effects of institutionalization
A6 Behavioural problems
A7 Disorders of thinking
A8 Emotional problems

Theme 2, Psychological Features of the Mentally Ill Individual, was more specific with regard to the physical and psychological features of mental illness. It was concerned with respondents' conceptions of how mentally ill individuals think, feel and behave and, given these perceived features, whether this type of individual ought to be held responsible for their behaviour or not. The following ten 'B' categories represent this second theme:

B1 Odd/bizarre behaviour
B1.1 Lack of coping skills
B1.2 Difficulties in communicating
B2 Degree of rationality dependent upon severity of illness
B2.1 Lack of insight/awareness
B2.2 Mentally ill people see themselves as rational
B3 Extreme/exaggerated/inappropriate emotions
B3.1 Emotional thought disorder
B4 Degree of responsibility dependent upon severity of illness
B4.1 Degree of responsibility dependent upon degree of rationality

Theme 3, Treatment for the Mentally Ill Individual, focused upon the issue of how such an individual ought to be treated and cared for, and was composed of the following four 'C' categories:

C1 Drugs overprescribed
C1.1 Drugs a means of control/suppress symptoms/mask causes
C1.2 Drugs supportive to therapy/multidisciplinary approach
C2 Use of psychological therapies only

Theme 4, Punishment for the Mentally Ill Individual, concerned whether or not punishment is an appropriate course of action to be taken against this type of individual. The following five 'D' categories represent this fourth theme:

D1 Punishment dependent upon degree of responsibility
D2 Punishment dependent upon degree of rationality
D3 Should be punished like any other offender
D4 Punishment not seen as beneficial to any mentally ill individual
D5 Other labels used for punishment

It is worth noting that a small number of respondents supported a medical perspective of mental illness in the sense that the cause of mental illness/schizophrenia was seen to be physical (A1), and that behavioural problems (A6) and disorders of thinking (A7) could be controlled through the use of drugs, a physical form of treatment. For example, one psychiatric nurse tutor remarked, 'Psychotic illnesses are much more organically based . . ., and a psychiatric nurse claimed, 'I think you need drugs if the symptoms are very bad to get the person to a state where you can work therapeutically. You need to suppress the physical symptoms.'

There are two points in particular worthy of mention here. First, there are sound ethical reasons for using drugs if they can break the cycle of stressor depression for the person. Second, there are less sound reasons for using drugs if they are used to control and manipulate the person so that they are in a state whereby the health practitioner can work therapeutically. There seems to be an underlying assumption that if the person's symptoms are masked or suppressed, then the real self or person becomes available for therapy. The use of drugs may have effects which health professionals are unaware of and, therefore, the real self or person may likewise be suppressed due to the effects of drugs, hence therapy may be of little value either before or after treatment.

Those respondents who supported a medical/physical perspective of mental illness/schizophrenia tended to equate the mind with the brain and to use the two terms interchangeably. Rose (1987) would corroborate this unity of the two terms 'mind' and 'brain' and advocate that any event or activity which can be described in biological brain language must also have a description in psychological mind language. However, there is an important way in which the languages of the mind and brain are incommensurable; the information content of a person's speech does not translate into statements about molecules or cells, even though both speech and molecules are aspects of the same unitary phenomenon. Speech carries sets of meanings which are influenced by social, cultural, economic, religious and experiential factors, and which are not reducible to biological parts. Further, conceptions of mental illness involve conceptions of what is normal; norms are not biologically based, they entail interpersonal agreement, shared meanings, assumptions, beliefs and evaluative judgements about what is acceptable behaviour and acceptable ways of thinking in different societies and cultures.

A number of respondents conceived of mental illness/schizophrenia as being defined by society (A3), as involving the effects of labelling (A4 and A5), that difficulties in interpersonal communication prevail (B1.2) and that the causes of mental illness can include a multitude of social as well as biological and psychological factors (A2). There is a sense in which some respondents adopted an eclectic perspective of mental illness because all aspects of an individual's experience were held to be possible causes of mental illness/schizophrenia. However, implicit within this eclectic perspective is a strong emphasis upon a social viewpoint which argues that mental illness is socially constructed, that the meaning and use of language are important and that the wider social influences are contributory factors. The social perspective also reminds us that all symptoms and behaviour have to be considered as taking place within a social context; it is here where the boundary between what is normal and abnormal is determined.

Some respondents conceived of mental illness/schizophrenia very much in behavioural terms (A6) and supported the notion of odd behaviour (B1), lack of coping skills (B1.1) and difficulties in communication (B1.2) as features of mental illness which can, perhaps, be treated through behavioural therapy. For example, a psychiatric nurse remarked, 'The main difference is in the way the behaviour manifests itself . . . it's usually more unpredictable, it can't be defined in normal terms.' The emphasis here seems to rest upon the actions of the individual; either they are appropriate, acceptable and conform to society's expectations and norms or they do not. If the actions of the individual are not socially acceptable, this raises the question of whether they ought to be changed and, if change is recommended, then ought this to be brought about through treatment, therapy and/or punishment? Further, who decides that a change in behaviour is necessary? For some respondents punishment can serve to change behaviour into something more socially acceptable and/or make the individual realize they have done something wrong (D3). According to a psychiatric nurse, 'Occasionally if you get a very undesirable behaviour and you want to stop it or change it, then punishment can have that effect.' Another psychiatric nurse claimed, 'Punishment is the only thing that makes them realize they are doing wrong. Trying to reason with them doesn't always work.' The respondents who supported the idea that the mentally ill/schizophrenic individual is not always rational and responsible, and yet would advocate some form of punishment in order to make the individual more aware that he/she has done something wrong, are reflecting a degree of inconsistency and confusion. The problem with this type of reasoning is that, if the mentally ill/schizophrenic individual is not rational, is experiencing disorders of thinking or believes him/herself to be rational and right and that everyone else is irrational and wrong, then is there any purpose in punishing that individual? In other words, will he/she understand and accept the reasons for punishment in the same way that the administrator of the punishment accepts and advocates it?

A number of respondents used alternative labels for what other individuals might construe as falling under the general heading of punishment (D5). As one psychiatric nurse remarked, 'I wouldn't call it punishment. We do implement Policy 20 in this hospital which is seclusion for the patient. It's not punishment because I don't think you should punish the mentally ill person ...' A second psychiatric nurse commented, 'Very rarely would I advocate punishment. I would rather advocate extinction, negative reinforcement or denial.' It is evident that the meaning and use of language are central to the interpretation of the term 'punishment'.

For some respondents, punishment for the mentally ill/schizophrenic individual was seen to be dependent upon whether he/she is responsible for his/her own actions (D1), and/or upon whether he/she is rational or not (D2). As one psychiatric nurse tutor remarked, 'If a person is responsible for their behaviour then they should be punished ... If they are rational I believe they are responsible, and if they are responsible they should be punished.' The different perspectives of the appropriateness of punishment emphasize the complexity of the term, and to enhance any understanding of its application to the mentally ill/schizophrenic individual, then other complex terms and conditions need to be considered – for example, rationality and responsibility.

Interestingly, disorders of thinking (A7) were seen to be a central distinguishing feature of mental illness. According to one psychiatric nurse, 'Mental illness is some sort of malfunction of the thought processes.' A psychiatric nurse tutor remarked, 'I think rational thinking is a problem area . . . they perceive life differently, understand and relate differently to the world around them.' In most cases respondents had in mind schizophrenia when referring to thought disorder. However, to use the term 'thought disorder' only makes sense if respondents acknowledge a subjective and inferential basis, because thought disorders cannot be observed; nor does it follow that thought is disordered simply because speech is disordered. Further, it would have been more consistent had those respondents who supported a physical cause of mental illness/schizophrenia spoken of neural disorder rather than thought disorder, which would then match a descriptive and causal perspective of mental illness.

The idea that the degree of rationality is dependent upon the severity of the illness (B2) was strongly supported by the respondents. For example, a psychiatric nurse tutor commented, 'It depends on the type of the mental illness; for instance, with a neurotic type of illness such as acute anxiety the person will be rational, but if schizophrenia or a depressive illness is the problem then that person may not be as rational.' A psychiatric nurse remarked, 'With depression the person is absolutely rational but totally lacking in emotion. With schizophrenia they are very emotional and at times very irrational.' Two important points emerge from these kinds of claims about rationality. First, it could be argued that the type and severity of the mental illness may be dependent upon or influenced by the degree of rationality. In other words, the question arises, does diminished rationality cause mental illness or does mental illness cause diminished rationality? Second, the idea that rationality and the emotions are separate appears to be implicit within many of the respondents' comments; few respondents actually acknowledged category B3.1, emotional thought disorder. It is important that the interrelationship between thought and emotion is recognized in order to enhance the understanding of mental illness. As Schacter (1971) suggests, the quality of the emotions depends upon how the external world and the internal state of the person are cognitively interpreted. Similarly, Mandler (1975) supports the notion that emotions are influenced by the cognitive evaluation or 'meaning analysis' of the current state of affairs.

The suggestion that emotional problems (A8) are a distinguishing feature of mental illness was strongly supported by the respondents. Further, many respondents were more specific and referred to extreme, exaggerated and inappropriate emotions (B3) as being a feature of mental illness. Indeed, one psychiatric nurse believed that mental illness should really be referred to as 'emotional illness'. The strong support for this category and the lack of support for emotional thought disorder (B3.1) re-emphasize the necessity for psychiatric health professionals to become more familiar with the relationship between thought and emotion, and to recognize that the individual must have thought about or been cognitively aware of the circumstances or events that stimulated an emotional reaction.

There seems to be a complex interplay between rationality, the type and severity of the mental illness and responsibility. A large number of respondents held that the degree of responsibility was dependent upon either the severity of the mental illness (B4) or the degree of rationality (B4.1). For example, a psychiatric nurse tutor thought, 'Schizophrenics are probably not responsible most of the time, whereas with a neurotic illness the person would be responsible for quite a lot of the time.' A second psychiatric nurse tutor remarked, 'If people are thinking logically they are responsible really.' This complex interplay of terms and their meanings is further complicated by the emotions; consequently, what becomes difficult to discern is to what extent each of these factors influences the other. In other words, to what extent do the severity of the mental illness, the degree of rationality and the emotional state interact with each other and, in turn, influence decisions about responsibility and punishment? The terms 'free will' and 'determinism' are often used to enhance the understanding of responsibility. For example, if a person is determined or influenced by external factors to behave in particular ways then he/she is not usually held responsible. Conversely, if a person is behaving on the basis of free will and is exercising choice and making decisions, then he/she is usually held to be more responsible. The question arises, how responsible is the person if he/she is acting freely but on the grounds of disturbed thoughts and/or emotions?

When respondents were asked about their conceptions of personality disorders two main links were made: either a personality disorder was seen as a form of mental illness, or personality disorders conjured the idea of an 'evil' individual. It is not the intention here to discuss respondents' conceptions of evil, but when probing questions were asked of the respondents more questions and confusion were generated. It seemed to be the case that respondents had little knowledge about personality disorders, hence their uncertainty about the meaning of the term and its relationship with other terms. It is likely that this lack of knowledge and uncertainty derive from the fact that student psychiatric nurses do not consider personality disorders to any great extent in their professional education, and from the fact that such disorders pose a number of theoretical and practical problems for the legal profession which neither moral philosophers nor psychiatrists can seemingly resolve.

The opportunity was given to respondents to reflect upon their own professional education and experience, and to evaluate the curriculum for its appropriateness in understanding the term 'mental illness'. A number of opinions emerged. First, some respondents held that their professional education presented a medical perspective of mental illness with emphasis upon a descriptive set of criteria, that is, the signs and symptoms. A medical perspective was thought to be too restrictive and simplistic, to the extent that social and psychological aspects were largely ignored. Such a perspective was deemed neither to match ward experience nor to enhance the relationship between theory and practice. Second, a number of respondents felt that the knowledge base was not sufficiently broad, in-depth or 'academic'. It was not seen to facilitate critical thinking, common sense or any evaluation of complex concepts such as rationality, responsibility and personality disorders. Further, the specific subject of psychology was thought to be inadequate and to provide no foundation in different psychological approaches, and it was thought that ward experience of 'madness' did not fit with the theoretical psychology of the 'normal'. Third, some respondents perceived experience to be the most important factor in relation to conceptualizing and understanding mental illness.

Professional psychiatric education needs to place far more

emphasis upon the complex concepts identified as causing confusion, and needs to synthesize commonsense knowledge and experience with more formal theoretical knowledge. This ought to enhance an understanding of mental illness and related issues, and facilitate critical thinking around highly complex interdependent concepts such as rationality, the emotions, responsibility and punishment. Commonsense knowledge is taken to involve the individual's beliefs, attitudes and values, the influence of the social context, the meaning and use of everyday language and experience in a social world. It is evident that the psychiatric health professionals involved in the research utilized commonsense knowledge in order to conceptualize mental illness.

References

Berenson, F. M. 1981. *Understanding Persons*. Sussex: Harvester Press.
Concise Oxford Dictionary. 1987. Oxford: Oxford University Press.
James, J. 1977. Ethnography and social problems. In R. S. Weppner (ed.). *Street Ethnography*. California: Sage.
Mandler, G. 1975. *Mind and Emotion*. New York: John Wiley.
Rose, S. 1987. *Molecules and Minds*. Milton Keynes: Open University.
Schacter, S. 1971. *Emotion, Obesity and Crime*. New York: Academic Press.

PART III

Clinical

The delivery of care has always been a central theme when considering the various perspectives which can be taken regarding nursing. The evolutionary process has seen many changes in the theory and application of professional knowledge. The nursing process and the utilization of models has greatly influenced the way nurses perceive their relationship with patients. The days of viewing the person as a pathology to be cared for only in physiological terms have been left behind. Introducing concepts such as autonomy, partnership and individuality has helped to move the patient from a passive recipient of nursing care to a position where active participation in the decision process is seen as the norm.

Despite these advances in trying to instigate patient parity there are still occasions when the nurse has a role to play as an advocate. Paul Witts (Chapter 10) has investigated this vital aspect of care and presents us with an analytical insight into the development of advocacy through to its place as a central concept in clinical care. The author makes a pertinent argument for the placing of advocacy as a key element in nursing education. Furthermore, Witts makes the appeal that advocacy should be underpinned by the rationale found in ethics and psychology.

Liz Hanson (Chapter 11) tackles the sensitive issue of stress levels amongst persons with cancer. This chapter is firmly based upon research findings and it illustrates the importance of understanding the concepts of stress if an effective basis for care is to be achieved. The very notion of cancer is fraught with fear regarding death, suffering and the unknown in general. If we are to even approximate towards an understanding of the fear and anxiety which persons with cancer suffer then it is necessary to consider the mechanisms involved in stress formation. The rationale which Hanson presents us with can help to achieve this end.

Helen Ellis (Chapter 12) takes us to the very essence of the clinical ethos by discussing the philosophical and pragmatic considerations to be found within the concept of care. This valuable contribution examines the themes which major theorists have made in trying to present the tenets involved within the practice of caring. A key element within the discussion concerns the possible area of conflict between 'cure' and 'care' in practice. Ellis succinctly develops various threads in a manner which elucidates a complex issue and which will help nurses to analyse their contribution to caring in the light of contextual factors. This chapter will present all practitioners with a stimulating basis for reflecting upon their own 'care-giving' as a dynamic process.

The next contribution may initially seem misplaced in a section which deals primarily with clinical issues. However, Catherine Williams, Jon Barry and Keith Soothill (Chapter 13) present a stringent argument for the notion of nursing wastage having a direct influence upon clinical matters. The authors argue that nurse wastage is not merely a problem for management but can also have an effect upon the delivery of care. The issue is examined from interesting perspectives, with consideration being given to the views not just of nurses working within the Health Service but also of those who have left it. This provides a balanced analysis of a far-reaching issue particularly in the light of recruitment problems and demographic changes.

The advent of Project 2000 has presented the profession with a structure which can revolutionize the nature of nurse education. However, this also has implications for a number of traditional groups responsible for certain aspects of care-giving. Emily Griffiths (Chapter 14) considers the role of the nursing auxiliary with particular reference to the proposed changes involved with Project 2000. The introduction of the new support worker presents a stark innovation to the traditional role of the auxiliary. Griffiths presents a research-based chapter which vividly illustrates the feelings of auxiliary nurses working at a 'grassroots' level.

In the final contribution to Part III, Kevin Kendrick (Chapter 15) discusses the importance of ethical analysis and understanding within the research process. It is fervently argued that nursing is a participatory profession, therefore research must reflect the realities of practice. The notions of personhood and partnership remain central to the discussion, which helps to provide a valid introduction to research together with the philosophical underpinnings of the profession. The emphasis is placed upon ethical analysis and research, which provides a firm foundation for our final Part on management.

CHAPTER TEN

Patient advocacy in nursing

Paul Witts

Introduction

The duty of the nurse is to obey him [the doctor] and recognise his sole responsibility for treatment, and her own responsibility purely as an executive officer. Rightly or wrongly, we can't have every subaltern of genius discussing his superior's orders. Only one battle has been won in a century by the disobedience of orders. But let not the nurse think herself a Nelson!

(*Hospital Journal*, 31 July 1887: 163)

The position of the nurse in the delivery of health care is both unique and complex. An examination of this role reveals two fundamental components. One involves providing a continuous 24-hour support system for other health professionals, notably medical practitioners, in which the nurse takes on delegated functions such as the administration of medicines and the carrying out of other therapeutic directions (e.g. maintaining intravenous infusions or behaviour modification programmes devised by clinical psychologists). The other fundamental component is that in which the nurse becomes the prescriber of care regimes which seek to restore to the patient levels of independence which ill health or medical intervention may have disrupted (Henderson 1972).

A major part of this second component of the nursing role involves the nurse in acting as an advocate for the patient (International Council of Nurses 1973). However, the role of patient's advocate, in which the nurse acts to protect and promote the rights and welfare of the patient, is problematic. These problems arise from a number of sources, most particularly from historical values which characterize the nurse as subservient to the doctor and from the persistent tradition within health care which affords the medical profession with almost total decision-making primacy (Ilife 1983; Navarro 1978).

Problems from the past

Gamarnikow (1978) suggests that a major influence in the process of nursing's subordination to medicine has been the way in which the Victorian nursing reformers subsumed nurse–doctor relations under the rubric of male–female relations:

> The comfort and well-being of the ward largely depends upon whether the house surgeon and sister work well together or whether they swim in different currents. This will rest chiefly with the sister. Never assert your opinions and wishes, but defer to his, and you will find that in the end you generally have your own way. It is always easier to lead than to drive. This is a truly feminine piece of counsel, and I beg you to lay it to your heart.
> (*Hospital Journal*, 8 January 1898: 127)

Nursing was set up and defined as women's work (White 1978; Garmarnikow 1978) and a good nurse came to equal a good woman (see Nightingale 1881). This definition placed the nurse–doctor relation within a patriarchal structure characterized by the subordination of nursing to medicine. The occupational ideology of nursing consequently genderized the division of labour in which doctors were associated with science and authority, and women with caring (putting science into practice). In this way health care came to be based on gender-specific personal qualities. Nurses were defined in the first instance by their personal qualities and virtues. It was character that mattered – and character was intimately linked with femininity. For Nightingale, femininity consisted primarily of moral attributes and qualities:

> To be a good nurse one must be a good woman, here we shall all agree ... What is it like to be 'like a woman'? 'A very

woman' is sometimes said as a word of contempt: sometimes as a word of tender admiration . . . What makes a good woman is the better or higher or holier nature: quietness – gentleness – patience – endurance – forbearance – forbearance with patients, her fellow workers, her superiors, her equals . . . As a mark of contempt for a woman is it not said, she can't obey? – she will have her own way? As a mark of respect – she always knows how to obey? How to give up her own ways?

(Nightingale 1881)

Nightingale, as one of the main nursing reformers, insisted on the existence of a close link between nursing and femininity, the latter being defined by a specific combination of moral qualities which differentiated men from women (Rathbone 1890). Indeed, the success of nursing reforms depended primarily, according to Nightingale, on cultivating the 'feminine' character, rather than on training and education.

The account so far has been an attempt to show how patriarchal ideology, and more specifically the views of Victorian medical men and nursing reformers, came to characterize the role of the nurse and the status of nursing within the health care system. The role and status of the nurse remained almost unaltered throughout the first part of the twentieth century. Changes which have come about since the early 1960s have been mainly concerned with nursing management structures, theoretical and small-scale practice development (Baly 1980; Abel-Smith 1975). However, the themes of good woman = good nurse as a subordinate worker in relation to medicine are still highly relevant in an analysis of nursing in the 1990s.

The experience of nursing today

The majority of nurses today are women (around 90 per cent) (Nutall 1983) and nursing is still generally regarded as women's work (Rayner 1984: Oakley 1984), with the possible exception of psychiatric and mental handicap nursing where the image of the male nurse as custodian and attendant is still strong (Stuart and Sundeen 1983). Kalisch and Kalisch (1983) comment that the image of the nurse in Western culture has remained unchanged over the past 30 years, and, additionally, a cross-cultural study of some 30 different languages discovered that the term 'nurse', while rated as being 'good', was also rated 'weak' and 'ineffective' (Austin *et al.* 1985).

However, while the image of nursing might have remained relatively unchanged over the years, the last 20 years have seen a number of theoretical and practice developments within nursing as a health discipline (Pearson 1983).

Most people, including nurses, tend to define nursing as looking after sick people with the aim of reducing their suffering and nursing them back to health. However, the increasing complexity of modern medicine and the needs of the people who use the NHS demand a more sophisticated approach. Advancing medical technology, with its increased capability to prolong life, the changing needs of an ageing population and the development of specialities allied to medicine (i.e. dietetics, physiotherapy, occupational therapy) indicate the need for a greater flexibility, sensitivity and expertise on the part of the nurse. Modern definitions of what nursing is are both numerous and diverse inasmuch as they reflect the relationship of nursing as a 'jack-of-all-trades' support system to medicine and its allied occupations. However, a central theme amongst the majority of nursing theorists is one which seeks to specify those aspects of the nursing function which are unique to the nurse and are not merely delegated to nurses by doctors and other health workers. One of the most notable of these definitions of nursing is that given by the American nurse, Virginia Henderson, and it is one which seeks to emphasize the nurse's role as one which is person-centred, empowering of the patient, and restorative:

> The unique function of the nurse is to assist the individual, sick or well, in the performance of those activities contributing to health or its recovery (or to peaceful death) that he would perform unaided if he had the necessary strength, will or knowledge. And to do this in such a way as to help him gain independence as rapidly as possible.
>
> (Henderson 1969)

Citing such broad and polished definitions of the nurse's role might give the impression that nurses are free to develop their art without hindrance. But this would be to forget that the medical profession is still the dominant force within modern health care

(Navarro 1978; Doyal 1979). Some of the constraints under which nurses work have been highlighted by the Royal College of Nursing's report, *Standards of Nursing Care* (1980), which looked at the nurse as overseer and coordinator of all the work concerned with patient care. While nurses are charged with this role under the codes of professional organizations such as the United Kingdom Central Council for Nursing, Midwifery and Health Visiting (UKCC), and the International Council of Nurses, it must nevertheless be acknowledged that the nurse has no formal control over any other staff group or service. Such a broad conception of the nurse's role within health care is representative of an incursion into the areas of responsibility for patient treatment and care which medicine has made its own and which are specified in law (Navarro 1978). This historic and legalistic legitimation of nursing by medicine is one which still informs the delivery of health care in the United Kingdom. Although nursing theorists, such as Orem (1980), comment that 'nurses are the designers of nursing care', it is still the doctor who establishes the link between nurse and patient, and who defines the relationship between them by prescribing what is done (by way of treatment). Melnyk (1983) comments: 'if this situation is accepted, then nursing and the relationship of the nurse to the patient require an external authority to define, legitimate, and energize them, and the nurse is little more than an extension of the physician . . .' Despite the work of nursing theorists and the official accounts of what nursing (in theory) is, Ferguson (1984) concludes that in reality nurses 'do generally abide by the medical diagnosis and follow a medical regime'.

However, although the majority of nurses might abide with the medical diagnosis and regime, practitioners such as Pearson (1983) have attempted to develop the role of the nurse as an autonomous practitioner (independent of medicine) in relation to those groups of patients whose primary need is that of nursing, rather than medical, care. Such developments are few and far between and have met with medical opposition (Salvage 1985). Other specific instances of nurses attempting to develop the delivery of their care and voice nursing opinions which may run against those of the medical profession can be seen in the introduction of the 'nursing process' and nurses acting as patient's advocate. The intolerance of the nursing process by doctors can be seen in the following extract from the *British Medical Journal* in which Professor Mitchell echoes the sentiments of the Victorian medical men quoted earlier:

> Patient care cannot be done by committee ... the medical profession is alarmed at the suggestion that patients in a ward may be admitted by nurses without being under the care of a doctor, or that there may be nursing documents, subserving a nursing diagnosis and a nursing plan, which are independent from or even in opposition to the medical diagnosis and the medical plan. I do not believe that two people can be equally in charge of the same patient.
>
> Quo vadis?
>
> I hope that nursing and medicine can devise a synthesis which will address itself to the two key questions that Florence Nightingale identified – what is a nurse? And how should nurses and doctors work together?
>
> (Mitchell 1984)

In espousing a return to Nightingale's definition of a nurse and the relationship between nurses and doctors, Mitchell is clearly underlining the contemporary medical view that nursing should remain subservient (Salvage 1985; Clay 1987).

Situations where nurses challenge the professional judgement of doctors are becoming more frequent (Clay 1987). One example of this is the case of a senior nurse at Wrexham Park Hospital being dismissed after refusing to administer, without the patient's consent, an injection ordered by a doctor. Commenting on the affair in a medical journal, the doctor concerned wrote: 'Consultants must be in charge and be seen to be in charge ... authority should be delegated sparingly, preferably to other consultants ... challenges to consultant authority must be dealt with sympathetically but firmly ... the alternative is the risk of anarchy' (Maddocks 1982).

The preceding examples typify the current hostility and resistance of the medical profession towards nursing autonomy which appears to challenge their authority (Kennedy 1983; Oakley 1984; Salvage 1985). These challenges tend to arise from two main sources: individual nurses who challenge doctors on ethical and professional grounds, and nurses working in nurse education and practice development within higher education.

Individuals who challenge the status quo appear to gain little support from the nursing hierarchy, whose main emphasis is one of preserving tradition and a notion of service which has the effect of depoliticizing the nurse's position within the health care system (Muff 1982). The challenges from nurses in higher education tend to centre on the reorganization of care delivery with the transfer of nurse education into the universities and polytechnics. Although such ideas appear to be welcomed by government, the high cost they represent to health authorities and the Exchequer make them very distant and remote possibilities. Commenting on nursing autonomy, Pearson (1983: 42) writes:

> Autonomous decision-making at the clinical level is notable by its absence. The bureaucratically organized setting of nursing, both in hospitals and in community health, is such that decisions are made according to carefully developed protocols which attempt to cover every eventuality – a feature of bureaucracy.   (Weber 1947)

Despite the attempts of a small minority of nurses to challenge the medical domination of nursing and to promote autonomy for nurses, nursing remains subordinate to medicine and under the control of an entrenched bureaucratic hierarchical structure (Baly 1980; Dickinson 1982; Pearson 1983; Salvage 1985).

This situation is, in part, sustained by way of socialization of nurses in training and practice. Simpson *et al.* (1979) define the process of occupational socialization as one which includes the imparting of skills and knowledge to do the work of an occupation, of orientations that inform behaviour in a professional role, and of identities and commitments that motivate the person to pursue the occupation. The value system into which nures are socialized can be seen to emphasize hierarchy of authority, ritualistic behaviour and excessive role portrayal in everyday clinical practice (Stein 1978). Current day-to-day practice is subject to rule following, standardized activity, and a clear nursing hierarchy with firm allocation of supervisory responsibility (Davies 1976). Such standardization is an effective way of avoiding some of the stress and anxiety inherent in the nurse's work, and is partly, suggests Menzies (1960), a social defence system set up by the hospital nursing system 'to protect its members against the stress arising from their work'. Rigid routines are imposed to remove the need for stressful decision-making, and nursing schools socialize students into valuing routine (Pearson 1983). Stein (1978) describes the schools as being highly disciplined and aimed at inculcating subservience and inhibiting deviance. A fear of independent action can result from this, and consequently the clinging to hierarchical support systems becomes a needed and appreciated activity. Nurses throughout their training and in first post are constantly reminded that they are obliged to conform to statutory and local policy rules, which may, for example, deny them the right to refuse to take part in treatments they consider unethical. In 1982, nursing students in at least three hospitals were sacked for refusing to take part in sessions of electroconvulsive therapy (ECT), because they disagreed in principle with the use of a treatment the effects of which can be harmful, and whose operation is not scientifically understood (Salvage 1985). Nurses may well have their own strongly held personal moral beliefs, but because of the climate that exists in nursing which discourages criticism and can punish 'trouble-makers' with bad ward reports, reduced promotion prospects and dismissal, individual nurses on the whole choose to keep quiet and conform (Courtney 1985; Witts 1986; Henry 1986).

Nursing and social influences

Nursing has been described as an occupation which is subordinate to and legitimized by medicine. The doctor defines who is to be 'a patient' and the nature of the nurse–patient relationship by way of prescribing treatment. This relationship of nursing to medicine has been shown to have come about via the influences of patriarchal ideology and it has also been suggested that this ideology still informs 'the consciousness of women' as shown by some sociological and psychological studies. Conditions such as these point to the possibility of autonomous actions, such as those involved in patient advocacy, being minimized because of the overarching ideology of the health care system.

   That such ideologies do have potent effects on the behaviour of individuals, and specifically individual nurses, can be seen in the work of Milgram (1974) and Hofling et al. (1966). Milgram's studies on obedience demonstrate the lengths people will go to in following orders given by superiors or those in authority. Subjects were asked to take part in 'learning experiments' in which the researcher was specifically interested in the effects of punishment on verbal learning. The subject was allocated to the role of 'teacher' in these experiments and the accomplice to the role of learner. The 'teacher' was made aware of an electric shock generator which would be attached to the learner, and was told that for every error the learner made he must administer a shock increasing in voltage. The mock generator was equipped with switches clearly showing the voltage level of the shock it would give: these ranged from mild through severe to danger.

The disturbing results of these experiments were that most of Milgram's subjects used every shock level, including lethal voltage, on their learner victims. All the subjects used some of the shock levels. However, both the proximity of the learner and the distance of the researcher (variables employed in the study) reduced the willingness of subjects to use high shock levels – with the distance of the experimenter producing the greatest effects.

The teacher subjects did not act without feeling. On the contrary; they expressed tension, conflict of conscience, sympathy for the learner, dissatisfaction with the experiment and the research organization. But they continued to administer shocks.

Milgram's experiments have been criticized by some (see Orne and Holland 1968) for being artificial because of their experimental setting. Similar studies do exist, however, which have been carried out under more ordinary conditions within actual organizations. One such is that by Hofling et al. (1966) in which nurse subjects working in a hospital received bogus telephone calls from 'a doctor' (actually a researcher) requesting the nurse to give a particular patient a drug called 'Astroten' to be found in the ward drug trolley. The nurse was asked to get the bottle (which had a label clearly stating the maxium dose as 10 mgms) and to give the patient a dose of 20 mgms. A real doctor posted nearby stopped each trial, informing the nurse of the experimental nature of the situation after the nurse had poured out 20 mgms of the harmless placebo, or refused to accept the order, or tried to contact another doctor. Despite the dose being excessive, that prescriptions should never be accepted over the telephone (except in an extreme emergency) and that the prescription was given by an unknown person, 21 out of 22 nurses poured out the medication ready to give to the patient.

The above studies, together with findings by other social psychologists such as Sherif (1935), Asch (1955), Crutchfield (1955) and Zimbardo and Ruch (1973) on compliance and conformity, suggest that individual behaviour is rarely an individual response to a context. Rather, it is more often a response to social influence directed either through the socialization processes of childhood, adolescence and occupation or through the social influence of the behaviour of others in that context. We need now to examine how such influence is articulated within health care organizations.

To work as a nurse in a hospital or community setting is to occupy a role within an organization. Katz and Kahn (1966) describe a role as consisting of specific forms of behaviour associated with given positions that tend to develop from task requirements. Role behaviour, within the context of organizations, refers to the recurring actions of an individual, appropriately interrelated with the repetitive activities of others so as to yield a predictable outcome. In formal organizations, such as hospitals, many of the functionally specific behaviours comprising the system (e.g. doctor, nurse, sister, matron) are specified in written and coded presentations and emphasize the point that the role behaviour required is a function more of the organizational setting than of their own personal characteristics. An example of this depersonalization of the nurse is the strict enforcement within nursing of dress codes which amplify the traditional image of the nurse and are a symbolic representation of the nurse's role (see Allport 1933; Salvage 1985).

Katz and Kahn (1966) comment that members of a person's role set depend on that person's performance in as much as they are rewarded by it, judged in terms of it, or require it to perform their own tasks. Because of this dependence, they develop beliefs and attitudes about what the person should and should not do as part of that role. Such prescriptions and proscriptions held by members of a role set are designated role expectations and they define the role and the behaviours expected of the person who holds it.

The content of role expectations consist mainly of preferences with respect to specific acts – things the person should do or avoid doing (e.g. that nurses should always seek the permission of a doctor and seek the approval of a senior nurse). However, role expectations may also refer to personal characteristics or style, ideas about what the person should be, should think, or should believe. Nursing, as we have seen, is an occupation which has a potent historical ideology which equates nurse as 'good woman' and possessor of such 'feminine virtues' as service, obedience and submission to superiors. These factors, coupled with the ways in which women see themselves and in which they are expected to behave, can be seen in the continued socialization of nurses in such a role via nurse training (Salvage 1985; Clay 1987; Pearson 1983), their continuing lack of careerism (Simpson et al. 1979), relatively low inclination towards acquiring training, low economism and low union solidarism (Brown 1976; Barron and Norris 1976). So role expectations are not restricted to job descriptions, but are a result of ideologies, socialization generally and occupational socialization in particular (Milgram 1974).

Role expectations are communicated to members of organizations not only via informational channels but also through messages which are intended to bring about conformity to role expectations. These messages can be of many kinds: instructions about preferred behaviours and those to be avoided, information about rewards and penalties contingent on role performance (e.g. nurses who do not carry out medical instructions such as electroconvulsive therapy will be dismissed), and evaluation of current performance in relation to role expectations (e.g. nursing students' ward reports, annual employee evaluation and promotion interviews).

Such attempts at influence imply consequences for compliance and non-compliance and can take the form of rewards or sanctions. However, the concept of legitimacy, and its acceptance by organizational members, makes the actual use of negative sanctions infrequent in many organizations. Members obey because the source of the command is legitimate and its form and subject matter are appropriate to the source. In addition to the motivational forces aroused by role expectation and other cues, intrinsic satisfaction derived from the content of the role may provide an important source of intrinsic motivation towards role performance.

The reliability of role behaviour is the requirement intrinsic to human organizations (Merton 1957) and every organization faces the task of somehow reducing the variability, instability and unpredictability of individual human acts (Katz and Kahn 1966). That organizations are successful in achieving this reduction is symbolized in the wearing of uniforms, the adoption of certain styles and formalities in interpersonal relations, and that behaviour in organizations shows a selectivity, restrictiveness and a persistence which cannot be observed in the same persons when they are outside the organization. Members of formal organizations respond to visible environmental pressures and can be motivated by shared values. However, the dominant organizational solution to the problem of achieving reliable performance and compliance is to promulgate and enforce rules of conduct. Five conditions can be identified conducive to producing compliance in an organization (Katz and Kahn 1966):

(1) a societal background of normative socialization processes;
(2) recognized and appropriate symbols of authority;
(3) clarity of legal norms and requirements;
(4) specific penalties and sufficient police power; and
(5) expulsion or threat of expulsion of non-conformers from the system.

Compliance with authority is basic to what Tannenbaum (1974) has described as hierarchical control in organizations and which is a universal feature of organizations.

Although the structure of hierarchies can differ in shape and numbers between organizations, what hierarchy does always seem to denote is that there is a firm system of superior/subordinate relationships. Mayo (1949; and McGregory 1960) outline some of the assumptions which lie behind the concept of hierarchy:

Society consists of a horde of unorganized individuals; every individual acts in a manner calculated to secure his/her self preservation or self-interest; every individual thinks logically, to the best of his/her ability, in the service of his/her aim.

the average human being has an inherent dislike of work, and will avoid it if he can; therefore most people must be directed, threatened or coerced to make them work; the average human being prefers to be directed, wishes to avoid responsibility, has relatively little ambition, and wants security above all.

Rowan (1976a) points out that although evidence exists that might be supportive of such assumptions, if they are viewed from an informed psychological perspective they form a classic example of the 'self-fulfilling prophecy': if persons are treated as if they are irresponsible then they will tend to behave in an irresponsible way. Several studies exist on the effects of hierarchy on people. Aiken and Hage's (1966) study on welfare agencies which varied along dimensions of 'orientation to rules', 'emphasis on hierarchy' and 'job codification' showed such factors to be highly and positively intercorrelated. Moreover, they were accompanied with feelings of inadequate professional competence, low self-expression, failure to influence others and low participation in agency affairs. Lawrence and Lorsch (1967), comparing four successful and four less successful organizations with complex problems, found that the less successful firms were more rigidly hierarchical, had managers who felt less influential and successful, had high levels of suppressed disagreement within departments, and were unable to produce creative answers to their problems. Blau and Scott (1966) comment that hierarchical organization, because it restricts the free flow of communication, is unsuitable for solving fresh problems: 'The tendency for hierarchical organizations to be inflexible in the face of new problems results from the barriers on two-way communication. Orders come down but there is no feedback from below' (Shipman 1968).

In their meta-analysis of research in this area, Payne and Pugh (1971) conclude that: 'The general effect of job level on job or need satisfaction is fairly clear. Across most types of companies need satisfaction increases directly as level in hierarchy increases.'

Katz and Kahn (1966) summarize the situation when they comment:

> We are led by these analyses to an attitude of great respect for formal hierarchical organization. It is an instrument of great effectiveness; it offers great economies over unorganized effort; it achieves great unity and compliance. We must face up to its deficiencies, however. These include great waste of human potential for innovation and creativity and great psychological cost to the members, many of whom spend their lives in organizations without caring much for the system (except its extrinsic rewards and accidental interpersonal relationships) or for the goal toward which the system effort is directed. The modification of hierarchical organization to meet these criticisms is one of the great needs of human life.

Having briefly outlined the effects of social influence on individuals and the means by which this influence is articulated in organizations (e.g. hierarchy and role), the suggestion is that nurses, particularly those working in general hospitals, practise health care within strictly defined roles and hierarchies of authority (see Salvage 1985; Pearson 1983; Clay 1987). I now want to juxtapose this situation with a review of the background and requirements of the particularly innovative role of the nurse as patient's advocate, followed by an account of how a working environment might be designed to facilitate such innovation.

The nurse as patient's advocate

The nurse's primary commitment is to the patient's care and safety. She must be alert to take appropriate action regarding any instances of incompetent, unethical or illegal practice by any member of the health care team, or any action on the part of others that is prejudicial to the patient's best interests.

(International Council of Nurses 1973)

Fewer concepts are mentioned with more frequency in discussions of the broadening role of the nurse and the need for increased political awareness in nursing than that of the 'nurse as advocate'. The term 'advocacy' implies that nurses should be educated, motivated and facilitated to assist patients in transcending any barriers to their needs while they are undergoing health care. A nurse is an advocate in the sense that she acts as an intermediary between the patient, his/her family, medical practitioners, other health care personnel and agencies, his/her ultimate aim being the cooperation of all for the patient's benefit (Tschudin 1986). Further definitions exist. Kohnke (1982), adopting a behavioural view, states that 'the role of the advocate is to inform the client and support him in whatever decision he makes'. Gadow (1980) describes advocacy from a philosophical perspective whereby the actions of the advocate reflect a philosophy of caring and support: '[individuals] should be assisted by nursing to authentically exercise their freedom and self-determination.' So rather than the patient advocacy role in nursing being exclusively confrontational/conflict-oriented (as the above ICN quotation might imply), it is also concerned with creative and innovative approaches to person-centred care (Jones 1982). This latter formulation coincides with the main tenet of modern nursing care theory: that the nurse appreciates each patient as an individual with a unique background and a particular set of needs (see, for example, Riehl and Roy 1980).

Despite the apparent importance of the concept of advocacy to nursing theory, philosophy and practice, in a review of the UK literature this author could find no mention of the utilization of the concept of patient advocacy in any nursing curriculum (see Henry 1986; Clay *et al.* 1983; Courtney 1985; Witts 1986). However, a curriculum aimed at fostering the development of advocacy in nursing has been outlined by Eileen Jones (1982), an American nurse, and consists of six main themes:

(1) the nurse must have a thorough appreciation of each client as an individual with a unique background and particular set of needs;

(2) the nurse should be enabled to perform creative behaviours carefully chosen in order to bolster the patient's independence as the chief decision-maker in his/her health care;

(3) the nurse should be able to modify her tactics in the overall strategy of health promotion according to the unique set of behaviours presented by each patient;

(4) the nurse should be able to demonstrate that she can assist her patient in coping with the difficulties he/she experiences as a group member; furthermore, she should exhibit behaviours geared towards assisting groups with problem-solving;

(5) the nurse must be able to articulate, on both practical and theoretical levels, her role as one member of the health care team, so as to identify the unique elements that exist only in cooperative efforts with other helping persons; and

(6) the nurse-advocate should be able to create new patterns of health care delivery that are based on principles of client-centred care.

This curriculum outline represents a radical revision of nurse education and care delivery with an emphasis on enabling nurses to be constantly innovative to meet the unique needs of each patient. It also assumes that the environment in which such nursing practice takes place facilitates nurses being autonomous and innovative (Kohnke 1982; Pearson 1983).

Nurse education and practice in the UK do not prepare or specifically set out to enable patient advocacy. Research suggests that nurses do bring with them their own moral awareness and that they are prepared to act on this in certain circumstances (cases of nurses refusing to assist with ECT tend to underline this) (Witts 1986). The impression gained from this author's research (Witts 1986; see also Courtney 1985) is that nurses tend to take on advocate roles according to the extent to which their working environment facilitates such behaviours. How, then, can we characterize such an environment?

Environments for advocacy

Nursing has been characterized as a hierarchically organized occupation which is ideologically dominated by medicine and historical nursing values. We have also seen how the nurse's role is one which is heavily proscribed. This situation, it has been suggested, is one which promotes conformity and, consequently, can inhibit innovative approaches to nursing care delivery such as patient advocacy. Patient advocacy can be seen to be innovative in as much as it involves the nurse in new behaviours and the enactment of novel nursing strategies within the context of each unique nurse–patient relationship (see Kohnke 1982). Consequently, can we characterize an environment which would support and facilitate advocacy as a kind of innovation?

West *et al.* (1986) comment that the ability to innovate 'is a quality shared by most professional and managerial workers (and probably all workers), and that given the appropriate facilitating environment such innovativeness is likely to be enacted in the work environment'. Drawing on their own previous research, they proceed to outline major contextual psychological features which facilitate individual innovation within organizations. Not surprisingly, perceived freedom has consistently been shown to be of major significance in predicting innovation in organizations (see West 1986; King and West 1986; Amabile 1984; Peters and Waterman 1982). Freedom at work can be characterized as the extent to which an individual feels s/he can act independently of superiors; set his/her own work targets and objectives; choose the methods for achieving work targets and objectives; and the extent to which choice can be exercised over who to deal with to carry out work duties. West *et al.* (1987) comment that 'there is intuitive reason for seeing discretion as of particular importance in predicting innovation since it is unlikely that much innovation will be introduced and applied if individuals or groups perceive little latitude open to them in their role performance'.

Freedom in decision-making was found by Amabile (1984) to be the most frequently cited environmental obstacle (when it was absent) to creativity in her study of Research and Development staff. Freedom can be both an objective feature of the work environment and a perceived characteristic and therefore mediated by personality and attitude. Latitude in relation to the use of time is another important aspect of freedom. Amabile (1984) found that time pressure was the fourth most frequently cited environmental obstacle to innovation in Research and Development settings.

Referring to research linking an individual's social support network with stress and psychological health at work, West *et al.* (1986) comment that 'a combination of social climate factors and personal support will be important influences on innovation in organizations and will influence the effects of most other factors on innovation' (see also Hirsch 1981). Group influence will also affect innovation by:

(1) the extent to which the group reinforces risk-taking and attempts at innovation;
(2) the cohesiveness of the group, which will determine the extent to which an individual believes s/he can introduce and attempt to apply a novel idea without personal censure; and
(3) the specific support of the group for the individual.

Leadership style is another important factor. Kanter (1982) and others (e.g. Peters and Waterman 1982) comment that the likelihood of innovation occurring is increased where the leadership style is participative and collaborative. Criticism of the 'elevator mentality' of hierarchical organizations dominated by restricting vertical relationships in relation to innovation, motivation and morale can be found throughout the organizational, psychological and nursing literature (see Kanter 1982; Rowan 1976b; Pearson 1983; Little and Carnivali 1976).

Feedback is also cited as an important environmental facilitator of innovation in organizations (see West *et al.* 1987; Kanter 1982;

Peters and Waterman 1982). West *et al.* comment that the amount and type of feedback received, both in general and in relation to innovation, are likely to have an impact on innovation within the organization.

Conclusion

The overwhelming majority of nurses, rather like doctors, receive little or no rigorous ethical education beyond a limited amount of 'professional ethics' (Henry 1986; Clay *et al.* 1983). Additionally, the concept of nurse as patient's advocate is rarely present in nursing curricula. This situation denies the largest health care profession a form of education which has the potential to enable nurses to improve even further the quality of care they offer to patients. However, despite this lack of formal education, studies have shown that nurses do act as the patient's advocate and have developed understandings of ethical issues (Courtney 1985; Witts 1986). If advocacy and ethical understanding are present in the informal and unstructured ways these studies suggest, then the possibilities for the role of the nurse as patient's advocate, in the presence of developed educational support and organizational development, offer many potential benefits for patient care and for nurses themselves. With increased awareness and ability in the areas concerning patient advocacy will come an increased political awareness, which may enable nurses to be more assertive in safeguarding a health care system dominated by inappropriate management policies.

Advocacy considered as a form of innovation, as a feature of excellence in performance, is part of the overall picture of 'quality of care'. Advocacy, as an event, has both psychological and ethical implications for the nurse and the patient. While the moral, philosophical and ethical issues in health care and nursing have been established for some time, the psychological context and implications of nursing and promoting quality of care are not as well understood. Willis (1986) makes the point that, while nurses should, quite properly, continue their research into defining and measuring standards of care with regard to physical and medical activities, it should be psychologists, both occupational and clinical, who measure the quality of psychological care. Developing a greater understanding in this area seems essential in an attempt to define what quality of care really means. At the moment it is relatively easy to say what bad care is (the uncaring nurse is fairly easy to spot), but it is difficult to define what goes to make good-quality care. More work in this area of defining and measuring the quality of care is necessary and its importance cannot be overstressed, especially when one considers that the process of recovery from illness has been construed by some researchers as being, essentially, a matter of restored psychological well-being after medical or surgical treatment (see Johnston and Lee Jones 1979; LeShan 1984). When we have been able to form a clearer picture of what constitutes this notion of quality of care, we will be better able to comment on performance in nursing (for there is a sense in which quality of care is a reflection of performance) and go on to examine stressor and moderator effects on nurses and the quality of care they provide.

The process of recovery from illness and restoration to health is one which is shot through with moral and ethical values. Such a view can be traced back to Aristotle (see *The Nicomachean Ethics*) and is reflected in the many statements on the role of the nurse. The aim of these ethical values, when applied to health care, is to promote basic concepts such as personal autonomy, independence and self-determination among patients, and all these form part of the meta-ethic of psychology and, indeed, the social sciences as a whole. When we consider the notion of quality of patient care, we are of necessity committing ourselves to a discussion of ethics and moral values as they relate to both physical and psychological well-being. In this way advocacy can be seen to have profound consequences for the quality of psychological care.

References

Abel-Smith, B. 1975. *A History of the Nursing Profession*. London: Heinemann.
Aiken, M. and Hage, J. 1966. Organizational alienation. *American Sociological Review* 31.
Allport, F. H. 1933. *Institutional Behavior*. Chapel Hill: University of North Carolina Press.
Amabile, T. M. 1984. Creativity motivation in research and development. Unpublished manuscript, Department of Psychology, Brandeis University.

Asch, E. S. 1955. Opinions and social pressure. *Scientific American*, Reprint No. 450.

Austin, J. A., Champion, V. L. and Tzeng, O. C. S. 1985. Cross cultural comparison on nursing image. *Journal of International Nursing Studies* 22(3): 231–9.

Baly, M. 1980. *Nursing and Social Change*, 2nd edn. London: Heinemann.

Barron, R. D. and Norris, G. M. 1976. Sexual divisions and the dual labour market. In D. L. Barker and S. A. Allen (eds), *Dependence and Exploitation in Work and Marriage*. London: Longman.

Blau, P. M. and Scott, W. R. 1966. *Formal Organizations: A Comparative Approach*. London: Routledge.

Brown, R. 1976. Women as employees. In D. L. Barker and S. A. Allen (eds), *Dependence and Exploitation in Work and Marriage*. London: Longman.

Clay, M., Povey, R. and Clift, S. 1983. Moral reasoning and the student nurse. *Journal of Advanced Nursing*, 8: 297–302.

Clay, T. 1987. *Nurses, Power and Politics*. London: Heinemann.

Courtney, M. 1985. Nurses' perceptions of patients' quality of life. Unpublished manuscript, Department of Health Studies, Sheffield City Polytechnic.

Crutchfield, R. S. 1955. Conformity and character. *American Psychologist* 10: 191.

Davies, C. 1976. Experience of dependency and control in work: The case of nurses. *Journal of Advanced Nursing* 2(5): 273.

Dickinson, S. 1982. The nursing process and the professional status of nursing. *Nursing Times*, Occasional Paper, 2 June.

Doyal, L. 1979. *The Political Economy of Health*. London: Pluto.

Ferguson, M. C. 1984. Undergraduate nursing curriculum building: an exploration into the 'sciences'. *Journal of Advanced Nursing* 9: 197–204.

Gadow, S. 1980. Existential advocacy. In S. F. Spicker and G. Gadow (eds), *Nursing Images and Ideals*. New York; Springer.

Gamarnikow, E. 1978. The sexual division of labour: The case of nursing. In A. Kuhn and A. Wolpe (eds), *Feminism and Materialism: Women and Modes of Production*. London: Routledge & Kegan Paul.

Henderson, V. 1969. *The Nature of Nursing*. London: Collier Macmillan.

Henry, C. 1986. Perceptions of the concept of the person: a developmental view. PhD thesis, Department of Education, University of Leeds.

Hirsch, B. J. 1981. Social networks and the coping process: creating personal networks. In B. J. Gottlieb (ed.), *Social Networks and Social Support*. Beverly Hills: Sage Publications.

Hofling, C. K., Brotzman, E., Dalrymple, S., Graves, N. and Pierce, C. M. 1966. An experimental study in nurse–physician relationships. *Journal of Nervous and Mental Disease* 143: 171–80.

Iliffe, S. 1983. *The NHS: A Picture of Health?* London: Lawrence & Wishart.

International Council of Nurses. 1973. *Ethical Considerations in Nursing Practice*. Geneva: International Council of Nurses.

Johnston, M. and Lee Jones, M. 1979. Evaluating the case of post-surgical patients in the community hospital. In D. J. Oborn *et al.* (eds), *Research in Psychology and Medicine* Vol. 2. New York: Academic Press.

Jones, E. 1982. Advocacy: a tool for radical nursing curriculum planners. *Journal of Nursing Education* 21(1): 40–5.

Kanter, R. M. 1982. *The Change Masters.* New York: Simon and Schuster.

Katz, D. and Kahn, R. L. 1966. *The Social Psychology of Organizations* 2nd edn. New York: John Wiley.

Kennedy, I. 1983. *The Unmasking of Medicine.* London: Paladin Books.

King, N. and West, M. A. 1986. Experiences of innovation at work. Unpublished manuscript, Social and Applied Psychology Unit Memo No. 772, University of Sheffield.

Kohnke, M. F. 1982. Myths and realities about advocacy–clinical research–abuse. *Journal of the New York State Nurses' Association* 13(4): 22–8.

Lawrence, P. R. and Lorsch, J. W. 1967. *Organization and Environment.* Harvard: Harvard University Press.

LeShan, L. 1984. *Holistic Health.* Wellingborough: Turnstone Press.

Little, D. E. and Carnivali, D. L. 1976. *Nursing Care Planning.* Philadelphia: Lippincott.

McGregor, G. 1960. *The Human Side of Enterprise.* New York: McGraw-Hill.

Maddocks, P. 1982. *The Consultant,* December.

Mayo, E. 1949. *The Social Problems of an Industrial Civilization.* London: Routledge.

Melnyk, K. A. M. 1983. The process of theory analysis: An analysis of the nursing theory of Orem. *Nursing Resident* 32: 3.

Menzies, I. E. P. 1960. Nurses under stress: A social system functioning as a defence against anxiety. *International Nursing Review* 1(6): 9.

Merton, R. K. 1957. *Social Theory and Social Structure.* New York: Free Press.

Milgram, S. 1974. *Obedience to Authority: An Experimental View.* New York: Harper & Row.

Mitchell, T. 1984. The nursing process. *British Medical Journal* 288: 216–19.

Muff, J. 1982. *Socialization, Sexism and Stereotyping – Women's Issues in Nursing.* St Louis: C. V. Mosby.

Navarro, V. 1978. *Class Struggle, The State and Medicine: An Historical and Contemporary Analysis of the Medical Sector in Great Britain.* Oxford: Robinson.

Nightingale, F. 1881. Letter to the probationer–nurses in the 'Nightingale Fund' Training School, at St Thomas's Hospital, 6 May. Nightingale Collection, London School of Economics.

Nuttall, P. 1983. Male takeover or female giveaway? *Nursing Times,* 79, 12 January: 10–11.

Oakley, A. 1984. What price professionalism? The importance of being a nurse. *Nursing Times,* 12 December: 24–7.

Orem, D. 1980. *Concepts of Practice*. New York: McGraw-Hill.

Orne, M. T. and Holland, C. C. 1968. On the ecological validity of laboratory deceptions. *International Journal of Psychiatry* 6: 282–93.

Payne, R. and Pugh, D. 1971. Organizations as psychological environments. In P. B. Warr (ed.), *Psychology at Work*. Harmondsworth: Penguin.

Pearson, A. 1983. *The Clinical Nursing Unit*. London: Heinemann Medical.

Peters, T. J. and Waterman, R. H. 1982. *In Search of Excellence: Lessons from America's Best Run Companies*. New York: Harper & Row.

Rathbone, W. 1890. *History and Progress of District Nursing*. London: Macmillan.

Rayner, C. 1984. What do the public think of nurses? *Nursing Times*, 29 August, 80(35).

Riehl, J. P. and Roy, C. 1980. *Conceptual Models for Nursing Practice*. New York: Appleton-Century-Crofts.

Rowan, J. 1976a. *Ordinary Ecstasy: Humanistic Psychology in Action*. London: Routledge & Kegan Paul.

Rowan, J. 1976b. *The Power of the Group*. London: Davis-Poynter.

Royal College of Nursing. 1980. *Standards of Nursing Care*. London: Royal College of Nursing.

Salvage, J. 1985. *The Politics of Nursing*. London: Heinemann Nursing.

Sherif, M. 1935. A study of some social factors in perception. *Archives of Psychology* 187.

Shipman, M. D. 1968. *Sociology of the School*. London: Longman.

Simpson, I. H., Back, K. W., Ingles, T., Kerckhoff, A. C. and McKinney, J. C. 1979. *From Student to Nurse: A Longitudinal Study of Socialization*. Cambridge: Cambridge University Press.

Stein, L. 1978. The nurse–doctor game. In R. Dingwall and J. McIntosh (eds), *Readings in Sociology of Nursing*. Edinburgh: Churchill Livingstone.

Stuart, G. W. and Sundeen, S. J. 1983. *Principles and Practice of Psychiatric Nursing*. St Louis: C. V. Mosby.

Tannenbaum, A. 1974. *Hierarchy in Organizations*. San Francisco: Jossey-Bass.

Tschudin, V. 1986. *Ethics in Nursing*. London: Heinemann.

Weber, M. 1947. *The Theory of Social and Economic Organization*. New York: Appleton Century-Crofts.

West, M. A. 1987. A measure of role innovation at work. *British Journal of Social Psychology* 26: 83–5.

West, M. A., Farr, J. F. and King, N. 1986. Innovation at work: Definitional and theoretical issues. MRC/ESRC Social and Applied Psychology Unit Memo No. 814, University of Sheffield.

White, R. 1978. *Social Change and the Development of the Nursing Profession*. London: Henry Kempton.

Willis, D. 1986. Keynote address to the BPs Occupational Psychology Conference, University of Nottingham, January.

Witts, P. M. 1986. Moral recognition in clinical nurses. Unpublished manuscript, Department of Health Studies, Sheffield City Polytechnic.

Zimbardo, P. G. and Ruch, F. L. 1973. *Psychology and Life*. New York: Scott Foreman.

CHAPTER ELEVEN

Assessing the stress in persons with cancer: an exploration of the main perspectives of stress in relation to their psychological care

Liz Hanson

The problem regarding the lack of psychological care of persons with cancer has been gathering greater attention over the last ten years approximately. I aim to help students and qualified nurses to begin to address this problem in their clinical practice (in both the hospital and community settings), via a critical analysis of the differing perspectives regarding the assessment of stress. This leads to the rationale for the adoption of a humanistic model of stress for the psychological care of persons with cancer.

The following areas relating to the concept of stress and persons with cancer will be discussed:

(1) a review of health care literature on the lack of psychological care of persons with cancer and the principal reasons for this occurrence;
(2) the importance of the assessment phase of the nursing process;
(3) the complex nature of the concept 'stress' and the differing perspectives of stress.

Review of health care literature relating to the psychological care of persons with cancer

A review of key studies of communication between nurses and persons with cancer leads to the central criticism of the psychological support role of the cancer nurse and also his/her ability to detect and monitor the possible causes of concern for persons with cancer. From her study of communication processes in a radiography outpatients' department, Bond (1978) concluded that nurses give a low level of attention to the social and psychological aspects of illness. Her findings revealed that nurses engaged in few interactions lasting more than approximately 3 minutes with persons not requiring physical care. Maguire found in his earlier study (1978) that there was only 1 out of 20 interactions in which nurses were concerned regarding the well-being of persons with cancer. Maguire argued that one of the main reasons for the failure to detect hidden psychological morbidity amongst persons post-mastectomy, was that nurses did not routinely inquire about their psychological adjustment.

In his later work, Maguire (1985) labels this phenomenon 'distancing tactics', as nurses assume that persons with cancer will disclose their problems. Thus, they rarely inquire directly regarding their psychological state. Bond (1982) similarly refers to the nurses' use of diverting tactics if a person with cancer risks disclosure about an emotional problem. For example, attempts to brush the problem away with premature/false reassurances, that is, jolly the person along, or to ignore the person's words and change the topic of conversation or even to avoid entering into conversation with him/her. Bond (1978) reports in her study that if a person with cancer had an emotional outburst which influenced other persons with cancer, the nurses would move the offending person and ask him/her to control such outbursts. Tait *et al.* (1982) and Ray *et al.* (1984) argue that the above techniques effectively block communication regarding psycho-social aspects of a person's care.

The above studies put forward the overwhelming view that some nurses, albeit subconsciously in some cases, attempt to maintain an emotional distance. Bond (1982) explains that some nurses take the view that they are acting in the best interests of the person with cancer – the rationale being that the less the problem is discussed, the less upset the person will become. Maguire (1985) supports this argument as he states that some nurses believe it is unwise to 'go looking for problems' by directly asking about a person's psychological welfare. This is due to the fact that this may lead to the person with cancer asking 'difficult' questions (for example, 'Am I going to die?' 'Is the treatment really working?'). Maguire argues that many nurses fear that the person with cancer may reveal strong emotions, which causes reciprocal distress in the nurse concerned. Thus, in order to avoid such a situation, he notes that both persons with cancer and nurses appear to conspire to pretend that the former are coping well emotionally. As a result, nurses tend to ignore crucial verbal and non-verbal cues which persons with cancer give about their problems.

Following from the above, it can be argued that cancer nurses are not acting as support agents for persons with cancer. Baum and Jones (1979) found that few individuals with cancer talk with nursing staff about their psychological well-being. Bond (1978) noted that half of the sample of persons with cancer in her study who were anxious and/or depressed did not express their feelings to nursing staff. Maguire (1978) reported that, of the persons post-mastectomy affected by depression, few disclosed their problems to anyone concerned with their care. However, it is significant that approximately 90 per cent of the persons with cancer in Bond's study (1978) stated that they would have wanted a discussion regarding their overall situation. Yet, they admitted that they did not feel the nursing staff were appropriate. In Holmes and Dickerson's study (1987), most persons with cancer linked feelings of isolation with an inability to talk with the nurses. Bond (1982) concludes that it is likely that persons with cancer rely upon others as an outlet for their emotional difficulties.

Bullough's American study (1981) presents interesting parallels, as she found that approximately 80 per cent of the sample of persons with cancer in her study were supported by personal friends and family. Of these individuals, only 38 per cent received professional support in conjunction with family/friend support. Only 25 per cent of the sample said that nurses were a significant source of support. Only 2 per cent of the sample identified a professional (that is, nurse or doctor) as the sole source of support. She concludes that nurses have not yet established themselves in the public mind as a group that can and does give emotional support to persons with cancer.

Johnston's study (1982) reveals that fellow patients play a significant supportive role. She found that other patients are more accurate in estimating the number of worries a person with cancer has and tend to be more sensitive in detecting which worries a person has, than are nurses with responsibility for the person. She also found that nurses overestimate the number of worries the person with cancer has and are also more likely to deal with worries that individuals with cancer do not have.

The key British studies outlined above (Bond 1982; Maguire 1978; Maguire *et al*. 1980, 1985), consider that most nurses are not yet equipped to give emotional support to persons with cancer because they find it extremely difficult and stressful to do so. Vachon *et al*. (1978) found that the stress amongst nurses working with persons with advanced cancer was only slightly less than the stress experienced by new widows, and higher than for women commencing radiation treatment for cancer of the breast. It is clear, therefore, that the stress levels of nurses is a significant factor affecting their patterns of communication.

From the above literature, it appears that cancer nurses are failing to give persons with cancer support regarding their emotional needs. Tait *et al*. (1982) regard this as a major drawback and conclude that this lack of support is usually associated with a much poorer social and psychological outcome for the person with cancer.

The literature in this field (Maguire *et al*. 1980, Maguire 1985, Macleod Clark 1981, Ray *et al*. 1984, Bond 1982) points to the inadequacy of current nurse education in providing training in communication skills. As Bond (1982) states, communication tends not to be a subject that is taught, but is simply regarded as an accumulation of experience. As a result, commonsense methods are often employed, with tactics and routines learnt through observation and experience. She criticizes this unbalanced approach as it cuts off possible alternative practices and learning strategies.

Bridge and Clark (1981) emphasize that communication is a skill which, like any other type of skill, requires to be carefully learnt before it can be effectively used. They state that communication skills need to be introduced in basic education and developed further in post-basic courses. Tutors need to examine the proportion of teaching time devoted to meeting the physical needs of persons with cancer in comparison with the time given to their psycho-social needs. They see the urgent need for an even balance between the two needs.

Maguire *et al.* (1980) emphasize the importance of nurses working on cancer wards to have training in the psychological aspects of cancer. They argue that the nurses would then be able to develop specialist communication skills in interviewing and assessing persons with cancer and remember to pay attention to the psychological and social areas of an individual's history. This directly leads into the next section regarding the importance of the assessment phase of the nursing process.

The assessment phase of the nursing process

I endorse Maguire *et al.*'s focus upon the effective assessment of the psycho-social status of the person with cancer. Maguire *et al.* (1980) found that a specialist nurse who assessed persons with cancer in an outpatient department detected latent psychiatric symptoms in 90 per cent of those persons who subsequently developed psychiatric problems. The remaining nursing staff, who had not received any specialist training, failed to detect any psychiatric symptoms in these persons.

It can be seen that the assessment phase of the nursing process constitutes the first crucial step in the problem-solving approach. It is essential that any needs or problems are identified at the outset before nursing care is enacted. This may appear at first to be common sense to the reader. However, my own study (Hanson 1991) found that some nurses, when interviewing persons with cancer, gave detailed information regarding treatment and its side-effects, without first exploring the individual's perceptions of his/her treatment and suitably adjusting the information given as appropriate. Welch-McCaffrey (1984) likewise argues that nursing assessment is essential because before the cancer nurse treats a problem he/she needs to identify it. She emphasizes that cancer nurses must always be concerned about making judgements based on assumptions rather than deliberative assessment.

Various strategies have been put forward to help nurses in the assessment of a patient's psycho-social well-being. Morrow *et al.* (1978) devised a Psychosocial Adjustment to Illness Scale which consists of seven areas of adjustment: health care orientation,

vocational environment, domestic environment, sexual relationships, family relationships, social environment and psychological
distress. Bond (1982) views this model as a systematic assessment
of a patient's adjustment to illness. However, I agree with Bond
that it is complex for use in nursing practice. It also would require
a significant amount of training input for nurses to use it
effectively. Bond recommends Izsak and Medalie's scale (1971) as
much simpler to use. They map out the physical, psychological
and social progress of persons with particular types of cancer and
cover recognized key topics. As a result, they ensure that
appropriate areas of concern are attended to. Also, an individual's
progress is easily compared with the set scale.

I argue that, although Izsak and Medalie's scale is useful for
assessing the psycho-social status of persons with cancer, it does
presume a certain amount of knowledge and skills and therefore is
not intended as a useful starting point for students and newly
qualified nurses. I regard it as essential that nurses begin to
develop their assessment skills systematically. This would initially
take the form of exploring the nature of stress and the central
psychological theories put foward to help us to unravel this
phenomenon. This leads into the next section regarding the nature
of stress and the differing perspectives of stress.

The concept of stress and the major psychological perspectives of stress

The actual concept 'stress' is extremely complex and subject to an
endless variety of meanings in our current society. The *Concise
Oxford Dictionary* gives the following definitions: 'constraining
or impelling force'; 'effort, demand upon physical or mental
energy'. I argue that, in order to gain a clearer understanding of
this phenomenon, it is important to explore the key psychological
theories put forward to explain its meaning.

The response-based model of stress

This first model, expounded by Selye (1957), is commonly
adopted by health care professionals, in particular, medical staff,
as it focuses clearly upon physiological factors. Selye argued that it
is necessary to look for a particular pattern of responses which

can be taken as evidence that the person is stressed. The response is then treated as the stressor or as its defining parameter. Thus, the occurrence of the response represents the occurrence of stress, which may act as a stimulus for producing further responses.

Selye's central view of stress is the idea of non-specificity of the physiological response of the body to any demand made upon it. In this way, the physiological response is not dependent on the nature of the stress or species as there is a universal pattern of defence. Selye described this defence reaction in terms of the 'general adaptation syndrome' (GAS). If the stress continues, resources dwindle and collapse and finally disease states occur which are the cost of defence.

Selye further showed that the physiological response is dominated by two major psycho-endocrine systems: the sympathetic adrenal medullary (SAM) and the pituitary adrenal cortical (PAC). This assumes that there is an important functional balance between the two branches of the autonomic nervous system which govern the activity of the internal organs – for example, cardiac smooth muscle, digestive function. Thus, Selye's definition of stress is clearly in physiological terms, as he stated that stress occurs when the controlling mechanisms are strained in the maintenance of the internal environment of the vital areas.

Selye illustrated his medical model by explaining what happens to the body in an emergency reaction, that is, a stress situation. He stated that there is a clearly defined sympathetic activity which is an adapted response in a demanding situation. Using Selye's model, Cox (1978) explains that stress can be assessed in terms of its physiological effects – for example, increased catecholamine secretion, increased corticosteroid activity, increased blood glucose levels, increased heart rate and blood pressure, dryness of mouth and throat and dilation of pupils. He also argues that more general health effects can be seen as a response to stress – for example, headaches and migraines, ulcers, cardiovascular disease, sweating, dizziness, amenorrhoea, diarrhoea, insomnia, nightmares, frequent urination, asthma.

This list gives specific physiological indicators of stress, such as pulse and blood pressure, as well as more generalized symptoms of stress which relate to physical illness. I argue that it is essential that physiological indicators of stress are not assessed in isolation from the psycho-social factors affecting the individual with cancer.

This happens because Selye's model does not provide for the entire concept of stress. Indeed, it leads to the physiological orientation presented by Bond (1982) and Maguire (1985). My main criticism of Selye's response-based stress model is that it fails to reveal an interaction between physiological and psychological factors. Clearly, both factors are involved, but as Lazarus (1966) stated, the most important factor to consider is the individual's perception of the situation as stressful or not. Selye's model loses sight of the individual because it is a general theory which focuses on 'scientific generality', with the result that accuracy with respect to any individual is sacrificed.

Mason (1968) also revealed an explicit weakness in Selye's concept of non-specificity of the body's response to stress, arguing that specificity is evident. Mason proposed that there are different responses to different stresses as people differ. In prticular, catecholamine excretion rates differ. Likewise, heart and respiratory rates differ, as one individual may respond more or less to a stressful situation than another. Mason (1968) concluded that the physiological reaction is much more complex than Selye first thought. I note also that an increased corticosteroid activity, for example, may reflect the cancer patient's disease and effects of treatment, as opposed to being an indicator of stress. It is therefore important that physiological indicators are assessed in conjunction with the physiological effects of the individual's illness and treatment.

Cox (1978) proposes more generalized responses to stress in the form of behavioural and cognitive effects of stress – for example, excessive eating, drinking or smoking, drug taking, impulsive behaviour, lack of concentration, forgetfulness, trembling, nervous laughter, impaired speech, excitability, restlessness. In my study (1991), the cancer nurses spoke of the relevance of a change in behaviour in relation to assessing stress in persons with cancer. For example, 'going over the top', extremely high in spirits; individuals who are extremely quiet and often do not respond to questions or mix with other people; individuals with cancer who may be unusually chatty or complain about lots of things/something non-specific. Most nurses mentioned if a person with cancer was not sleeping at night. Several nurses explained that they may get up and ask for a cup of tea and/or smoke a cigarette or shut themselves off in the dayroom. One nurse explained that at night their symptoms are heightened, thus they feel worse. Most nurses mentioned the opposite of Cox's first behavioural indicator, that is, the person with cancer *not* eating.

Most nurses also spoke of the importance of non-verbal cues. These focused upon physiological cues, that is, body language – for example, crying, wringing hands, looking sad, 'rejection face' (that is, 'come and follow me is written in their faces'), door closed when usually open, holding your attention longer than is needed, looking very worried, fidgeting. I also observed 30 individuals during their nursing admission assessment and found that most exhibited stress from their non-verbal cues – for example, frequently rubbing their hands together; looking down frequently when talking; giving small smiles; repeatedly brushing their fingers through their hair; speaking very quickly, repeating some words and using 'ah's' and 'um's' at intervals. One person's voice was very quiet and almost inaudible at times. Several individuals tended to laugh very loudly and quickly after they had finished talking.

I am careful to point out that the non-verbal cues of some individuals substantiated their implicit verbal reports of stress. However, in other cases, non-verbal cues were in opposition to a person's 'cheerful' verbal communication. Thus, it is important to reiterate that non-verbal and behavioural cues are not always assessed in the entire context of the individual with cancer and are not evaluated as separate variables.

Thus, to conclude, it can be seen that the response-based model of stress focuses upon a physiological approach which gives an overall pattern of effects. Whilst physiological and behavioural cues (including body language) are important in the assessment of stress, it is essential that they are considered with reference to each person with cancer.

The stimulus-based model of stress

A stimulus approach to stress is based upon a medical/engineering model and considers which external stressors in the environment lead to the stress response. Welford (1975) suggests that stress occurs whenever the demand for adaptation made on an organism departs from a moderate level. This illustrates that low levels of demand on an individual can be as stressful as high levels of demand. Most organisms, including man, have evolved to produce optimum adaptive performance under conditions of moderate demand.

A stimulus approach to stress is concerned with attempting to identify situations which can reliably be described as stressful to man. For example, Cox (1978) puts forward the following demands in the work situation which can be viewed as stressful stimuli: within the physical environment, excessive noise or complete silence; excessive heat or cold; poor illumination or glare; extremes of humidity; atmospheric pollution.

Holmes and Rahe (1967) attempted to quantify the degree of stress associated with life events. They constructed a scale of 43 life events. The authors found that death of a spouse was consistently rated highest and so was given a value of 100. All other events were given proportional values based on this value – for example, divorce 73, marital separation 65, jail term 63, death of close family member 63, personal injury or illness 53, marriage 50, fired at work 47, marital reconciliation 45, retirement 45. The authors reveal that the scale has shown that people in the United States, western Europe and Japan tend to rate life events in almost exactly the same way.

The cancer nurses in my study (1991) put forward their perceptions of the main causes of concern for persons with cancer which can be equated with stressful stimuli. They were as follows: prospect of death; stigma; effect on family; feelings of helplessness; effect on life-style; treatment and its side-effects; altered body image; pain. The nurses stated that these factors caused stress in the majority of persons with cancer. I am careful to note, however, that, similarly to the response-based model of stress, the stimulus model is a macro, general theory which fails to take into account individual differences. The cancer nurses gave specific examples of individuals with cancer for whom the above factors had caused them to experience stress but for differing reasons. For example, the effect upon the family was commonly explored as a main source of stress. One nurse recalled a person with cancer who was extremely worried regarding her disabled husband at home. Another nurse explained that an individual with cancer was worried about her daughter who was heavily pregnant and without work, to the point that she was unable to give herself time to consider her illness. From these examples it can be seen that stress varies according to the individual and his/her unique situation. This leads into the third model of stress.

The transactional model of stress

I argue that cancer nurses require a much more humanistic approach to the concept of stress as applied to persons with cancer. The transactional model of stress acts as a suitable humanistic framework for nurses to assess stress, as it takes into account the notion that each person is an individual with unique needs. It clearly reflects the philosophy of the nursing process and the importance of treating each patient as an individual.

The transactional model was developed by Lazarus (1966), who stated that stress occurs when there are demands upon the person that tax or exceed his/her adjustive resources. Thus, he views stress as being an interaction between the individual and the environment. The individual is recognized as an active agent, as opposed to the passive being reflected in the medical approach and in particular in the response and stimulus theories of stress. In this way, stress may constitute a mixture of personal factors and factors within the environment, but the crucial element remains the individual's perception of him/her self and particular situation. This may sound common sense, but this factor is often ignored by the above theories of stress. These models tend to overlook the individual and give emphasis to physiological factors, so that man tends to be viewed almost as a machine. The emphasis upon the active role of the individual reflects the current move within nursing philosophy towards self-care and personal responsibility for health, away from the traditional medical view of the patient as a passive being.

Lazarus (1978) emphasizes that we must treat the person as an active agent of change on the environment as well as respondent to that environment. He argues that we need to give as much attention to describing transactional relationships as to their causal determinants. Lazarus notes that these relationships are characterized as much by change and flux as by stability and consistency. Similarly, the cancer nurses in my study regarded signs of stress as changing over time; for example, 'they vary from person to person and it also depends on the time the person catches them and vice versa'.

As regards indicators of stress within a humanistic framework, Lazarus considers the importance of a person's own verbal reports of stress – the premise being that the individual is the expert on him/herself. The cancer nurses in my study reiterated this view.

They regarded it as essential to know the person with cancer in order for him/her to be able to confide their worries. The role of intuition was explained by several nurses in relation to assessing stress in individuals with cancer – for example, 'just a feeling', 'you just know – it's difficult to put into words'. It can be seen that this phenomenon relates to the complex role of cognition in perceiving stress acknowledged by Lazarus. I argue that the cancer nurse is likely to intuit an individual's stress correctly if he/she knows the individual well, as opposed to making assumptions regarding the person's stress.

Lazarus (1966) accepts that there are occasions when an individual may be unaware of the true nature of his/her stress owing to the subconscious use of defence mechanisms such as denial. For example, in my study one nurse recalled a person with cancer who was unaware that she was denying the stress associated with her diagnosis of cancer as she adopted a cheerful front. In this situation, Lazarus explains that it is important to take other indicators into consideration – for example, non-verbal and behavioural cues – to see if there are any revealing differences. Thus, I argue that it is essential to adopt a holistic approach in which the cancer nurse gives central consideration to a person's verbal reports of stress, but also relates these to the individual's physiological and behavioural cues.

There were nurses in my study who, similarly to the literature above, valued the views of the person's family, as they appreciated that (in most cases) they know the person well. As a result, they are more likely to detect any changes in his/her psychological state. This information, when fed back to the nursing staff, gives them a greater awareness and subsequent understanding of the person concerned. Thus, the nurses emphasized the importance of communicating effectively with a person's family/significant others to create a mutually supportive network.

If nurses are to adopt Lazarus's transactional model of stress in which an individual's appraisal of a situation is central, it follows that they need to fulfil their psychological support role. This is because nurses need to give due consideration to the verbal reports of persons with cancer regarding their perceptions of stress, in order to assess their psychological well-being. Similarly to the literature above, the cancer nurses in my study noted the value of listening to the person with cancer; of sitting down and talking with him/her; of creating an informal atmosphere; of maintaining the impression that he/she is always available if needed, so that the individual is able to trust the nurse and feels able to confide any worries as and when necessary.

The cancer nurses in my study explained that, despite their awareness of the importance of their support role, it was difficult to achieve in reality. This was owing to the lack of appropriate education regarding counselling and specialist communication skills and lack of formal support for themselves. In addition, the nurses regarded the practical constraints of workload and staffing levels as adding substantially to the existing problem.

Thus, to conclude, I do not claim to have answered all the significant problems explained above. However, I have attempted to provide an outline of the current situation regarding psychological care of persons with cancer and the role of the cancer nurse. In order to begin to address this situation, I have focused upon the assessment phase of the nursing process. This is because it provides the first crucial stepping stone towards the ultimate goal of creating and/or maintaining psychological well-being in persons with cancer. The exploration of differing psychological perspectives of stress led to the discussion of the implications of the prevalent emphasis upon the response- and stimulus-based theories. I have argued that, in order for the cancer nurse to assess stress in persons with cancer more fully, he/she needs to adopt a humanistic framework. The transactional model of stress (Lazarus 1966) is recommended as an approach in which the individual, together with that individual's perceptions of a situation remain of paramount importance.

Acknowledgement

The author wishes to thank the Department of Health for the support given to undertake the research mentioned in this chapter.

References

Baum, M. and Jones, E. M. 1979. Counselling removes patients' fears. *Nursing Mirror* 148(10): 38–40.
Bond, S. 1978. Processes of communication about cancer in a radiotherapy department. Unpublished PhD thesis, University of Edinburgh.

Bond, S. 1982. Communications in cancer nursing. In M. Cahoon (ed.), *Recent Advances in Cancer Nursing*, pp. 3–31. London: Churchill Livingstone.

Bridge, W. and Macleod Clark, J. 1981. *Communications in Nursing Care*. London: HM and M, Chapters 1, 8.

Bullough, B. 1981. Nurses as teachers and support persons. *Cancer Nursing* 4(3): 221–5.

Cox, T. 1978. *Stress*. London: Macmillan.

Hanson, E. J. 1991. An exploration of the taken for granted world of the cancer nurse in relation to stress and the person with cancer. Unpublished PhD thesis, University of Lancaster.

Holmes, S. and Dickerson, J. 1987. The quality of life: design and evaluation of a self-assessment instrument for use with cancer patients. *International Journal of Nursing Studies* 24(1): 15–24.

Holmes, T. and Rahe, R. 1967. The Social Readjustment and Rating Scale. *Journal of Psychosomatic Research* 11: 213–18.

Izsak, F. and Medalie, J. 1971. Comprehensive follow-up of carcinoma patients. *Journal of Chronic Diseases* 24: 179–91.

Johnston, M. 1982. Recognition of patients' worries by nurses and by other patients. *British Journal of Counselling Psychology* 21: 255–61.

Lazarus, R. 1966. *Psychological Stress and the Coping Process*. New York: McGraw Hill.

Lazarus, R. 1978. Stress-related transactions between person and environment. in L. A. Pervin and M. Lewis (eds), *Perspectives in International Psychology*, pp. 287ff. New York: Plenum Press.

Macleod Clark, J. 1981. Communicating with cancer patients: communication of evasion. In R. Tiffany (ed.), *Cancer Nursing Update*. London: Baillière Tindall.

Maguire, P. 1978. The psychological effects of cancer. In R. Tiffany (ed.), *Oncology for Nurses and Health Care Professionals*, vol. 2. London: Harper & Row.

Maguire, P. 1985. Barriers to psychological care of the dying. *British Medical Journal* 14 December, 291: 1711–13.

Maguire, P. *et al.* 1980. Plan into practice. *Nursing Mirror*, 24 January: 19–21.

Mason, W. 1968. In T. Cox, *Stress*. London: Macmillan, 1978.

Morrow, G. R. *et al.* 1978. A new scale for assessing patients' psychosocial adjustment to medical illness. *Psychological Medicine* 8: 605–10.

Ray, C. *et al.* 1984. Nurses' perceptions of early breast cancer and mastectomy and their psychological implications and the role of health professionals in providing support. *International Journal of Nursing Studies* 21(2): 101–11.

Selye, H. 1957. *The Stress of Life*. New York: McGraw Hill.

Tait, A. *et al.* 1982. Improving communication skills. *Nursing Times* 22–29 December: 2181–4.

Vachon, M. I. S. *et al.* 1978. Measurement and management of stress in health professionals working with advanced cancer patients. *Death Education* 1: 365–75.

Welford, A. T. 1975. In T. Cox, *Stress*. London: Macmillan, 1978.
Welch-McCaffrey, D. 1984. Oncology nurses as cancer patients: an investigative questionnaire. *Oncology Nursing Forum* 11(2): 48–50.

CHAPTER TWELVE

Conceptions of care

Helen Ellis

If we can understand how complex and intricate, indeed how subjective caring is, we shall perhaps be better equipped to meet the conflicts and pains it sometimes induces. Then too, we may come to understand at least in part how it is that in a country that spends billions on caretaking of various sorts we hear everywhere, the complaint 'nobody cares'. (Noddings 1984: 12).

The word 'care' is, more often than not, attached as a suffix to the word 'nursing'. Yet many people in all walks of life claim ownership of the word and both lay people and professional people use the term to denote what it is that they are doing when they are working with ill or dependent people. The aim of this chapter is to describe some of the facets of caring as it relates to nursing. Care and caring for people within the context of nursing are complicated and at time confusing concepts. This chapter will discuss the validity of defining care, describe a variety of definitions of the term and look at the reciprocal nature of caring. Caring and curing will be related to each other through a discussion of the expanded/extended role debate, and finally the personal cost of caring for nurses will be highlighted as an issue which is rarely given thought but which is integral to the caring role of the nurse.

Care in the context of nursing

Dunlop (1986: 665) argues that 'while it seems possible that nursing is *a* form of caring, it seems much less reasonable to claim it as *the* form of caring. Such a claim does scant justice to other people workers'. This chapter is specifically concentrating upon professional nurses and their delivery of care to clients who have entered the health care system as it exists in the United Kingdom today. In order to discuss the meaning of the term for nurses we need to consider the fundamental difference between lay and professional caring. Kitson (1987) did just this by comparing and contrasting the two forms of caring. She demonstrated that the two are fundamentally alike, sharing the 'main attributes which are commitment, knowledge, skills and respect for persons'. The point at which lay caring and professional caring differ is reached when the person in need of care requires special care skills, a particular physical environment, and a carer with deeper knowledge and understanding of the problem. Nurses are professional carers providing commitment, resources, knowledge and skills.

Attempting to determine what we mean when we use a certain term in nursing is a fairly recent exercise for nurses. A deeper interest in the fundamental concepts underlying nursing practice has been generated by the importation of academic nursing theory from the United States of America. Nurse theorists in the USA have developed many models and theories which attempt to explain the role of the nurse, her professional function and the specific skills required for professional nursing. Meleis (1985), in looking at the many nursing models/theories which emerged in the USA since the 1950s, placed them within a social and political framework in order to clarify the direction of nursing interests. The early theorists such as Henderson and Orem attempted to answer the question, 'What do nurses do?' (Answer – they meet people's needs.) Evolving out of these theorists' ideas came the next question, 'How do nurses meet people's needs?' (Answer – they interact.) The most recent question to emerge is 'Why do nurses do what they do?' This fundamental question was answered in terms of looking at the outcomes of nursing care upon client outcomes – which, incorporating a prerequisite for knowledge and skills and the right attitude to clients, could form the basis of professional caring.

For all the arguments about nursing models and their use in British nursing, they have stimulated nurses to take a closer look at nurses and nursing. Many nurses theorists have also stimulated interest in the clarification of concepts pertinent to and of relevance to nursing, such as reassurance, dependency and anxiety. Although it has become an accepted part of our nursing culture that the four main concepts for nursing are Man, Health, Environment and Nursing, the concept of care remains central yet little researched. The American Nurses' Association in 1965 identified the essential components of nursing as 'care, cure and co-ordination'. The caring aspect was to be more than the concept of 'to take care of' as in the traditional physical care approach, it was also to include 'to care for and care about'. The *Report of the Committee on Nursing* (Briggs 1972) in the UK highlighted this same issue for British nurses when it stated that 'nursing and midwifery are the major caring professions'. The report did not deny that other professional health care workers also 'cared', but was at pains to point out that for nurses caring was pre-eminent and central. The report recognized the immense variety in nursing when it argued that the range of human and technical skills required in nursing and midwifery is very wide. Not one type of nurse is required but many – and hence not one form of caring but many.

Indeed, we have a 'duty to care'. The increasingly litigious society in which we live has stimulated nurses to become aware of their responsibilities, duties and actions, not only in a social sense but in a legal sense. The term 'duty of care', although essentially a legal term, highlights the importance of understanding what our 'care' is. A nurse's duty of care encompasses the professional, moral, ethical and sociological duties of care that exist within the nurse–patient relationship. The legal test of whether a duty of care exists was laid down in the case of Donoghue v Stevenson, where manufacturers were held to owe a duty of care to the ultimate consumer. By analogy the nurse is the manufacturer of care and the patient the consumer. The caring relationship, or the caring acts, begin with the nurse. The increasing awareness of the term 'duty to care' within nursing's consciousness should stimulate us to look closely at the concept of care within a nursing context and to understand the implications of caring for both nurse and patient.

It is simply not enough to claim that as nurses we care. As only one of the caring professions it is rapidly being made clear that in order to justify our actions we have to understand and declare the fundamental nature of what we are doing. Nurses must be able to define what they mean by 'caring' and indeed if caring is truly their function. In responding to the American espousal of caring as the central tenet for nursing, Gaut (1981: 18) felt that this was simply use of jargon to give more authority to the role of the nurse. She asked, 'could it be possible that caring is really nothing more than a slogan to provide a rallying point for nurses involved in a movement towards professionalism and role identification? It is possible that caring is a key idea in many nursing slogans but at the same time it seems to be found more and more in nursing literature and as a principle for action, a case in point of arguments and in certain cases a doctrine for belief.' She goes on to say that the concept of caring initially used as a slogan has through time been given the role of a justifying principle or a norm for various statements about nursing with little explication of the concept.

Defining care

It has to be remembered that nurses in the USA had been developing a theoretical, nursing base for their practice for many years and by 1979 Watson had developed her theory of nursing as a basis for nursing and Leininger had begun her work on the transcultural aspects of caring. In 1981 the proceedings of the first National Caring Conference were published. Leininger (1981: 3) addressing the conference stated the fundamental problem: 'although nurses have linguistically said that they give care and they talk about nursing care activities still there has been virtually no systematic investigation of the epistemological, philosophical, linguistic, social and cultural aspects of caring and the relationship of care to professional nursing care, theory and practice.'

Leininger unequivocally declared that caring is the central and unifying domain for the body of knowledge and practices in nursing. She believes that nurses should study the concept of care for the following reasons.

(1) The construct of care appears critical to human growth, development and survival for millions of years. Leininger takes an anthropological viewpoint when she asserts that caring must have been around since the beginning of mankind and that caring was the critical factor that helped mankind through its social and cultural evolution.

(2) A second reason is to clarify care-giver and care-receiver roles

in different contexts. She feels that we know little about how care is given and received in different cultures and throughout history. If we knew a little more it might help us define our nursing role more clearly today.

(3) A third reason for studying caring is to maintain and preserve this attribute for future generations. She feels that there are many forces acting to devalue caring in our world today. Examples are the dehumanizing use of technology, the increasing number of homicides, political and economic restraints that reflect a lack of care for others. She believes it is the role of the nursing profession to place an increased emphasis on caring and on making known caring attributes.

(4) The fourth reason for studying care is to study it in relation to nursing care.

Increasingly nurses are attempting to define or clarify the concept of care. Perspectives vary from the philosophic (Griffen 1983, Roach 1982), the anthropological (Leininger 1981), the psycho-social (Watson 1979) and practice (Benner 1984) viewpoints. Global definitions of caring have been developed, but for the nurse practitioner and educator such definitions do not provide many guidelines. Such a definition is that given by Mayeroff (1971) who offers 'caring, as helping another grow and actualize himself, is a process, a way of relating to someone that involves development, in the same way that friendship can only emerge through mutual trust and a deepening and qualitative transformation of the relationship'. Leininger's (1981: 9) definition offers more scope as she defines caring as 'those assistive, supportive or facilitative acts toward or for another individual or group with evident or anticipated needs to ameliorate or improve a human condition or way of life'.

By 1979 in America, Watson had developed ten carative factors in an attempt to develop a caring basis for all nurses. She describes caring as being formed of such factors as a humanistic, altruistic value system; the instillation of hope and faith; empathy; a helping–trust relationship; interpersonal teaching; the provision of a supportive/protective physical and/or mental environment. Watson's approach has been grounded in psychological and sociological theories borrowed to describe the work of nurses. From a philosophical viewpoint, Bergman (1983) cites Roach's (1982) unified caring model as a model to unify health and human needs. The components of the model are compassion, competence, confidence, conscience and commitment. These five 'C's' arguably are subsumed within Griffen's (1983) two major aspects of caring in nursing: an activities aspect and the attitudes and feelings underlying them. Griffen argues (1983: 291) that the two aspects are complementary and she states: 'the "activities" of caring defined as assisting, helping and serving are mediated through the nurse–patient relationship which is a particular sort of personal contact'.

Both Griffen (1983) and Kitson (1984) have discussed various issues related to caring, namely, moral and personal issues in caring, emotional components and temporal and spatial aspects. Given the diversity of situations within which nursing takes place, caring could take on different meaning for different groups of nurses. Benner (1984) develops the thesis that caring is a moral art and is 'primary for any health care practice'. By uncovering good examples of nursing practice she clearly demonstrates the nursing–caring role of clinical nurses. The caring role of the clinical nurse develops into its mature form from its early stages of the novice nurse through to the expert practitioner.

It is clear from the above brief descriptions of care and caring that defining the concept for nursing is not easy. Care has many dimensions and can be approached from many viewpoints.

The contexts of care

Attempting to define caring in a generic manner is useful to set the scene. However, the meaning of caring for nurses will constantly change and be in need of reassessment. Henderson (1980: 245) points this out when she muses that 'because I believe that we cannot possibly understand nursing in any age unless we see it as an aspect of the social scene, I must wonder whether the essence of nursing can be stated except in relation to the society in which it exists'. Social change and concomitant changes in nursing have led to a fundamental shift in the perception of the nurse's role. As we generically reassess our roles and functions, the changing nature of the delivery of health care within many and varied settings also forces us to reassess the nature of nursing within specific contexts.

There is an increasing trend towards specialisms in nursing

practice, which is encouraged by specialist forums within which nurses can learn and debate about their own specialty. Nurses will need to clarify what they mean by caring in the specialist sense – how they care within their own setting. This is not an argument to split nursing into fragmented parts, as generically nurses will probably share the same basic tenets of caring. It is how they are manifested in the particular clinical setting that will be of interest. Because an important aspect of caring is 'presencing' – i.e. the carer must be in the presence of the cared-for – the emphasis on the context of caring increases. This point is raised by Benner (Benner and Wrubel 1989) when she cites Brown's (1986) study of patients' perceptions of caring; she highlights one of the central aspects of caring, that 'caring is always understood in a context'. Benner's earlier work in 1984 does imply that good nursing care becomes clear if the context of the care and the actions involved are described. Nursing care becomes clear within the context.

Caring frameworks

Nurses are giving a lot of thought to the nature of the delivery of care to their patients/clients. Over the past 10–15 years nurses have progressed in fits and starts from a wholly accepted stance of task allocation through to patient allocation and the concept of total patient care. The concept of total patient care has recently become subsumed into the term 'holistic care'. It is worth pausing here to ask if nurses have once again fallen prey to Gaut's doctrine of belief? Although nurses have argued that they give total patient care, it was clear that in practice this did not happen. Many research studies highlighted nursing's inadequacies in the field of interpersonal skills and psycho-social attributes. Also it was rarely asked if the patient wanted to receive total patient care.

Francis (1980) quite clearly put the case as to why the concept of total patient care might be a misnomer. She based her argument upon Tonnies' (1887) work, which attempted to look at the bases of human association. Two relationships were put forward, namely a relationship between patients and their families and the relationship between patients and hospital staff. The first relationship, between patient and family, is a primary one formed over time through daily and intimate knowledge of the other. The second relationship arises from 'conscious planning and reasoned intent', and is a secondary relationship which patients enter into with only a small part of themselves. Francis points out that hospitalization places a person in a world of secondary relationships; even the nurse has her own primary relationships elsewhere. Therefore, the premise arises that nurses should not and indeed cannot turn secondary relationships into primary relationships. The increasing emphasis on interpersonal skills such as empathy, counselling and communication skills must avoid the kind of caring relationship that Salvage (1990) describes as the 'quasi-psychotherapeutic kind'.

The reciprocity of care

There has been little attempt by nurses to clarify the interpersonal aspect of caring, but the development of a humanistic approach to patient care has led to an increased awareness by nurses that interpersonal skills play an important and decisive role in the care of their patients. The humanistic approach is exemplified by Noddings' (1984) discussion of caring, whereby the carer (the nurse) is motivated towards the cared-for (the patient), respects his personal freedom (autonomy) and views the cared-for as a person and not an object. Noddings argument (1984: 9) supports Mayeroff's assertion that 'to care for another person in the most significant sense is to help him grow and actualize himself'. This self-actualization lies at the heart of many nursing models, in both the physical and the emotional sense. It is reflected in Orem's theory of nursing in that self-care is the crux of nursing. Orem describes three systems of nursing.

(1) The wholly compensatory system – which is needed when the patient's capacity for self-care is temporarily or permanently destroyed. In such situations caring is manifested through acting for and doing for the patient.
(2) The partly compensatory system – which is used when the patient can help himself a little. The caring act is demonstrated through doing for the patient and helping the patient to do for himself.
(3) The supportive–educative system – which is used for those patients who need only support and guidance. Caring here lies within the encouragement of the patient's own autonomy.

Noddings argues that to accept the gift of responsiveness from the cared-for (the patient) is natural for the carer (the nurse), but to demand such responsiveness is both futile and inconsistent with caring. This altruistic viewpoint supports the premise that the nurse will gain satisfaction from watching and observing the increased freedom/autonomy of their patients. The patient may reciprocate with gifts and words but the heart of reciprocation in the caring act for nurses will lie in the patient's increased independence and happiness.

In the nursing environment, care has tended to be something which nurses deliver to the patient. Despite the increasing interest in the concept of care, it is notable that little thought is given to the recipient of care. This is reflected in the sense that we do not have a specific word meaning 'the recipient of care' in our language. It is increasingly important that nurses examine the viewpoint of the recipients of care and also what the act of caring does to the patient. Griffen's (1983) philosophical analysis of caring in nursing points to caring having an activities and an attitude aspect. However, nursing has traditionally emphasized the activities aspect, and to some extent does so today. This has been recognized, and increasing emphasis is being placed on the attitudinal aspects of nursing care. The attitudes aspect completes the act of caring both from the carer's perspective and from that of the cared-for. Noddings (1984: 19) emphasizes this point when she points out that 'to the cared for no act in his behalf is quite as important or influential as the attitudes of the one caring'.

The caring act cannot be completed unless the cared-for is aware of the caring. The patient 'feels the difference between being received and being held off or ignored. Whatever the one caring actually does is enhanced or diminished, made meaningful or meaningless in the attitude conveyed to the cared for' (Noddings 1984: 61). It would appear that patients in hospital are aware of being cared for and not being cared for. Harrison (1990) described her experiences in hospital, experiencing both an 'absence of caring' and 'caring' from the nursing staff on her ward. Caring nurses were described as taking time, listening, being genuinely interested in the patient as a person and able to share of themselves. The uncaring nurses appeared to be interested in completing tasks, did not listen to patients' concerns and did not inquire about their patients' perceptions and feelings.

Benner and Wrubel (1989) highlight the reciprocal nature of

caring when they argue 'that caring is a basic way of being in the world and that caring creates both self and world'. They go on to say that 'expert caring has nothing to do with possessing privileged information that increases one's control and domination of the other. . . . expert caring liberates and facilitates in such a way that the one caring is enriched in the process'. Benner's (1984) study of the development of clinical perception outlines how a nurse develops through five stages from novice, to advanced beginner, competent nurse, proficient nurse and finally the level of the expert nurse. The conclusion drawn from interviewing expert nurses and studying examples of nursing behaviour at the expert nurses' level, was that the expert nurses demonstrated the central role of caring, of a committed, involved stance in nursing practice. This involved the acquisition of an extensive knowledge base and its application through time to actual practice. Caring in the context of nursing can therefore be developed, over time, with the support of colleagues and matured with experience. The implications for education and research are enormous. If caring is a central definitive role for nurses, how can we teach this? How can the student nurse learn to care?

Caring and curing

The debate concerning the caring and curing functions of health care workers has been around for many years. Florence Nightingale (1860) clearly defined the caring function of the nurse as distinct from the curing functions, although she was clear that nature and not medical staff cure! In the case of both the medical and the surgical patient the nurse was there to 'put the patient in the best condition for nature to act upon him'. Luckman and Sorenson (1980) describe associated but different responsibilities for the care and cure components of health care.

The physician has a primary function to 'cure' and a secondary function to 'care' which is best carried out in cooperation with the nurse. The nurse has a primary function to 'care' and a secondary function to 'cure' which is best carried out in conjunction with the physician. Furthermore, curing is most effectively done within an environment of caring. It is the creation of such an environment that is the challenge of creative nursing.

The collaboration between caring and curing is increasingly becoming blurred for nurses today. There remains a strong commitment to cure rather than care, from past educational and clinical frameworks taking the medical perspective. The contextual constraints imposed by economic and organizational forces within hospital settings have also led to nurses increasingly accepting delegated functions to the detriment of their caring function.

The intensive care unit epitomizes the conflict facing nurses. In an intensive care unit both nursing and medical staff are present. Operating within the framework of their own philosophy and professional standards, both groups deliver 'care' to the patient. Telfer (1984: 11) described an intensive care unit as 'a unit catering for the needs of patients who require constant individual nursing attention throughout twenty four hours and the immediate availability of medical help'. This description uses the phrase not 'nursing care' but rather 'nursing attention'. It reflects the medical model of diagnosis, treatment and cure within the phrase 'medical help' and thus highlights the confusion over the nature of the nurse's role within such a setting. There is a lack of consensus about the meaning of these phrases and in particular what is represented by the term 'care' in the highly technological environment of modern units. Intensive care units have been classified under the heading 'rescue work' by Jennett (1986) in an attempt to correct the polarization of the concepts of care and cure that appears to occur within the intensive care setting. Because of the obvious high degree of medical input and technological systems within intensive care units, it has been argued that nurses who work in such a setting are not carers (nurses) but rather technicians. It is seldom realized, but a great deal of caring from both activities aspects and the attitudes aspects goes on. Jennett pointed out (1986: 77) that 'an intensive care unit is a place – not a technology; much of what goes on there is nursing care'.

Expanded and extended roles for nurses

The caring and curing functions of nurses have been articulated through the debate within the nursing profession over the extended/expanded role of the nurse. This debate is in many ways a reflection of nursing's search for a definitive caring role as opposed to a curing role. There is a different perception to be given to the terms 'extended' and 'expanded'. According to Zornow (1977), extension is seen as 'elongating specific already assumed functions to fill perceived gaps'. MacGuire (1980) suggests that extension refers to the situation where nursing expertise is not vital and the additional tasks incorporated in the widening of the role are essentially medical (curing). Expansion is a fundamentally different concept, which is concerned with a deepening and development of the role, drawing on those skills and areas of knowledge that are uniquely nursing (caring). MacGuire in her literature search on the subject discussed two models lying behind views about the development of extended and expanded roles in nursing. The model underlying the concept of the extended role depicts nursing and medicine as two distinct disciplines – a care versus cure dichotomy. People working within this model are concerned that nursing functions will be lost from the new role in favour of the assumption of medical tasks. The model underlying the expanded role of the nurse argues that there are 'health' care and 'illness' care needs with separate types of skills, and different sorts of interventions needed. Who does what is immaterial provided they are trained for the task, competent, acceptable to the patients and achieve the same standards.

MacFarlane (1980) suggests that such innovations as the extension of the nurse's role require the nurse to acquire basic diagnostic skills for which she is not at present trained (but for which she could be trained), but also that the occupier of extended roles practises on the basis of a medical model of care. She argues that it may also be appropriate to expand nurses' roles in other contexts to improve nursing in its purest sense, by building up nursing knowledge and equipping nurses to provide nursing expertise for those who need it. The danger appears to be that extension of the nursing role may be emphasized at the expense of expansion. It is not the intention of this chapter to give an in-depth analysis of the extended/expanded role debate, but it is of relevance when we discuss the meaning of care for nurses working in high-technology areas such as intensive care units. The emphasis in the nursing literature today is on the uniqueness of nursing, and the return to our clinical nursing base. The traditional role of the nurse was related to the provision of physical care for patients and the carrying out of medical orders. There was little emphasis on psycho-social care and interpersonal skills. The advent of nursing theory in the UK in the 1970s, coupled with an increasing number of British studies which highlighted the need for greater interpersonal skills, and an increased use of psychological and sociological theory, led to a swing of the pendulum. The emphasis is now on the psycho-social skills required to meet the needs of the whole person. Nurses still care, but from a holistic perspective.

The debate has been very heated at times on both sides and has created a tug of war for nurses working in the clinical environment. A strong attack on the extended role of the nurse was made early in the debate by Hall (1964), who felt that the medical aspect of nursing had grown so that something had to go. 'What went was the nurturing process which now the nurse in turn delegates to less well prepared persons.' She observed that nurses have shed the essentially 'nurturing' aspects of their role to practical nurses, but that the doctors have not yet established a cadre of practical doctors;

> They don't need them . . . they have nurses. Interesting too is the fact that most nurses show by their delegation of nurturing to others that they prefer being second class doctors to being first class nurses. If she feels better in this role, why not? This is the prerogative of any nurse. One good reason why not for more and more nurses is that with this increasing trend, patients receive from professional nursing second class doctoring and from practical nurses, second class nursing. Some nurses would like the public to get first class nursing.

Debate over the extended role of the nurse has led to a demand that nurses get back to their caring roots and expand their skills through the use of psychological and sociological theories, rather than act as the doctors' handmaiden in the extension of their skills. This debate must be tied into the increasing calls for autonomy in nursing, which in turn is attached to another push to professionalization. The problem is that technology is not about to go away. Patients requiring expanded nursing skills may well require the support of technology. Technology, however, tends to be related to the extended role of the nurse side of the debate. Reports from various centres of higher education over the past few years have indicated that nurses leaving university with their honours degree and RGN qualifications have frequently taken positions as staff nurses in the care of the elderly setting, because they were able to give more nursing care. The implication is that nurses, in order to care, did not get involved with technology as manifested by acute areas in general hospitals. If nurses answer the call to expansion only, how then can they care for patients who require technological support?

The answer may lie in taking a contextual approach. Nurses working in specific contexts must define how they care – and this definition must include how they care for the patient attached to technology. In a study on the impact of new technology on workers and patients in the health services (Fitter 1986) this point was indirectly raised through one of the issues of concern to the researchers – namely, whether the balance of activities between the caring and curing roles is changing for nurses. The study addressed the important question of whether the increasing use of technology has led to an emphasis on curing at the expense of caring activities, or whether the technology has freed nurses' time so that they can devote more time to their caring role. This study tended to emphasize the dichotomy between care and cure from a professional role viewpoint. If we believe that caring is context dependent, it would be pertinent to ask 'How do nurses care in a cure/technological environment?' In a study entitled 'Technological caring: a new model for critical care', Ray (1987) outlined five themes of human caring experiences in critical care. One of the themes was titled 'technical competence' and Ray indicated that 'caring is technology'; 'caring is technological competence'. Once the nurse had become familiar with the technology – i.e. had grown and become mature within the intensive care setting – she could concentrate upon the patient and the family.

The personal cost of caring

Ray (1981: 29) points out that our health systems appear to be incongruent with caring as a professional ethic and argues that 'given the structural value system, economic competition and the entrenchment of health care settings with the medical model of of diagnosis, treatment and ultimately cure, caring values are submerged'. Conflict is being created within the nursing profession. If nurses claim that caring is one of their central functions, it needs to be promoted within educational, clinical and management settings. The reductionist approach to health care and the introduction of market principles must force nurses to ask, what cost caring?

Apart from the economic, social and political costs of caring, there is a personal cost to be weighed in the balance. Mayeroff (1971) has emphasized that caring is not always agreeable; that it is sometimes frustrating and rarely easy. This is recognized implicitly and explicitly by the increasing number of workshops and study sessions relating to 'caring for the carers'. Harrison (1990) reiterates a widely held view within the nursing profession that, in order for nurses to be caring with their patients, they must feel cared for and valued by their colleagues and the hospitals in which they work. The good nurse is expected to be selfless, tireless and completely altruistic. Their own needs come last. Burn-out has been related to nurses not being able to give care in the fullest way they could wish. This may be due to the economic and bureaucratic situations in which they have to work, but it is also linked to a lack of positive rewards and recognition for their actions and efforts.

Parse (1981: 130) has defined caring as 'risking being with someone towards a moment of joy'. She defines 'risking' as being exposed to possible injury. Through reaching out towards the patient the nurse may be exposed to hurt and rejection. 'Being with' the patient may be at great risk and personal cost to the nurse. Many nurses may have experienced the effect of nursing a patient whom they could not like or were revolted by through their illness or physical condition. If we accept that caring on the part of the nurse can be exhibited through attitude, actions and indeed no action, in a nurse–patient relationship which exhibits antagonism, rejection or injury can the nurse truly care? The nurse may feel that she 'ought to care' for the patient, but inability to do so through either rejection or personal dislike may lead to strong feelings of guilt and ambivalence. Noddings (1984), in a discussion of guilt in the caring relationship, felt that we redefine our caring with regard to principles – the nurse may simply carry out procedures on the patient, not with the patient, reduce personal contact to a minimum and encourage other nurses to be with the patient. In fact she has stopped caring.

Conclusion

There will never be a conclusion to the changing conceptions of caring. Technology is increasingly being used in hospital and community settings to assist nurses in their everyday actions. Older ideas about caring will give way to new ideas and debate will continue. Caring is now entrenched in the professional nurse's persona and yet we are only beginning to identify and describe what caring means to nurses, their patients and their families. Global definitions of caring are useful for they do have the function of allowing nurses within specific clinical settings to agree or disagree with the general statements they contain. It is perhaps too simple to say that nurses care and doctors cure. There is certainly recognized overlap between the two roles, and the advent of new technologies for monitoring and supporting patients will increasingly blur the distinctions for many nurses working in specialized clinical areas such as intensive care units. Not surprisingly, the extended/expanded role debate consequently has a high profile within intensive care units. Caring and technology can work together as long as the nurse's caring functions are clear and have the necessary value placed upon them. Unfortunately, it is easier to objectively and categorically state nurses' functions with regard to technology. It is harder to do so with the caring – as caring is to do with individual people.

The concept of care should increasingly be looked at from the context within which it occurs. Much work lies ahead of the nursing profession in order to define caring in specific contexts and the first steps have been taken by researchers such as Morrison (1989), who has begun by examining nurses' self-perceptions of caring. In the light of organizational and management imperatives such as quality assurance issues, resource management and cost–benefit analyses, it is increasingly necessary for nurses to be clear about their pre-eminent role of caring. Do we care? Do we want to care? Do our patients want us to care?

References

American Nurses Association 1965. *Educational Preparation for Nurse Practitioner and Assistants to Nurses*. New York: American Nurses Association.

Benner, P. 1984. *From Novice to Expert: Excellence and Power in Clinical Nursing Practice*. California: Addison Wesley.

Benner, P. and Wrubel, J. 1989. *The Primacy of Caring: Stress and Coping in Health and Illness*. California: Addison Wesley.

Bergman, R. 1983. Understanding the patient in all his human needs. *Journal of Advanced Nursing* 8: 185–90.

Briggs, A. 1972. *Report of the Committee on Nursing*, Cmnd 5115 (Chairman Professor Asa Briggs). London: HMSO.

Brown, L. 1986. The experience of care: the patient's perspective. *Topics in Clinical Nursing* 8: 56–62.

Dunlop, M. J. 1986. Is a science of caring possible? *Journal of Advanced Nursing* 11: 661–70.

Fitter, M. 1986. *The Impact of New Technology on Workers and Patients in the Health Services (Physical and Psychological Stress)*. Consolidated Report MRC/ESRC, Social and Applied Psychology Unit, University of Sheffield.

Francis, G. 1980. 'Gesellschaft' and the hospital: is total care a misnomer? *Advances in Nursing Science* 2(4): 9–13.

Gaut, D. A. 1981. Conceptual analysis of caring: research method. In M. Leininger, *Caring: An Essential Human Need*. New Jersey: Charles B. Slack.

Griffen, A. P. 1983. A philosophical analysis of caring in nursing. *Journal of Advanced Nursing* 8: 289–95.

Hall, L. E. 1964. *Project Report*. The Soloman and Betty Loeb Center and Montefiore Hospital. New York: Loeb Center for Nursing.

Harrison, L. L. 1990. Maintaining the ethic of caring in nursing. *Journal of Advanced Nursing* 15: 125–7.

Henderson, V. A. 1980. Preserving the essence of nursing in a technological age. *Journal of Advanced Nursing* 5(3): 245–60.

Jennett, B. 1986. *High Technology Medicine*. Oxford: Oxford University Press.

Kitson, A. L. 1984. *Steps towards the Identification and Development of Nursing's Therapeutic Function in the Care of the Hospitalised Elderly*. Unpublished DPhil thesis, New University of Ulster.

Kitson, A. L. 1987. A comparative analysis of lay and professional (nursing) caring relationships. *International Journal of Nursing Studies* 24(2): 155–65.

Leininger, M. 1981. *Caring: An Essential Human Need*. New Jersey: Charles B. Slack.

Luckman, J. and Sorenson, K. C. 1980. *Medical–Surgical Nursing*, 2nd edn. Philadelphia: Saunders.

McFarlane, J. K. 1976. A charter for caring. *Journal of Advanced Nursing* 1: 187–96.

MacFarlane, J. 1980. *Essays on Nursing.* King Fund Paper.

MacGuire, J. M. 1980. *The Expanded Role of the Nurse.* London: Kings Fund.

Mayeroff, K. 1971. *On Caring.* New York: Harper & Row.

Meleis, A. 1985. *Theoretical Nursing Development and Progress.* Philadelphia: Lippincott.

Morrison, P. 1989. Nursing and caring: a personal construct theory of some nurses' self perceptions. *Journal of Advanced Nursing* 14: 421–6.

Nightingale, F. 1960. *Notes on Nursing: What it is and What it is not.* Edinburgh: Churchill Livingtone. 1980 reprint.

Noddings, N. 1984. *Caring: A Feminine Approach to Ethics and Moral Education.* Berkeley: University of California Press.

Orem, D E. 1985. *Nursing: Concepts of Practice,* 3rd edn. New York: McGraw-Hill.

Parse, R. P. 1981. Caring from a human science perspective. In M. Leininger, *Caring: An Essential Human Need.* New Jersey: Charles B. Slack.

Ray, M. A. 1981. A philosophical analysis of caring within nursing. In M. Leininger, *Caring: An Essential Human Need.* New Jersey: Charles B. Slack.

Ray, M. A. 1987. Technological caring: a new model for critical care. *Dimensions of Critical Care Nursing* 6(3), May–June: 166–73.

Roach, Sister M. S. 1982. A framework for nursing ethics. A paper delivered at the 1st International Congress in Nursing Law and Ethics, 13–17 June, Jerusalem, Israel.

Salvage, J. 1990. The theory and practice of the new nursing. *Nursing Times* 86(4): 42–5.

Telfer, A. 1984. Choosing the right number. *Nursing Mirror* 158: 11–12.

Tonnies, F. 1887. *Gemeinschaft und Gesellschaft.* Translated by C. Loomis as *Community and Society.* E. Lansing: Michigan State University Press, 1957.

Watson, J. 1979. *Nursing: The Philosophy and Science of Caring.* Boston, Mass.: Little Brown.

Zornow, R. A. 1977. A curriculum model for the expanded role. *Nursing Outlook* 25(1): 43.

CHAPTER THIRTEEN

Nursing wastage from the nurses' perspective

Catherine Williams, Keith Soothill and Jon Barry

Introduction

Wastage is an emotive term. In the dictionary the meaning of waste is peppered with pejorative terms such as: unproductive, desolate, useless expenditure (Chambers 1988). On the whole it is regarded as a negative word. To waste is quite simply a bad thing. Having considered how emotionally loaded is the meaning of the word, one has to ask why it is generally used instead of the less emotive term 'turnover', particularly with regard to the service sector. Rarely do you hear talk of the *wastage* rates of factory workers in industry where the notion of 'turnover' is routinely used. So, in contrast to the emotively charged term of 'wastage', turnover is defined as 'the number of employees starting or finishing employment at a particular place of work over a given period'. Turnover is a clean, clear definition of a situation. So, while 'turnover' is essentially factual in thrust, 'wastage' is a judgemental term, incorporating ideas of uselessness, loss and unprofitability. Just as the poet, William Wordsworth (1807), spoke of echoes – 'Like – but oh, how different' – so being part of the turnover of the NHS has different connotations to being part of the wastage of the NHS. From a nurse's standpoint it is important to see the difference. Indeed, our aim here is to try to understand the nurses' point of view.

Language has been called 'the garment of thought',[1] and it is important to try to tease out the underlying thinking when words are used. Words used judgementally imply that one group is making a judgement of another group. And here is the rub for nurses. Nurses always seem to be the ones who are being judged.

The language is instructive. Ask what 'nursing wastage' means. When talking about the topic to acquaintances, many thought that nursing wastage meant all the equipment, dressings, etc. that nurses wasted! Certainly the term 'wastage' is one which nurses readily internalize. It has intimations of sin, guilt and letting down the service. Nursing retains enough of the notions of a vocation to suggest that nurses who leave are rejecting their calling. So all this adds to the pressure which nurses already suffer in trying to conform to the popular image of the caring, all-giving nurse (see Chapter 2 on 'The Media Representation of the Nurse') without being regarded as a waste if she takes a break from nursing or turns her ambitions to the apparently greener grasses of other occupations. The crucial point, though, is that 'wastage' is too readily seen as a problem created by nurses leaving – they're to blame – rather than generating any attempt to begin to consider more fundamental structural reasons within the working environment which may actually create the problem.

Identifying the problem

Wastage is such a loose term that some basic distinctions need to be mentioned, although trying to clarify what wastage actually means is considered elsewhere (see Chapter 16 on 'Managing Nurse Wastage'). It can be used to describe the loss in hours the NHS suffers from sickness, absenteeism and low morale, all contributing to decreasing nurses' work capacity. The NHS loses countless hours in this way, but it is really a different issue from what we are considering here. Sickness, absenteeism and low morale are exhibited by nurses who, in broad terms, either cannot or choose not to leave. Although vitally important and arguably caused by the same kinds of problems as nurses give as reasons for leaving the organization, discontent which manifests itself in these other ways must be treated as a separate issue. Our concern is essentially with turnover from the nurses' perspective.

However, from all points of view nursing turnover/wastage has two sides to it. Too little causes a static and possibly dulled workforce, too much causes a constantly moving and possibly insecure workforce. From the nurses' viewpoint there is less recognition that a very low turnover can itself product problems; in such circumstances, promotion opportunities may rest only on the scope offered by 'natural wastage' such as retirement. However, it is when turnover becomes somehow recognized as 'unnatural' that a whole range of problems of a different order begin to emerge. It is within this context that our own research on 'nursing wastage' developed.

In 1985 a then Chief Nursing Officer of a district health authority in the North West of England[2] contacted one of the authors expressing some concern about the numbers of nurses who seemed to be leaving the authority. A small study (Hockey 1987) showed that many nurses in the district echoed this concern, indicating a wide range of issues which underpinned some of their discontent and dissatisfaction regarding their work as a nurse. However, it soon became evident that at a local level the whole question had political dimensions and there was serious contention whether there was indeed a problem of nurse turnover. In brief, senior managers were less inclined to view the staffing situation as serious, while nurses did.

At this time in the mid-1980s the problems of the nursing profession were much less public. Despite the fact that approaching half a million nurses are employed within the National Health Service, many issues surrounding nurse turnover had not been considered in a systematic way for over a decade. In fact, the Review Body for Nursing Staff, Midwives, Health Visitors and Professions Allied to Medicine had commented in its second report in June 1985 that *'in the management's view* only a very small proportion (of nurses) left the NHS for reasons of dissatisfaction' (our emphasis). This was said at a time when some local health authorities were beginning to recognize that they were experiencing difficulties in the recruitment and the retention of nurses. We felt that it was clearly time to hear what *nurses* had to say.

Our work (Mackay, 1988a,b, 1989; Francis, Peelo and Soothill, Chapter 4 in this volume) has been to identify some of the recurring themes which emerge when you talk to nurses or ask them to respond to questionnaires. Since then we have developed this work further by considering in detail the views of some nurses who had left this authority over the previous three years.

Reasons for leaving

Focusing now on this follow-up study of nurses in the North West of England, we discuss elsewhere (Soothill *et al.* 1990) the considerable advantages of following through the same set of nurses in a longitudinal study rather than the more usual cross-sectional research design when nurses are questioned about their attitudes at one particular point of time. Again we argue elsewhere (Williams *et al.* in press) that nurses' attitudes are dynamic rather than static. In other words, the situations of nurses change over time – in both expected and unexpected directions, reflecting both conditions internal to nursing (such as changes in pay and conditions) or events external to nursing (such as a partner moving job to another area, having a baby, etc.) – and, as a consequence, their view of their situation will change as new evidence of their life chances emerges. More specifically, we found in considering the outcome of stated intentions that people change their mind about whether they intend to leave or not (Soothill *et al.* 1990) and also that they are likely to shift their views as to whether they regard nursing as a vocation, a career or just a job (Williams *et al.* in press).

Health authority records indicated whether or not the nurses in our sample had left within the three-year follow-up period.[3] However, it was more difficult to trace the physical whereabouts of nurses for the purpose of probing more systematically their reasons for leaving.

Ninety persons returned the questionnaires we despatched. An analysis of their responses (Williams *et al.* 1991a) gives the flavour of how nurses disperse into a range of activities when they leave a particular health authority. In fact, two-thirds (66 per cent) remained in nursing after they left. Of the total sample, 40 per cent left to move to other health authorities within the NHS for a wide variety of reasons, from promotion to discontent. A further 26 per cent decided that nursing outside the NHS was the best option for them. Of the remaining one-third (34 per cent), most were not now in paid employment and were child-rearers, students, retired, ill, disabled or registered unemployed. Some of these outcomes, such as retirement and some ill health, are inevitable. However, leaving for reasons of ill health may not be straightforward. Some, for example, who have suffered from the after-effects of illness felt that they could have worked in a different area of nursing and that no effort was put into finding them alternative work or part-time work until they were completely recovered. Similarly, childrearing is also an acceptable loss providing the parent has chosen to be a full-time parent rather than feeling that she has been coerced into that position by lack of adequate child-care facilities.

The smallest group of 11 per cent represent those who had left nursing altogether and had moved into other occupations. These former nurses were doing a variety of activities from setting up a snail farm, secretarial work, gardening, painting, dressmaking, running a child-minding service to working in shops.

The follow-up shows the diversity of activity after leaving, but the most striking aspect of the follow-up study was that in essence all the groups were saying remarkably similar things and expressing dissatisfaction at staff shortages, lack of resources, the workload getting in the way of them doing their work properly, the lack of personal development opportunities in their own training and careers, the management of the NHS, non-existent child-care facilities and difficulties around shifts for parents, and a feeling of not being appreciated and valued both financially and by their managers and government.

This sad and rather depressing tale of woe emerged not only from responses to the questionnaire but also from a series of interviews conducted with a sub-sample of the 90 persons who had returned completed questionnaires. Out of the 39 leavers interviewed, none had had a formal leaving interview and only one or two had had an informal leaving interview. There seems to be a total lack of interest in the reasons why these nurses left. The reasons entered on the computerized personnel records that we had access to were often at serious odds with what the nurses said at the interview. In fact, this discrepancy is not altogether surprising, for however efficiently leaving interviews may be conducted there are always likely to be some differences between the reasons given to the health authority for leaving and those which may be given to more intimate associates (for further discussion on this point, see Chapter 16 on 'Managing Nurse Wastage'). A variant of this process is what we term the 'official' and 'unofficial' reasons for leaving.

'Official' reasons are indeed the reasons given to officials. The reasons given in their letter of resignation are usually safe polite reasons that would not offend or jeopardize a future refrence. In contrast, the 'unofficial' reasons, which are more likely to be expanded at length to close intimates, may paint a rather different picture. Again, there is a danger in believing that these accounts represent some kind of 'objective truth', for one needs to appreciate that one often needs to justify one's actions to loved ones. Actions are not always so straightforward and rational as one often tries to portray them. Hence, the usual pattern is to 'gild the lily' so that one emerges in one's own unedited account in a somewhat better light than, say, an account given by a disinterested bystander who knew all the facts. Nevertheless, 'unofficial' reasons given to intimates are much more likely to contain the genuine passion which may accompany leaving decisions. Such passion has usually been sanitized from the 'official' letters of resignation which nurses know may remain on file. We felt that by gaining confidence and trust in terms of guaranteeing anonymity and confidentiality our interviews got much closer to unpackaging the 'unofficial' reasons for leaving which may usually be given only to the nurses' more intimate associates.

Certainly the 'unofficial' reasons told at interview were much more passionate and often described shocking attitudes from those senior to them and poor conditions at work. The interviews complemented the responses to the questionnaire. The top three reasons given for leaving in the questionnaire were centred upon working conditions and combined workload preventing nurses giving their best, staff shortages and the constant struggle with underfunded resources (see Table 13.1). The second group of three issues focused on the personal prospects of the individual and encompassed wanting to widen experience, wanting a new challenge and a general concern about a lack of promotion prospects. Issues around management, stress and child-care were also prominent as reasons for leaving and aspects requiring improvement.

Beyond the surprising point already mentioned that pay was *not* a primary issue emerging from our research, it was also not the work that nurses routinely do which caused upset. Only three people ticked 'a dislike of nursing work' among the possible options listed on the questionnaire, showing that it was not the actual content of the work that caused nurses to leave. Quite simply, it was the conditions on the ward or in the clinical situation that were causing the passionate discontent voiced both in our questionnaire and in our interviews that provoked these nurses to look for greener pastures. The more detailed responses emerging from the interviews are given elsewhere (Williams *et al.* 1990a,b,c), and here we just give a flavour of the responses for illustration.

Table 13.1 Top ten reasons for leaving

	Overall % (N = 90)	Top reasons			
		1st (%)	2nd (%)	3rd (%)	Total (%)
Workload prevents giving of best	40	4	10	67	21
Staff shortages	37	3	9	10	22
Constant struggle with underfunded resources	31	3	0	7	10
Wanting to widen experience	31	11	6	0	17
Wanting a new challenge	31	2	8	6	16
Lack of promotion prospects	29	2	2	7	11
Management style of organization	27	0	4	0	4
Hours not suiting home life	26	4	3	7	14
Stress too high	24	6	7	2	14
Bad atmosphere at work	24	8	1	2	11

The passion displayed was quite disturbing. A midwife in her late twenties said:

'My first reason [for leaving] was understaffing . . . the staff was diminished, we missed meal breaks because no one came to relieve you, coffee breaks in the mornings just didn't exist . . . It's not worth going to work, working as hard as you do, staying late, not getting time back and getting all that aggro at work . . . I just thought I can't exist like this.'

A recently qualified RGN answered the interview question angrily:

'Well you'll have heard it all before, not enough resources, not enough time, not enough back-up . . . you've not enough time to do your job properly. The current way that I am being treated has knocked all the stuffing out of me because I'm not allowed to do my job properly.'

What is important to stress is that these kinds of criticisms, of which the above two give just an indication, are concerned with upsetting elements of the job which are preventable. In other words, they are not talking about matters are an inherent part of the job like bedpans, faeces and vomit. Nurses seem to accept these unalterable facts of human frailty. In contrast, they are criticizing aspects of the job that can and should be changed. The criticisms of the job are ones of NHS finance and management. Hence, they are concerned with unpleasant features of the job which are *in principle* avoidable. In short, money, management training, drive and initiative could alleviate many of these kinds of problems in a remarkably short time.

In considering why people leave, it is also instructive to consider the complementary question of why people decide to take up nursing (Williams *et al.* 1991b). In fact, we asked our sample of leavers, 'What made you decide to take up nursing as a profession?' and gave them a list of ten possible reasons, asking them to tick as many as applied. Interestingly, not one person ticked 'the money', indicating the general attitude of nurses to their pay. More than half (56 per cent) of our sample were under 30 years of age, so this is not a throwback to the era when it was thought that if nurses were paid *too* much, then the *wrong* sort of person would come into nursing, but an up-to-date statement that none of our sample chose their career for money. The two factors ticked by most people were 'opportunity to work with people' (64 per cent) and 'to be part of a caring team' (62 per cent). These clearly reflect that the two main factors that decided these people to take up nursing are based on an interest in the *content* of the actual work. Nursing is very person-centred and demands considerable interpersonal skills. In fact, these two factors link in with the top three reasons our sample gave for leaving – 'workload prevents giving of best', 'staff shortages' and 'constant struggle with underfunded resources'. While at first glance a relationship may not be immediately obvious, it became increasingly clear when the questionnaire returns were supplemented by the interviews we conducted that many of our sample quite simply felt that they were no longer part of a caring team, nor were they able to give to patients what the patients needed and wanted. The heavy workload, staff shortages and lack of resources were getting between the nurse and the patient and also between nurses themselves. The individualistic philosophy so enthusiastically encouraged during the 1980s is totally disruptive in operation on the wards:

'It was really happy and we had a real good team. That's what's missing, a team; everyones individuals on a ward now, we're not part of a team . . . there's no loyalty. I mean they haven't even got loyalty to each other, so how can they have loyalty to team . . . so it's dog eat dog, a matter of survival.'

Curiously, however, the scope for the thrusting and ambitious individual within nursing – perhaps willing to overthrow to some degree the traditional values of working as a team – seems equally limited and limiting within the NHS. So it is noteworthy that the second group of three reasons in the top six (see Table 13.1) focus on issues around the personal prospects for a career in the NHS for the individual nurse. This concern was again vividly captured during some of the interviews. A young man who had left nursing completely indicated some of the frustrations:

'I said I'd love to get a job on here and I would love to do my specialty training. But first of all you get told that sorry we've got no more money on the unit for new staff nurses, but just by chance you did get on, then they would never let you go on the specialty course because they don't second anybody and if you do get on a course, a job's not guaranteed, so where is all the career structure? If you've any sense of the future you want some sort of plan for the next few years, don't you?'

Similarly, a specialist health visitor left:

'because I felt stunted and restricted and because of a loss of opportunities and inability to go on study days. . . . It was really bad management, lack of career opportunities or even lack of interest from managers to pursue your career opportunities. You know, sort of keep everybody down, that's what came across to me.'

Earlier we noted how our leavers from the health authority we were studying moved to a variety of destinations. Not surprisingly, there were some differences in reasons given for leaving by the various groups (Williams *et al.* 1991a). So, for example, 'workload' was the primary reason for leaving the NHS for those still in nursing but now working outside the NHS. Among those in the unpaid group, retirement was the main stated reason for leaving. But, of course, behind this apparently benign reason there can be a multitude of accounts. Certainly a number had retired early because they were fed up at work and disillusioned by the problems within the health service. Among those who had taken a job outside nursing, a higher proportion had indicated 'stress too high' as a reason for leaving. Nevertheless, what seems to bind all the groups together is not the work but the broader issues surrounding the job. This is encapsulted by the saying – 'Nurses love their work but hate their job'.

Now, what of those who had left this health authority but remained working within the NHS? For these people the main reasons for moving health authorities were centred on career and personal development: 'wanting a new challenge', 'wanting to widen experience' and 'lack of promotion prospects' characterized the reasons cited by these nurses. Is this response saying that the nurses staying within the health service are willing to put up with all the issues cited so frequently by others, providing they get their own promotion, wider experience and challenge within the NHS? In fact, the analysis shows that the other reasons are also real issues for them, but that career issues were more significant to those who continued to work within the NHS.

Deciding to stay

The importance of a career is reinforced by the 'stayers' we interviewed.[4] These nurses, who had originally intended to leave but had continued in post during the three follow-up years, generally remained discontented, although for some their situation had positively improved. The two who were the most discontented were two enrolled nurses. One quite simply said:

'Money and lack of opportunity . . . are keeping me here now.'

She felt that as an enrolled nurse there was little opportunity within the health service but that the possibilities for someone of her age (in her late thirties) outside the health service were even more limited. She had applied for a variety of jobs but the pay was always less. The other unhappy enrolled nurse had also applied for a number of jobs outside nursing and said:

'If someone came along with an interesting offer, then I'm
afraid my loyalties to nursing would not have the same power
as they used to have.'

Both these nurses had worked for the health service for some
considerable time, and, while very disillusioned and dissatisfied,
neither had finally left. They were both single and felt very
restricted by their mortgages. In effect, they felt trapped in their
jobs.

In contrast, two other enrolled nurses amongst the stayers
expressed all the familiar dissatisfactions about shortages and
resources but were now quite content within themselves. The
major difference between these two and the unhappy two were
that they had both got places on a conversion course. They were
very buoyant about their improved prospects. They felt enormously lucky they had got a place on a conversion course, as one
indicated that there had been only 10 places and 300 applicants
on her course. So these women had achieved major career
development and, although both were aware and remained
passionate about staff shortages and other issues, they now
intended to stay in NHS nursing.

The other five 'stayers' who were interviewed had also achieved
promotion and had very good prospects ahead of them. They were
now in management positions and conveyed a feeling of
satisfaction in their progress, although the future for some was
still negotiable. One woman who three years earlier had been
intending to leave this health authority but had stayed remained
clear about her intentions:

'I'm quite busy and I'm enjoying every minute of it. [The health
authority] have been very good to me, but I've worked hard for
[this health authority] and I like what I'm doing. But I'm
looking for further development now, and I want a full-time
management post . . . I have a degree of loyalty to [this health
authority] because they've been good to me but . . . you have to
put yourself first these days . . .   I want an I [grade]. I'll go
elsewhere in the end if they don't give it to me.'

So, quite straightforwardly, if the health authority gives this
woman what she wants with regards to promotion they will keep

her; if not, she will go – the message could not be clearer, although the outcome maybe more problematic.

By looking at those who had unexpectedly opted to stay we can see that most of them had achieved promotion, which contributed to their decision to stay. In contrast, the first two had not progressed in their career and were both unhappy, feeling trapped after looking round for alternatives. There is little doubt that career progression – or lack of it – appears to seriously affect the way people view their job and alters what they are willing to tolerate or not tolerate.

Current attitudes

The evidence from our study indicates the ambivalence that many nurses and former nurses feel about their job. Many really do love the notion of nursing and the opportunity it gives them to work with people and help them recover, die, or prevent ill health. Few who left wanted to leave nursing. But the confines of the job often seemed to get in the way of allowing them to do what they want and need to do.

The opinions of people leaving a workplace are a valuable resource and a window into the working environment. We have tried to see the situation from the nurses' perspective. So whereas managers, for example, often maintain that there are indeed enough staff to do the required work, this is not how it is generally seen by nurses. However, we are not concerned here with the truth or otherwise of their assertions. Sociologically the family point is made, as W. I. Thomas suggested long ago, that once people define situations as real, they are real in their consequences.

Certainly staff shortages, lack of resources and all the other major causes of turnover highlighted in our study need to be faced and not just sidelined as issues raised by a few malcontents. The message is too widespread. Sadly, empirical work by academics can often be too easily dismissed as unrepresentative, out-of-date or out-of-touch with what is actually happening. However, in the study of nurse turnover and retention, various studies are producing very similar results (Price Waterhouse 1988; Martin and Mackean 1988; Waite et al. 1989).

It is difficult to estimate the extent to which current problems with nursing are transitory or permanent. Certainly we have identified certain features of concern which, though expensive to eradicate or improve, are at least *in principle* possible to confront in a positive manner. However, it is sometimes hard to dismiss the notion that discontent may also be rooted much deeper in our extremely materialistic society. In a society which glorifies consumerism and the constant change of personal belongings, toys, stereos, fridges, cars, etc., it is not surprising that this attitude also seeps into employment. The *new* car is always going to be better, more fun and give more satisfaction, as is the *new* job. Reality is, of course, often different. New cars are involved in accidents and break down, as do new jobs. Hence, there is the argument that, until our society moves away from gross consumerism into valuing what you have and enjoying familiarity instead of looking to the shiny, new alternative, high turnover in jobs will continue to be the norm.

There may be some truth to this inherently conservative position that one should treasure what one has and that some nurses are caught up in the increasing spiral of consumerism. Furthermore, it would be foolish to deny that nurses are somehow immune to any major shifts in the cultural values of society.

Of course, there are also considerable regional differences which need to be considered. Turnover or wastage has different connotations and implications depending on where you stand in the NHS structure. In fact, Grocott (1989) has distinguished between 'pure wastage' (i.e. those leaving the NHS altogether) and 'internal transfers' (i.e. those moving within the NHS). He appears to consider only those leaving altogether as a problem and he does not discuss the sometimes unnecessary expense of nurses moving within the NHS. Grocott also challenges the notion of a 'demographic timebomb' and argues that with people re-entering nursing after career breaks and despite a decrease in learner intakes, the qualified workforce in the NHS is increasing. The corollary to his message is that individual health authorities may have problems but overall the picture is not so gloomy.

While Grocott's analysis must be of some comfort to those concerned with the overall problem, the situation often remains dire for the individual nurse. Our study, which focused on talking to nurses who all lived and worked in the North West of England, indicated how the local geographical context may be crucial. Generally, these nurses did not feel that there were jobs which were 'up for grabs' owing to staff shortages. Indeed, quite the opposite. A father of two children under 5 years, who had worked as a welder for four years, then did his RMN training and worked in the psychiatric field for two years and had just completed his RGN training, was finding it very difficult to find a job, saying:

'The only thing is that they're short of money as usual, and they're only employing staff on temporary contract. For some staff they're only on weekly contacts, so they don't know where they are, so morale is low because of that. ... They're desperately short of staff, but they won't employ any others because they've no money.'

The current situation is extremely paradoxical, confusing and ambiguous. The NHS Regional Manpower Planners' Group (Conroy and Stidson 1988) suggested that staff shortages would replace finance as the most significant block to providing an efficient service. However, certainly in the North West of England, finance remains the main factor. In brief, the nurses are there, the money isn't. This shortfall of money affects recruitment and retention in terms of providing meaningful careers for the majority of nurses within the workforce and, more immediately, in providing sufficient posts to counter the concerns of nursing staff and their unions.

The notion of the 'demographic timebomb' is based on the facts that between 1966 and 1976 births fell in the UK by 35 per cent. In that case we should be right in the middle of the 'timebomb', as 1984–94 are the years when there is a shortage of 18 year olds, and 1987–97 when newly qualified staff are in short supply. Yet paradoxically it is some of these rare newly qualified nurses who are having to go on the dole through a lack of jobs. Nurses today may well identify a conflict between what is being spoken about and their own experience.

The situation is certainly perplexing. The Labour Party and nurses in both our study and the recent IMS study (Waite *et al.* 1989) are saying staff shortages are a major problem in the NHS. In contrast, the government is denying that there are staff shortages. Grocott (1989) and the Pay Review Board say that overall there are more qualified staff, and the newly qualified nurses of Wales, Burnley, Bedfordshire, Manchester, West Dorset, Liverpool, Glasgow, Wigan and Calderstone are said to be having difficulties getting nursing jobs and are registering unemployed, or working in clinical areas they are not interested in (Friend 1990; Thompson 1990).

We seem to be caught in an Orwellian newspeak which is difficult to disentangle. Certainly there is a belief among nurses that staffing levels are being pruned to the minimum and that establishment figures are being driven to fit in with unrealistic financial targets rather than with patients' needs. As a consequence, vacancies may deliberately not be filled. The Orwellian touch is that when vacancies are not filled and the posts are eradicated, there is no staff shortage as the job does not exist any more.

The use of language is fascinating and we have pointed to how the pejorative term 'nursing wastage' rather than the more neutral 'nursing turnover' has connotations which tend to place the blame for staffing difficulties on to the nurse. We have portrayed the current concerns and discontent of nurses which often lead to a movement both to posts within nursing and to paid and unpaid employment outside nursing. We have hinted that the concerns about adverse demographic trends, while important, are used as a diversionary and screening tactic to avoid facing other fundamental issues. In short, staff shortages are due not to lack of personnel in many cases but to a lack of funding.

Managers are constantly being asked to restrict and cut back expenditure, yet we tend to forget that this can produce a downward spiral in morale which is difficult to reverse. Low morale, whether it leads to turnover or not, causes a drop in standards and lowers efficiency in nursing care. If more money, time and energy were spent addressing the issues that cause nurses to leave and move to another authority, into the private sector or out of nursing altogether, then it is possible that we could help to prevent people leaving work that they really enjoy because they cannot now stand the job:

'I can't imagine ever having a job that would give me the satisfaction that I used to have in nursing. I can't think that there is a job on this earth that would ever do that for me.'

– said by a woman who, despite wanting to be a nurse from childhood, has now left nursing altogether and has no intention of going back. She was unusual in deciding never to return to nursing, but typical in continuing to love the ideal of nursing. Nevertheless, perhaps she comes close to identifying some of the current conundrums within nursing as we grapple with the ideal and the realistic. Indeed, perhaps wastage is when the ideal is not realistic and the realistic is not ideal.

Notes

1 In fact, the historian, Thomas Carlyle, went further – 'Language is called the garment of thought: however, it should rather be, language is the flesh-garment, the body, of thought' (*Sartor Resartus*, i, 11).
2 This health authority has consistently wished to remain anonymous in all subsequent research publications.
3 In fact, this exercise was not so easy as this brief sentence suggests and the outcome for a number could not be traced (see also, Barry *et al.* 1989).
4 Recognizing that the 'leavers' maybe giving a somewhat distorted picture, we interviewed nine nurses who had altered their original intention of leaving the health authority and were still in post at the end of the three-year follow-up period. We were interested in what had persuaded them to change their mind about leaving.

Acknowlegements

The research team is most grateful for the grant from the Leverhulme Trust towards the financing of this project and to the health authority concerned for their help and cooperation.

References

Barry, J. T., Soothill, K. L. and Francis, B. J. 1989. Nursing the statistics: a demonstration study of nurse turnover and retention. *Journal of Advanced Nursing* 14: 528–35.
Chambers. 1988. *English Dictionary*. Edinburgh: W. & R. Chambers.
Conroy, M. and Stidson, M. 1988. *2001 – The Black Hole*. The NHS Regional Manpower Planners' Group.
Friend, B. 1990. Training for the dole. *Nursing Times*, 7 February, 86(6).
Grocott, T. 1989. A hole in the black hole theory. *Nursing Times*, 11 October, 85(41).
Hockey, J. 1987. A picture of pressure. *Nursing Times*, 8 July, 83(27).
Mackay, L. 1988a. Career woman. *Nursing Times* 84(10).
Mackay, L. 1988b. No time to care. *Nursing Times* 84(11).

230   CLINICAL

Mackay, L. 1989. *Nursing a Problem*. Milton Keynes: Open University Press.

Martin, J. P, and Mackean, J. 1988. *Can We Keep Nurses in the Health Service? A Study of Nurse Retention in Two Health Districts*. Institute for Health Policy Studies, University of Southampton.

Price Waterhouse. 1988. *Nurse Retention and Recruitment: A Matter of Priority*. Report commissioned by chairmen of Regional Health Authorities in England, Health Boards in Scotland and Health Authorities in Wales.

Review Body for Nursing Staff, Midwives, Health Visitors and Professions Allied to Medicine. 1985. *2nd Report on Nursing Staff, Midwives and Health Visitors*. Cm 9529. London: HMSO.

Soothill, K. L., Barry, J. T. and Williams, C. W. 1990. *Words and Actions: A Study in Nurse Wastage*. Working Paper No. 9, Lancaster University, Department of Applied Social Science.

Thompson, J. 1990. No vacancies. *Nursing Times*, 23 May, 86(21).

Waite, R., Buchan, J. and Thomas, J. 1989. *Nurses in and out of Work*. IMS Report No. 170, Brighton: Institute of Manpower Studies.

Williams, C. W., Soothill, K. L. and Barry, J. T. 1990a. *Leaving – We've heard it all before*. Working Paper No. 1, Lancaster University, Department of Applied Social Science.

Williams, C. W., Soothill, K. L. and Barry, J. T. 1990b. *How Could the Health Authority Have Kept You?* Working Paper No. 2, Lancaster University, Department of Applied Social Science.

Williams, C. W., Soothill, K. L. and Barry, J. T. 1990c. *Mothering and Nursing – Conflicting Interests*. Working Paper No. 3, Lancaster University, Department of Applied Social Science.

Williams, C. W., Soothill, K. L. and Barry, J. T. 1991a. Love nursing, hate the job. *Health Service Journal*, 14 February, 101(5238): 18–21.

Williams, C. W., Soothill, K. L. and Barry, J. T. 1991b. Targeting the discontented. *Health Service Journal*, 21 February, 101(5239): 20–21.

Williams, C. W., Soothill, K. L. and Barry, J. T. in press. Nursing – just a job? Do statistics tell us what we think? *Journal of Advanced Nursing*.

Wordsworth, W. 1807. Yes, it was the mountain Echo. Reprinted in *The Poetical Works of Wordsworth*, London: Oxford University Press, 1951.

CHAPTER FOURTEEN

Difficulties in provision of care for the elderly by auxiliaries – implications for the new support worker

Emily Griffiths

With the introduction of Project 2000, auxiliaries are to be replaced by the intended new support worker. She is not a nurse, but a 'helper' or 'aide' to the trained nurse. She is not an auxiliary, that grade of staff with very little or no training whose role, it is often suggested, is expanded beyond the desirable or the safe. The new support worker will be carefully trained and supervised in her work – or this, at least, is the hope.

Doubts have, however, been expressed about the impact of Project 2000 at ward level. It has been suggested that when the newly trained nurses, the 'knowledgeable doers', arrive on the wards they will succumb to the old way and follow inappropriate role models (Lee 1989). The attention paid to the training and future of the new support worker has been less than that focused on future trained nurses, but the fate of both are intertwined. Historically, much of the care for institutionalized elderly has been provided by the least qualified staff, and it would appear that this will continue to be the case, perhaps even to a greater extent (RCN 1989).

Care for the elderly often has a poor reputation. Clarke (1978) described the atmosphere of long stay and rehabilitation wards as that of 'getting through the work', with the emphasis on the provision of physical care and only good intentions to talk to the patients that were never put into practice. Hardie and Macmillan similarly describe the atmosphere on wards where many auxiliaries were employed as 'more one of getting through the work and finishing on time' than elsewhere (Hardie and Macmillan 1980: 115). In the research to be discussed this still appears to be the case.

The following research is based on interviews with 54 auxiliaries, including participant observation for 2–3½ hours with 24 of them. The fieldwork took place in 1989 in five hospitals of various sizes and locations in the North West of England. All but nine of the auxiliaries had worked on wards for the elderly or medical/orthopaedic wards. Six of them recently started their nurse training. One aim of the study was to try to explain the way in which the auxiliaries learnt their role and viewed supervision. The study is of particular relevance in view of Project 2000 as it is through the education and supervision of the new support worker that the greatest changes are anticipated. It is, therefore, these two areas which are looked at most closely.

The job

The key to understanding the auxiliaries' perception of their situation appears to be that they saw their main job as to 'get through the work'. In some respects they saw their work as like that in a factory, with a production line of patients to be washed, dressed, fed and toileted. Thomas (now doing his nurse training) described his experience as follows:

'I remember on a psycho-geriatric ward having to get up 20 to 30 confused old men and going down the line, getting them washed, dressed, to the dining room, and then the next one. Just a drudge really – I hated it.'

It was not that they saw this process as the best way to provide care. Many were in fact frustrated by it but felt that physical work, particularly 'dirty work' (washing and toileting patients), was their work. Norma commented,

'The auxiliaries get all the dirty work. I come on and am just expected to get on with it, without so much as a "good morning".'

All the auxiliaries working with the elderly saw direct patient care as their most important duty, to be done as first priority. 'Housekeeping' type tasks such as tidying lockers or bagging up linen were also a part of their job. On a ward where 'primary' nursing had been introduced, only the auxiliaries (renamed care assistants) did these housekeeping tasks. On other wards, trained staff, or those in training, helped the auxiliaries with this. These jobs were fitted in around direct patient care, with their execution constantly being interrupted by calls from trained staff to take someone to the toilet, pack their belongings and so forth.

Whether or not the auxiliaries were providing direct 'basic' nursing care, or what were ostensibly 'housekeeping tasks', such as tidying up the ward, the opportunities regularly arose to do more than the delegated tasks. For example, one auxiliary was told to bedbath a patient. From the observer's standpoint it appeared that the man also required pressure area care, bowel care, a shave, and repositioning to assist his breathing. An auxiliary on an orthopaedic ward was giving out drinks when she spotted a young man's first attempts to get into a wheelchair unaided and propel himself around the ward. In the first example the bedbath was given and other possible requirements left undone and uncommented on. In the second example the auxiliary provided assistance and explained to the man what the doctor had said he could do, warning him not to overdo it.

The limits to the care provided appeared to depend upon whether or not the 'extra' care was seen as 'common sense' and routine or a part of the trained nurses' work. In some cases what was work was clear cut. With the exception of only one auxiliary, the paperwork associated with care plans was seen as the trained nurses' prerogative. Attendance of ward reports on some wards was also only for trained staff. Patient education and provision of information for relatives was said to be a trained nurse's job. Giving information on ward routine, that is, 'what usually happens on the ward', was not, however. In the case of the auxiliary helping the orthopaedic patient, had a relative asked what the doctor had said they might well have been referred to a trained nurse. Dressing was usually not done by auxiliaries. The giving of enemas was no longer done by any auxiliaries. Some of the more experienced auxiliaries had difficulty understanding why they could not do the latter. They could see what needed doing and knew how to do it, but were not allowed to carry it out. On one occasion an auxiliary was seen to suggest to the trained nurse that the patient needed an enema. She then took the patient to her bed. The trained nurse gave her the enema and left immediately. Another auxiliary described how it upset her to see that patients needed, but were not getting, regular fluids via their ryles tubes. As she knew how to give them safely (or so she assumed, as she had been taught) and had been doing them for years, she would either remind a trained nurse to give fluids, or, if no one was about, do it herself, but not report it. Hazel (now doing her nurse training) described how when working as an auxiliary she had perceived herself as competent and was only now questioning whether or not this was so. The example she gave was that of doing bowel examinations prior to giving enemas:

'It's terrible the damage you could have done. It isn't sufficient, that little bit of training. No way was it sufficient for you to go around – let's face it – sticking your finger up someone's backside. . . . The number of times I did it because it was just expected of you.'

Only in retrospect did she feel that it was not a 'commonsense' thing to do. At the time, it was a matter of fact that things were done that way.

There were, however, situations where the auxiliaries did not see jobs as theirs but the trained nurses did. Edith described how difficult it was on a rehabilitation ward as 'there was nothing to do but talk'. Attempts by the sister to introduce twice-daily diversional therapy had been met with reluctance by the auxiliaries. Edith said it was not that she felt silly, as some auxiliaries did, 'chucking a ball about', but that some real knowledge of the patients' medical condition was needed to do it properly.

The patients

The auxiliaries talked very much about the 'job' and very little about the patients. The patients to them had two aspects: they were people who they were concerned about, but also the 'work objects' to whom they had to do things, as already illustrated.

First, to continue with the metaphor of factory work. Beynon and Blackburn (1972) described how the factory workers they looked at became frustrated when the line was interrupted, slowing them down, and how they gained satisfaction from achieving their targets. One of the main interruptions to the auxiliaries' work was caused by confused patients who were unpredictable and might disrupt their work with other patients, or undo work already done, for example, by getting up after being put to bed or otherwise failing to cooperate. As Ada said,

'Sometimes the patients do things that are unexpected and put me all behind – and everyone thinks I'm very slow anyway, and then I get irritable.'

Lucid patients could also 'put one behind'. On one ward a sister, who had only recently left, had encouraged patients to wait until the 'toileting rounds' before asking for the commode. 'Extra' requests – that is, those outside the routine – were seen as unreasonable. Therefore when a woman wanted to use the toilet before going to bed it caused an auxiliary to comment:

'You'd get finished early, but for her. She's spoilt.'

Although this attitude towards 'extra' work appeared extreme, this idea of some things being seen as 'extra' has been noted elsewhere (see Treacy 1987, in her study of student nurses). Bedfast patients who required only washing and changing were described as 'good', since they caused the minimum amount of 'extra' work and interruptions. Provision of care outside the usual order was also unpopular in that it also slowed one down. Hence Annette's comment.

'It's okay Ann [ward sister] letting patients lie in or giving them baths before breakfast, but it only means we've got to finish off the rest of the patients after breakfast, while they do something else.'

The patients were also seen as people. The auxiliaries cared about their work and wanted to do a good job. Only one interviewed had attempted to 'work to grade' during the dispute over levels of pay in 1989, as this involved limiting what they would do for patients. They wanted to do whatever they could to help care for them. Even so, there were difficulties for auxiliaries in forming relationships with patients. Again it was the confused patients who there was the most difficulty with. Hazel clearly illustrated this point:

'Where I was they were more confused than not confused. They'd no conversation, and when they did – sometimes you'd think, "Oh my God, they're away with the fairies". This might sound awful, but you weren't dealing with people.'

The auxiliaries could not judge confused patients by the same standards they would 'ordinary' relationships. Someone crying and upset who was confused did not appeal to the auxiliaries in the same way as a lucid person. Because they were confused it also meant that the auxiliaries were in a position of more power than they might be with people who could stick up for themselves. Again Hazel comments:

'You get a power struggle going on. I think it only happens in the care of the elderly. They can't always protect themselves. On orthopaedics I've never noticed that they have any sort of power, even though there are three or four auxiliaries on duty at a time. I think they are basically dealing with a younger sort of person, who can talk back, whereas with most of the elderly and confused elderly you don't get that. I think that auxiliaries there get a power that they have never had and get quite bossy. They're never talked back to. No one is going to say, 'Who do you think you are talking to?' as they would on a surgical ward. . . . You'd think, they're not a trained nurse, and anyway, they've no right to speak to me like that and tell me what to do. In a lot of cases this is what they do do. I've heard it said, "Do you want a bath Mrs So and So". "No I don't." "Well if you think you are getting off" . . . and they'd tell them off – I've heard it said.'

Another problem regarding many of the patients who are confused, partly suggested by the above, is that the auxiliaries can get used to treating patients as if they are confused, and then treat others in the same way. For example, they said that with the confused they treated them like children and had, on occasions, gone on to the next patient and treated him in the same way when he was in fact quite 'with it'. It was noted that distinguishing between people who were hard of hearing and confused in a brief encounter could be very difficult. Appreciation for what was done was a major source of satisfaction for the auxiliaries. This could come either from the patient or from relatives. The main frustration in working with patients who were not confused was the failure to say 'thank you'.

Roth (1978) argues that professionals providing care can achieve only a certain limited standard because of the lack of love for the patient felt by the professionals. This, he argues, might be present where care is provided by a relative. It must, however, be remembered that relatives caring for the elderly are faced with many problems, particularly where the elderly are confused, and that abuse by relatives can and does occur. There are also difficulties in caring for people in institutions that are specific to institutions; that is, which arise 'from the fact that the elderly people are different, have differing needs and standards than that of the institutional regime' (Payne 1988: 11). This is reflected in the auxiliaries' comments that the appropriate care of patients does not always fit in with the goal of getting through the work. The other problem arising is that, often, they could not treat patients as 'human' even if they wished to do so, and that this was carried over to other patients. Some of the difficulties and benefits derived from caring were similar to those involved in caring for people at home.

To summarize the argument so far, it is suggested that the auxiliaries play an important role in nursing the elderly. This role is not, however, only to carry out specific delegated tasks; it is much broader than this. The extent to which auxiliaries provide patient care beyond their formal role varies. It appears that the main factor in deciding whether they will provide more care is whether or not the task is seen as something that usually happens on the ward, and may or may not include what the nursing profession would argue is a trained nurse's role. The difficulties they encounter in work relate to problems in providing individual care in an institution and to dealing with individuals with whom even relatives might find it hard to cope.

So what is the impact of education and supervision on the auxiliaries' view of their role? It might be expected that education and supervision would influence their 'commonsense' approach, but research on student nurses has shown for example that, whilst they learn one way of doing things in the school, when arriving on the wards they have very much 'worker' status and learn a different and what they see as a more 'real' way to work. Despite being students they frequently receive minimal supervision (Treacy 1987). For the auxiliaries, formal attempts at education and supervision are much less important than for student nurses. Auxiliaries are to an even greater extent assumed to be workers rather than learners and so perhaps it is hardly surprising that the impact of education and training is slight.

Learning the ropes

When asked how much one needed to learn to do the job and how much was 'common sense', a typical answer was that given by Mary:

> '50% common sense, 50% learnt – or maybe 75% common sense.'

Nursing is traditionally seen as 'women's work', and caring for children or parents at home might be seen as similar to an auxiliary's role on the ward. All of the auxiliaries spoken to, who had recently started the job, rejected this view. Elizabeth, for example, found that the work at home was not helpful, other than teaching her not to be squeamish. Auxiliaries had to learn the hospital routine. Surprisingly and paradoxically, although it had to be learnt, they still saw it as 'common sense'. An example was having to use two flannels to wash people with, one for hands and faces and one for 'down below'. This was not done at home but was still 'common sense' once you have been told. This emphasis on learning the routine of a ward, rather than learning to care for people, which might in fact be similar to work done at home, is almost identical to the description of student nurses' experiences (Melia 1981; Treacy 1987).

The auxiliaries described being shown what to do, mostly by other auxiliaries. When asked what they had been 'taught' when starting on a ward, each mentioned activities such as lifting or bedbathing. They generally saw themselves, however, as being expected to 'pick things up as they went along'. Two women had been 'orientated' on their first day, but had been too anxious to remember anything. One had worked for several shifts with the same staff nurse and felt that she had learnt a lot from her. Overall, however, they had learnt by watching. They did not watch trained staff in particular, but whoever was at hand, usually another auxiliary, and questioned whoever was most approachable. Several had found their own 'mentors' in this way. For one woman it was an auxiliary who had started only a few weeks before her. The new auxiliaries described how learning through watching was very difficult, as everyone did the same tasks slightly differently. There were also apparent contradictions. For example, one of the sisters insisted that dirty linen should not be put on the floor. The newcomer then found that everyone did just that. The auxiliaries on that ward rapidly concluded that two types of behaviour were required, one to 'get through the work', and one for when sister was around.

For the auxiliary, as has been said earlier, it was the routine that had to be learnt rather than the nursing. The exception to this was those auxiliaries who had been employed for well over ten years. They had a series of teaching sessions from a charge nurse and had had to complete a booklet of competencies. What they described as important was not so much what they had learnt, but that at that time they were made to feel valued. The knowledge was relevant as they were expected to provide total patient care and their ideas were listened to. Although time may have made the memories happier, it did appear that the feeling of being valued and of the relevance of learning has altered. Many of the auxiliaries more recently employed had not been offered any 'classroom' teaching at all. 14 of the 54 had recently received some training in school and 8 had had some kind of lectures on the ward. (These figures include those employed for ten years or more who had had the lectures when they first started.) They described how they had felt thwarted, as what they had learnt and had been told they were competent to do they were no longer allowed to carry out. Two had recently been offered training but had refused it on the basis that they knew all they needed to do the job. Those who had not been on courses suggested that it would be interesting but irrelevant and this was largely endorsed by those who had recently been on them. Several who had done the courses were not sure what they had been about. In one hospital the auxiliaries were given booklets with a list of competencies to be signed when done satisfactorily under supervision. None of them had used the booklets. Asked what they had learnt that was useful, Rita said that the teacher suggested such things as raising the height of beds to prevent patients getting back into them! This and hints on walking patients from the physiotherapist were the only things mentioned. Clearly the theory/practice gap was as great or greater for these auxiliaries as for student nurses.

When asked what they *needed* to learn, the most frequently cited point was the meaning of abbreviations such as CVA. Several of the auxiliaries wanted to go on to do nurse training, and medical knowledge was of most interest to them and, notably, an understanding of the various illnesses. While in many respects auxiliary work could be described as nursing, nursing knowledge was not of interest to them. Knowing the routine was all the knowledge required for this job.

There was, to the auxiliaries, a clear split between what they did and what the student nurses learned about. The mention of training for Project 2000 caused anxiety, particularly among those who said that they were not very good at written work. They described how they did not teach student nurses, only 'showed them the routine'. The students were 'taught' only during formal teaching sessions.

In discussion with a tutor at one of the hospitals visited, it was commented that the aim of the auxiliaries' course was to teach them what they were not to do. Another said that really the aim was to make them feel important and interested in their job. It may be that, as the auxiliaries feel, they do not need teaching. However, this is presumably based upon the assumption by trained staff (not shared by the auxiliaries) that they are closely supervised. It is the auxiliaries' view of sueprvision that will now be considered in more detail.

Are auxiliaries supervised?

At the time of the fieldwork, auxiliary nurses had been 'regraded' and had received the lower of two possible grades, on the basis that they were supervised in their work. The auxiliaries did not feel that they were supervised, and some had 'worked to grade' for a short period. For example, some auxiliaries had refused to do a bedbath unless accompanied by a trained nurse. They had not continued to 'work to grade' for long, as they felt it was unfair to patients. The new auxiliaries especially were surprised by the extent to which they were just left to 'get on with it'. This was also, however, seen as one of the benefits of the job. Kate, for example, said she had worked for a time with a sister who was always checking up on her. It made her nervous and feel as though she was not trusted. Typically auxiliaries worked together, or on their own. There might be a trained nurse working in the same area as them, but not overtly observing their work.

Assuming that the supervision of the auxiliaries was not done, in that no one watched directly over them, it might be expected that they would be obliged to report back to someone on the work delegated. However, as has been shown, the paperwork associated with the nursing process was not used by the auxiliaries and at ward reports, even when the auxiliaries were present, attention was focused on the medical condition of the patients and not on the nursing care required or received. The auxiliaries themselves felt that, if they had the patient's medical diagnosis, that was all the information they needed. Only Thomas, who had worked in a hospice, had been encouraged by the sister to contribute to a ward report on spiritual or social matters, even if he had nothing on offer on nursing care. On one occasion during the participant observation, a report was given to an auxiliary who had just come on duty by a staff nurse. The auxiliary was specifically told to do various things, including encouraging a patient to eat her tea. Despite this, she still accepted the patient's first refusal to eat her meal. Again, it appears to come back to the auxiliary's belief that nursing knowledge is irrelevant. They have the routine.

The auxiliaries appeared in fact to have little use for the knowledge of trained staff. When asked in the first interview what they might ask trained staff about, Alice and Barbara both looked surprised. They said that they did 'report' things to staff, but that they did not 'ask' them anything. The other auxiliaries gave similar replies. Trained staff knew about dressings, drugs and medical information and required auxiliaries to report any changes to them. Without them they would not know what was going on. Although the auxiliaries were aware of the need to report things, the majority of those observed in their work did not appear aware of what to look out for and therefore report, so that they could not fulfil their good intentions.

Trained staff were rarely seen as either setting a standard or providing a role model. Penny was an exception to this. She had worked for several shifts with a staff nurse when she started and said she was one where you think 'I'd really like to be like her'. But Elizabeth, who had just started, was more typical:

> 'It's surely not right the way [a staff nurse] shouts at patients. I wouldn't like to speak to them like that.'

Another major difficulty mentioned several times was that trained staff contradicted each other. On one ward, for example, three staff nurses provided three sets of directions for handling skeletal traction, so that Sally said,

> 'You just have to remember who said what and do it that way when she's in the room.'

There were also inconsistencies in what was said and done. For example, auxiliaries were told it was important to talk to patients, but trained staff would then hand out jobs to anyone sitting down talking. It would seem that quality of care was important but, not paramount. Penny, despite being fortunate with her initial mentor, soon learnt:

> 'It didn't matter if your standards weren't immaculate, so long as you were quick and remembered to wipe the lockers as well as their faces.'

Auxiliaries also commented that new staff nurses started with new ideas, but in time they would 'get them trained' to their way of thinking. Whilst, formally, trained staff supervised the auxiliaries, on an informal basis it would often apear to be the other way around.

Conclusion

The situation described is one where there is a very strong culture amongst the auxiliaries as regards what is their work. Formal learning and supervision are not seen as relevant. Learning the 'routine' is seen as different from learning that requires knowledge of nursing care. Those more recently employed saw their job more as carrying out discrete tasks than providing total patient care. It has been suggested elsewhere that where auxiliaries work in a role clearly subservient to trained staff there is a risk of their 'potential alienation' (Robinson *et al.* 1989: 31). The training provided for them, and way in which the grade of their job was allocated, reinforces this. The difficulty appears to be that, particularly in the care of the elderly, auxiliaries are in fact the ones doing the nursing. The 'routine' is often nearly all the care the patients get. A study of hospital domestics showed that, when they were encouraged to do only their cleaning, much valuable patient care was lost, decreasing their job satisfaction and also increasing the potential nursing care required (Tonkin and Hart 1989). The effect of emphasizing these specific limits on the role of the auxiliary is likely to have a similar result. The loss of potential care from auxiliaries is however much greater.

The implications for the role of the new support worker can be summarized as follows. First, a clear distinction between her role and that of the trained nurse, which is intended, is likely to result in her feeling less valued and less motivated to care for all the patients' needs. Instead, only specific tasks may be done. Secondly, formal education of the support worker is likely to have little lasting effect on the ward. The impression received from colleagues on the ward will be far more real. Finally there is the possibility of supervision to consider. The evidence presented suggests that the auxiliaries, while feeling they were considered less and less as nurses, did not feel that they were more closely supervised. Where supervision was attempted, it was seen as inappropriate. The trained staff were not seen as having relevant superior knowledge concerning the work the auxiliaries did. In particular it was not apparent in relation to the two main problems faced by auxiliaries. These were providing care within the routine of an institution and dealing with people who could be very difficult to care for. It is not clear that this will be altered with the introduction of Project 2000. The desired outcome of Project 2000 is, one hopes, an improvement in patient care. For this to occur in care of the elderly, the full contribution of the auxiliaries must be understood. If their role is restricted in isolation of other changes, there is a danger that the result may be patients receiving less, not more, care.

References

Beynon, H. and Blackburn, P. M. 1972. *Perceptions of Work*. Cambridge: Cambridge University Press.

Clarke, M. 1978. Getting through the work. In R. Dingwall and J. McIntosh, *Readings in the Sociology of Nursing*, Edinburgh: Churchill Livingstone.

Hardie, M. and Macmillan, M. 1980. The Nursing Auxiliary in the National Health Service. Unpublished report, Edinburgh University.

Lee, T. 1989. 2000 Plus, the new nursing. *Professional Nurse* 5(3): 125–8.

Melia, K. M. 1981. Student nurses: aspects of their work and training: a qualitative analysis. Unpublished PhD thesis, University of Edinburgh.

Payne, M. 1988. Caring in residential homes. *Conference Paper*, British Geriatric Society Annual Conference, London.

RCN. 1989. *The Care of Elderly People – Provision after Griffiths and the NHS White Paper*. ACE/Focus Discussion Paper, London: Royal College of Nursing.

Robinson, J., Stillwell, J., Hawley, C. and Hampstead, N. 1989. *The Role of the Support Worker in the Ward Care Team*, Nursing Policy Centre 6, University of Warwick.

Roth, J. A. 1978. Care of the sick – professionalism versus love. In V. Carver and P. Liddiard, *An Aging Population*, pp. 354–60. London: Hodder & Stoughton.

Tonkin, G. and Hart, E. 1989. I love my work, I hate my job – a study of a hospital domestic. *ESRC Report*, University of Birmingham.

Treacy, M. M. 1987. In the pipeline – a quantitative study of General Nurse Training. Unpublished PhD thesis, University of London.

CHAPTER FIFTEEN

Considerations of personhood in nursing research: an ethical perspective

Kevin Kendrick

Act in such a way that you treat humanity, both in your own person and in the person of all others, never as a means but always equally as an end.

(Immanuel Kant,
Groundwork of the Metaphysics of Morals)

There has been a progressive increase in the amount of nursing research being carried out in Britain over the past 25 years. This is a promising trend which illustrates that nurses are becoming increasingly aware of the need to utilize research in their practice. The result of this has been that the delivery of care is now more likely to be based on insight and understanding rather than tradition alone. To a certain extent, this is a valid response to demands for nursing to become a research-based profession. If other professionals are seen to engage actively in research, then nurses must do likewise if a position of real parity is ever to be achieved.

Many different types of research methodology can be used as a tool for enquiry. To a large degree, the type of method used is often dictated by the nature of the research which is to be carried out and by the personal bias of the researcher. Although there is a choice available regarding what research method is used, the differences between them must be explored if clarity is to be achieved. In order to address the opposing perspectives which exist, consideration must be given to the philosophical differences which occur between quantitative and qualitative research.

Quantitative research

One of the most fundamental of philosophical issues can be found in the question, is social research a science? Quantitative researchers would undoubtedly agree that it is possible to apply the laws of the natural sciences to the social arena and establish causal relationships which are consistent with scientific enquiry. This perspective is sometimes referred to as 'empirical positivism' and it has a long tradition in the historical development of quantitative research.

The person accredited with introducing the notion is Auguste Comte (1798–1857), who believed that it was possible to have a science of society based on the principles of cause and effect which are found in the natural, physical sciences. This approach makes a number of assumptions about the nature and behaviour of persons. If positivism is considered in terms of logical progression, then the behaviour of people is said to be open to the same objective measurement as matter. If scientific rationale is to be considered valid, then it is necessary to quantify this matter in terms of some acceptable measurement. This type of enquiry has been largely adopted and accepted as a positive mechanism by medical scientists. There are many examples of causal relationships in the aetiology of disease processes; we are told that smoking cigarettes causes lung cancer, that atheroma causes heart disease, and that viruses cause influenza. All of these examples can be considered through scientific scrutiny and may be open to a certain amount of quantifiable observation. However, for the positivist it is feasible to take the methods used in this type of enquiry to establish causal links for human behaviour.

If we consider elements of nursing research which may be quantified, it seems reasonable to accept the notion that certain physiological parameters may fit the criteria for being considered as 'facts'. A person may have measurements taken of temperature, weight or blood pressure which can be taken as objective statements of physiological fact. The quantitative researcher who wishes to pursue a line of pure, positivistic enquiry would also argue that similar criteria could be devised to predict the behaviour of patients under certain circumstances. For example, the majority of people entering hospital put on their nightwear even during the day; this is in compliance with the unwritten code of the hospital ethos. This is a type of behaviour which can be observed and quantified without having to give any interpretation to the meanings that people associate with it. The end of this scenario is that nurse researchers who take this approach believe that it forms a valid foundation for reliable data.

The orientation which Comte instigated gained further support from the work of Emile Durkheim, who argued that science was concerned with the study of 'things' and that social observation should be carried out in the same way. He tried to illustrate that concepts such as religious belief or societal customs could be observed in the same way as objects in the physical world. The central theme which Durkheim tried to present was that social facts may impinge upon the individual's consciousness but that they still remain external and, therefore, may be studied by using objective criteria. Human behaviour is shaped and influenced by these social facts which contribute towards a collective way of thinking or acting. Durkheim produced a famous work on the nature of suicide to try and validate his positivistic stance. This presented an argument that suicide is not merely an act of individual consciousness but is influenced and caused by external social factors. This gave Durkheim a firm conviction that social phenomena are similar to natural phenomena in respect of the laws which govern their action. Given this fact, Durkheim maintained that the only valid criterion for producing research in the social realm is to use natural science methodology.

The concept of cause and effect is very much reflected in the philosophy of biomedical science, and to a certain extent this is acceptable because it is physical phenomena which are being observed. However, if we accept the perspective of philosophers like Comte and Durkheim then the same approach may be taken in observing human behaviour. This may be expressed in the following way:

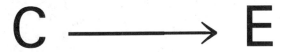

This is an acceptable model if 'C' represents a person sitting on a pin and 'E' represents the recoil due to pain. This simplistic representation shows that it is possible to explain human behaviour when it operates at the level of a reflex. The methods of causation become more complex when a number of factors are introduced into the equation. Let us consider the example given earlier of the person who enters hospital and puts on night attire in the middle of the day. Quantitative researchers would argue that the observation of this act is sufficient to validate it as data. The higher-order cognitions to do with why the person acted in this way and what meaning he/she can bring to illustrate their present state are thought to be unimporant in the search for scientific objectivity. The glaring problem with taking this approach is that the individual who is supposed to form the focal point of nursing or health research seems to have been left out of the equation.

If we leave a person out of the research process in terms of ignoring their cognitive elements then it would appear impossible to claim anything like an approximation towards understanding a given social reality. It is at this point that we can introduce the concept of qualitative research as an alternative perspective in research methodology.

Qualitative research

In sharp contrast to the philosophy of positivism, qualitative research places a great deal of emphasis upon the importance of interpreting meaning in the research process. This reflects the ethos of a philosophical theme called phenomenology.

Phenomenology is concerned with placing the person at the centre of the research process; persons are more than just a collection of atoms and molecules. Duffy (1985) continues this theme by arguing that persons cannot be viewed merely as objects. In the social arena, qualitative researchers take the stance that persons are not merely acted upon by social forces but that they react to them through a dynamic dialogue with fellow actors. If a researcher accepts that a person plays an active role in creating social reality, then research must be aimed at gaining insight and at interpreting the meaning which people give to social phenomena.

It is because emphasis is placed upon the importance of

meaning that qualitative research believes that the notion of values cannot be divorced from an enquiry which involves people. This is in contrast to the central theme of positivism which maintains that research must be value free if a position of true scientific objectivity is to be achieved. If phenomenology is used as the underpinning philosophy, then the main focus must be placed upon research which attempts to understand human behaviour from the agent's perspective.

From the perspective of phenomenology, there exists a fundamental difference between the subject matter of the natural sciences and that of persons. Physical matter does not have cognitive processes which are expressed through the conscious elements of the person. It is justified, therefore, to consider the reaction of matter when subjected to external stimuli. Matter is compelled to react in a preordained way because it cannot introduce any sense, interpretation or meaning to its behaviour. However, a person does have the facility to bring meaning to a given behaviour and to interpret and experience the construction of social reality.

Phenomenology research argues that attempting to quantify human behaviour is not possible through the use of scientific enquiry in the objective sense. If we consider the human condition in the same way as the physical sciences then we present a threat to the unique nature of individuality and freedom. It seems difficult to conceptualize a person as being at liberty to interact if the positivistic stance of being constantly under the influence of societal laws is to be understood in terms of the definitive. Howarth (1981) considers that positivistic research imposes a view of the person which is reminiscent of the reductionistic and materialistic perspectives which are favoured by the natural sciences. If an individual is seen through the perspective of positivism, then he/she is reduced to the unconscious level of elements used in the phsyical sciences. The term 'materialistic' is used because the person's cognitive processes are ignored in the search for an objective equation which will explain causal links in human behaviour.

What is starting to emerge here is similar to the stance which Henry (1987) takes in arguing that the concept of personhood is central to nursing and, therefore, must also take a dominant theme in any research which is carried out. This approach may be represented in the following way:

$$C \longrightarrow P \longrightarrow E$$

The important issue here is that the person has been placed firmly at the centre of any observable phenomena. The cause does not bring about an immediate effect; the person at the centre of the dynamic interprets whatever the information is through the avenue of cognitive processes. The effectual end of this scenario will be the result of a person bringing interpretation and meaning to a given situation.

Taking either a positivist or a phenomenological approach to research will strongly influence how it is conducted. Each philosophical theme will have an effect on the way in which measures are made or interpreted in a particular research project. However, it must be emphasized once again that natural science explanations of the world are based upon conceptions of things. In nursing research, it is essential to explore forms of knowledge more appropriately matched to conceptions of care. The main focus for the nurse researcher is interacting with persons within a health care environment. In this respect, the term 'person' is an evaluative oral term and is not used to describe an object or a thing in the world.

The process of research in nursing can strongly influence how we construe things. Because this process is concerned with two dominant elements – the concept of the person and the concept of care – then it is suitable to consider the ethical dimensions which can be introduced as a means of enhancing the relationship which is present between the researcher and persons involved in the study. The most essential ethical principle when undertaking nursing research must be an acknowledgement of 'respect for persons'.

Respect for persons

This is a central ethical doctrine which demands that any research involving people should place a great deal of emphasis upon the importance of autonomy, partnership and informed consent. If these concepts are acknowledged as playing a central role in the research process, then it suggests that the researcher accepts that persons have both an inherent worth and value. This is an excellent basis for enquiry because it means that persons are not merely being used as vehicles for substantiating the validity of a given theory. In terms of the approach which the philosopher Immanuel Kant would take, the researcher who has a respect for persons is using them not merely as a means to an end, but as valued ends in their own right. It is of the essence that nursing research should hold this principle at the centre of any project which involves persons and their care.

We have said that a respect for persons involves the acceptance of them having intrinsic worth and value. Harris (1985) argues that it also means that someone who has a respect for persons must show both a concern for their welfare and respect for their wishes. In health care ethics there is sometimes a degree of conflict between the wishes of the patient and concern for their welfare. For example, a person may express an intense desire to smoke following surgery of the stomach. The nurse realizes that this might result in a coughing episode which could rupture the wound. In this instance, the nurse would probably go against the patient's wishes in trying to maintain a respect for his/her physical welfare. This scenario is fraught with ethical issues regarding patient autonomy, paternalism and competency. There is no need to consider these concepts in detail as they were only introduced to show that conflict can occur between the expressed wishes of the patients and respect for their welfare. However, in nursing research it is unlikely that dilemmas of this nature will arise and the relationship between respect for a person's welfare and wishes should be both complementary and reciprocal.

Earlier in this chapter it was stated that the type of methodology employed will be influenced by the personal bias of the researcher and the type of data that are to be collected. The central theme of this chapter is concerned with presenting ethical and philosophical considerations about personhood in the research process. Because nursing research is concerned primarily with studying the delivery and effect of care, then the nature of ethical principles will be considered within a methodological framework which enables the nurse researcher to practise whilst formulating and collecting data; the research tool being referred to here is participant observation.

Participant observation: research as an adaptive partnership

Participant observation has a long history in social science research and involves the researcher joining in the everyday routines of those who are to be studied and observed. For the nurse researcher, this would involve joining the normal, natural environment of the ward. Although participant observation may be used by researchers with either a quantitative or a qualitative background, it is particularly favoured by those who adopt a phenomenological approach. However, like all methods of research, participant observation has both positive and negative aspects associated with it.

(1) Participant observation (PO) allows the nurse researcher to consider the patient's conception of objects and events by being a part of that person's activities during the hospital stay.

(2) PO is sometimes criticized because it is said that the researcher cannot gain access to the group's social reality because the presence of a stranger will inhibit normal social intercourse. This criticism is not valid in nursing research because the process is usually carried out by a nurse who is familiar with the norms, culture and values of the hospital environment.

(3) Because a nurse is already a part of the world which he/she wishes to study, then there is little likelihood of them imposing a false and detached reality upon the social world which they are seeking to understand. If a structured methodology was introduced, for example, a structured interview with a predetermined set of questions or a questionnaire with pre-set questions, then the researcher has already decided what is of importance. If a nurse researcher takes a number of prepared enquiries to a patient then a framework is being introduced which imposes personal research priorities upon those who are to be studied. When this is done, assumptions have already been made about how the patient perceives social reality within the confines of the hospital.

(4) Positivistic researchers claim that the data that are obtained from participant observation are unreliable. Objective scientific research involves using the same method of investigation upon the same types of material and that this should reproduce the same types of result. Very few social researchers would claim that the same degree of exactitude could be achieved in the

area of social research. However, they do claim that a certain degree of reliability is possible to achieve. Criticism is levelled at participant observation because its procedures are not made explicit, that the observations do not follow a systematic pattern and that the results obtained are rarely quantified.

(5) Participant observation relies greatly upon interpretive skills, and their value lies in providing useful insights into the meanings which persons put upon events which form social reality.

If the nurse researcher utilizes participant observation as a tool, then he/she is attempting to come face to face with the reality of the patient's experience. It is possible only to approximate towards an understanding of social reality; participant observation acknowledges this problem, but still enables the researcher to make valid observations. The researcher who adopts this approach must gain the trust of those who are to be observed. This demands that certain ethical principles are adhered to and the most effective means of achieving this is by viewing the person in a research programme as an equal partner in the understanding of our social world. This last point is of the essence when applied to nursing research.

Adaptive partnership

The notions of adaptation and partnership are not new to nursing theory but basing them firmly within a framework of ethical rationale and principles certainly is. The way in which people react to being in hospital can cover every aspect of the emotional spectrum. The nurse researcher can provide an avenue through which these issues can be addressed. In this way, a vital element of participant observation is advanced, the process of sharing information which reflects the meaning which patients put upon events relating to their present state.

Another proviso for partnership is that the nurse researcher must treat the patient as a complete equal. As Seedhouse (1988: 132) states:

the requirement to respect persons equally when working for health follows from the requirement to create and respect autonomy in all people, and from the work by philosophers establishing basic criteria for personhood. We regard people as valuable not only because of what each person can do, but essentially because of what each person is.

The requirement to treat people as equals is very important when considering the process of adaptation. A person in hospital has to adapt to a whole plethora of changing circumstances; treating the person as an equal demands that the nurse researcher complement the uniqueness of the patient by adapting knowledge to suit the patient's abilities and demands. If this approach is taken then it forms a foundation on which to base a plan of action which views the nurse researcher and the patient as equals in an adaptive partnership.

We have already discussed the rationale for utilizing participant observation in the process of nursing research. The next stage must be to consider certain ethical principles which must be recognized if the concept of the person is to remain central to the notion of research.

Ethics in nursing research

The concepts of autonomy and informed consent are of vital importance in nursing research. In certain respects the two terms are inextricable, but, in order to achieve clarity, the concepts will be considered separately before common strands and themes are drawn together.

Autonomy

In its purest form, the term 'autonomy' is used with reference to self-rule or self-government; Beauchamp and Childress (1982: 59) present the following interpretation.

> The most general idea of personal autonomy is still that of self governance: being one's own person, without constraints either by another's action or by psychological or physical limitations. The autonomous person determines his or her course of action in accordance with a plan chosen by himself or herself. Such a person deliberates about and chooses plans and is capable of acting on the basis of such deliberations, just as truly independent government is capable of controlling its territories and policies.

This interpretation of autonomy suggests a number of things. It implies that persons have the ability to express a dynamic and subjective orientation; furthermore, it suggests that autonomy is expressed through active participation within decisions. It also leads us to the position that an autonomous person is able to think about ends and to decide what means shall be utilized to achieve those ends. However, if we apply this to health care ethics it becomes evident that a person is unable to take any action in isolation because it is highly unlikely that any social factors are not involved and also that it will not affect somebody else. As an example, if a nurse researcher takes an action within his or her professional role, it is difficult to envisage this as not having some sort of effect upon other people within the health care environment, be they colleagues, patients or visitors. This brings us back to an earlier position: it is difficult to separate and isolate social actions from the meanings and consequences which they bring. Therefore, if all observable phenomena in the social realm are interrelated with factors such as judgements, interpretation and other subjective operations, then it is impossible to compartmentalize them in terms of a purely objective framework. The phenomenological researchers call this the relationship between the knower and the known (Henry 1987).

Autonomy is vitally important in nursing research if the patient is to be viewed as an end in his/her own right. This ties in completely with the notion of 'respect for persons' because it emphasizes that any person who forms the subject of a research project should be enabled to express autonomy within that context. In practical terms, this means that the nurse researcher must give the person as much information as he/she requires not only regarding the nature of the research, but also relating to the nursing care which is an inherent part of using participant observation in nursing research. The concept which is used to describe this process of information exchange is 'informed consent'.

Informed consent in nursing research

Herbert (1988: 1043) offers us a traditional interpretation of what is meant by the doctrine of informed consent:

an informed consent is that consent which is obtained after the patient has been adequately instructed about the ratio of risk and benefit involved in the procedure as compared to alternative procedures or no treatment at all.

It has already been said that the principles of informed consent and autonomy are largely interwoven. In terms of nursing research, this refers to the researcher's obligation to maintain the patient's dignity and integrity whilst attempting to achieve a partnership which will allow access to how a person perceives reality whilst in the hospital environment. The doctrine of informed consent is of vital and central importance to anybody involved in nursing research; a patient must be privy to the aims and objectives of how the programme will relate to him/her if the research is to be viewed as ethically valid. Faulder (1985: 32) comments on the importance of gaining a position of clarity over informed consent by stating:

> This is not obtuse pedantry. An important principle lies behind a deceptively simple formula; its words are burdened with shades of meaning which we must clarify in our own minds before we can use it.

If a person does not give a nurse researcher permission to take a certain form of action, then the researcher has no moral basis for instigating the action. It follows from this that it is vitally important that the patient understands, as far as is possible, the different permutations associated with the research. The nurse researcher, who is also practising, must ensure that the person is as fully aware as he or she wishes to be regarding a given nursing action. If this position is not adhered to, then it is not possible to say with certainty that a person has given a full and informed consent. If a nurse researcher performs a given action without the permission of the patient, then he/she performs an act which violates the individual. The consequences of such a situation can be grave and may even constitute negligence in legal terms (Kennedy and Grubb 1989: 225).

It is important that a great deal of emphasis is placed upon autonomy and informed consent during the research process in nursing. We discussed earlier the nature of qualitative and quantitative research and that it is the concept of the person which must form the focal point of whichever philosophical perspective is followed. However, if this is to be a formative endeavour then it must be underpinned with an ethical rationale such as that suggested here with autonomy and informed consent. Adopting this perspective provides us with the fundamental ethos of the relationship which should exist between persons in the research process, as Dyer and Bloch (1987: 12) have argued:

> It is the principle of partnership endowed with the qualities of mutual trust and human sincerity which may help health professionals aspire to the pursuit of the ethical principles which underlie informed consent.

The concept of freedom also plays a fundamental role in discussions concerning consent. It is not possible to do justice to a topic as vast as freedom in the confines of this discussion owing to its immense complexity; but it does merit some mention.

For the nurse researcher, freedom shoud be used to mean the liberty the patient has to do one thing rather than another. This is an integral element of enabling the person to express autonomy. This is another reason why the research process should be based on the interpretation of meaning; persons cannot be restricted by the clearly defined criteria of natural scientific enquiry, as Haring (1975: 135) informs us:

> the transfer of the natural scientific model to society is criminal in the eyes of critical theory. It represents the original sin of positivistic society.

Conclusion

This chapter has been concerned with the philosophical and ethical issues relating to persons in nursing research. If the people taking part in the research are fully informed of the ramifications associated with it and knowingly give their consent, then autonomy, individuality and dignity are being respected. Research in nursing can do much to enhance the care which people receive from practitioners; it can help deliver the nurse from being a dictator of practice to becoming a partner in practice with the patient. As Faulder (1985: 106) tells us:

Their trust must not be abused, nor their altruism. These human and moral considerations are more important than any scientific advance, and it is these obligations which impose the limits to science.

References

Beauchamp, T. L. and Childress, J. F. 1982. *Principles of Biomedical Ethics.* Oxford: Oxford University Press.
Duffy, M. 1985. Designing nursing research: the qualitative–quantitative debate. *Journal of Advanced Nursing* 10; 225–32.
Dyer, A. R. and Bloch, S. 1987. Informed consent and the psychiatric patient. *Journal of Medical Ethics* 13: 12–16.
Faulder, C. 1985. *Whose Body is It? The Troubling Issue of Informed Consent.* London: Virago Press.
Haring, B. 1975. *Manipulation: Ethical Boundaries of Medical, Behavioural and Genetic Manipulation.* Slough: St Paul's Publications.
Harris, J. 1985. *The Value of Life: An introduction to medical ethics.* London: Routledge & Kegan Paul.
Henry, I. C. 1986. Conceptions of the nature of persons. Unpublished PhD thesis, Leeds University.
Herbert, V. 1988. Informed consent – a legal evaluation. *Cancer* 46(4): 1043.
Howarth, C. F. 1981. The nature of psychological knowledge. In *The Structure of Psychology.* London: Allen & Unwin.
Kennedy, I. and Grubb, A. 1989. *Medical Law: Text and Materials.* London: Butterworth.
Seedhouse, D. 1988. *Ethics: The Heart of Health Care.* Chichester: John Wiley.

PART IV

Management

Recent concern about the problems of recruiting sufficient nurses for the future has highlighted nurse workforce planning as an essential activity for the nursing profession and for the health service in general. Nurse wastage is both a curious term and a curious phenomenon. Indeed, Jon Barry, Catherine Williams and Keith Soothill argue in 'Managing Nurse Wastage' (Chapter 16) that the issue of wastage is much more complicated than is generally recognized and that, at present, available information is not being properly or fully used to answer the important questions. They also discuss how specialized surveys can, when combined with information routinely collected on computer by personnel departments, produce important insights into this often puzzling phenomenon.

David Worthington's purpose in his chapter on 'Nurse Supply Modelling' (Chapter 17) is to introduce nurses and prospective nurses to the concept and potential value of nurse supply modelling in the current planning context. A clear discussion of this technical topic focusing on some of the important issues related to the practical application of nurse supply modelling leads to an assessment of its likely role and value to the nursing profession and to the health service, now and in the future.

During the last decade there has been much challenge to traditional working practices in many occupations. In most fields of employment the position of trade unions has come under increasing focus. Management always needs to consider its stance towards bodies whose task is to represent their members' interest. Certainly the actions of nurses' trade unions and professional organizations have had quite unprecedented media attention in recent years. Paul Bagguley's chapter (Chapter 18) examines the principal trade unions and professional organizations amongst professionally qualified nurses, and their diverse strategies for advancing the interests of the professional nurse. Using empirical data from a district health authority, he goes on to consider patterns of organizational membership and nurses' assessments of the service provided by their organizations. Finally, he engages in some speculation on the recent changes in nursing for organizations seeking to represent professional nurses.

Part IV concludes with the chapter by Stephen Ackroyd (Chapter 19) which focuses on the prospect of participative management in the NHS. First, he develops the important thesis that the management of public services is a different type of activity from management in most parts of the private sector. He then goes on to consider the development of the NHS, applying the three patterns of public sector management he has identified to the case of the hospital service in the NHS. He points to the progressive alienation of senior nurses from key managerial functions, which, he argues, has contributed to a drop in morale amongst nurses. Ackroyd maintains that the nurse, as the person who shapes the interface between the organization and its clientele, must become the key contributor to a new system of cooperative management.

CHAPTER SIXTEEN

Managing nurse wastage

Jon Barry, Keith Soothill and Catherine Williams

Introduction

'Nurse wastage' is a popular phrase these days – not only among health authority planners but also among journalists, social scientists and, in particular, nurses themselves. But what exactly is nurse wastage and how do we measure it? Is it a problem and, if so, how can it be reduced? One might have hoped that questions like these had nice simple answers and that someone, somewhere, had everything under control; in short, that nurse wastage was being properly managed.

Unfortunately, as we argue in this chapter, at present this is not the case. However, this is not surprising. The organizational and social problems with managing nurse wastage in a large and diffuse body like the National Health Service are immense. However, we believe that the problems are not insurmountable and that, technically, with the advent of the computerization of personnel records, vast improvements are possible.

There have been many articles expressing concern about the problems of recruitment in the NHS (e.g. Dickson 1987; Hancock 1986). This is especially true in light of the current and projected shortfall of 18 years olds eligible to enter nursing. Coupled with these recruitment concerns have been worries about the high level of turnover among nurses already employed (Price Waterhouse 1988; Martin and Mackean 1988; Waite et al. 1989). However, there has also been at least one conflicting article (Grocott 1989), which argues that wastage is not a problem because, while numbers of new learners are declining, the total workforce is actually increasing; in other words, that more previously qualified nurses are going back into nursing.

During this chapter we try to unravel the complicated issue of nurse wastage. We argue that, without a proper understanding of the problem, effective management is impossible. We begin with a brief discussion of nurse wastage and offer ideas about how it might be defined in different situations. We follow this analysis by examining whether wastage is a major problem today and if so, which aspects are most important. Finally, we discuss the implications of our findings for nurse managers.

Nurse wastage

Before a manager can decide whether nurse wastage is a problem and, if so, what to do about it, it is essential that he or she is clear about what wastage actually means. Unfortunately, a clear definition is not always obvious. In this section, we give our own definition of nurse wastage and discuss ways in which numerical summaries can be formulated. Finally, we discuss the effects of different types of wastage on the individual district and regional health authorities and on the NHS as a whole.

In the academic literature, nurse wastage has mostly been used as a general term to describe the number of nurses leaving in some given time period. That is, it has been taken as another word for nurse turnover. However, we feel that wastage encompasses more than this narrow definition.

The term 'wastage' implies that something is being unnecessarily thrown away. In our case, this 'something' includes, first, the training and experience that the nurse has gained; and, secondly, the cost of recruiting new staff. There are some other, less obvious, forms of wastage that can take place while a nurse is still in post. For example, wastage could also be considered in terms of absenteeism or lack of commitment due to becoming disillusioned with the job. That is, potential work is being wasted because a nurse is not happy with what she is doing. Another 'hidden' form of wastage occurs when a shortage of specialized nurses causes unqualified or non-specialized nurses to be employed in these specialized positions. Inevitably, the result of this is to reduce the standard and efficiency of working. However, while these other forms of wastage are of undoubted importance, here we will restrict ourselves to considering only the first two forms of wastage mentioned above – that is, looking at wastage in terms of wasted training and the cost of recruiting new staff. We will return to these ideas after we have looked at the standard ways in which health authorities (HAs) calculate summaries of wastage.

At present, most health authorities calculate wastage in six-monthly or yearly periods. This is done by dividing the number of leavers in the period by the average number of nurses employed during the period. Finally, this figure is multiplied by 100 to give wastage as a percentage. This is, however, not the only way to summarize nurse wastage numerically. For example, Bartholomew (1976) suggests using the time taken for some fraction of a cohort of nurses (say, all those in post on 1 January 1990) to leave employment or, conversely, the proportion of a cohort who survive for some specified period (e.g. 80 per cent of the above January cohort may have stayed for at least one year). One advantage of Bartholomew's suggestions is that they give a feel for whether the main turnover takes place among a small or a large proportion of the nurses. With the standard method currently used it is impossible to determine this.

Returning to the two types of wastage mentioned earlier, we can see that, even with these definitions, matters can become quite complicated. For example, as Grocott (1989) mentions, we can consider wastage in at least three strata. Grocott suggests that wastage can be divided into district (those leaving the district HA), regional (those leaving the regional HA) and national (those leaving the NHS altogether) levels. Grocott makes the point that, as far as the NHS is concerned, a nurse is not wasted if she joins an HA in another district or region and, similarly, as far as the region is concerned, a nurse is not wasted if she moves to an HA within the same region.

Certainly Grocott's analysis has been helpful in disentangling these various levels and he uses this approach to challenge whether there really is a problem of wastage. Indeed, Grocott claims that the total workforce within nursing is increasing and that the cries of the possible dire effects of a 'demographic timebomb' whereby nurse recruitment may be in jeopardy owing to the decreasing numbers of 18 year olds in Britain may well be exaggerated. Whether or not one accepts his full argument, it still stems from his analysis that the problem of nursing wastage is a relative one. So, for example, it is highly dependent on region, for no one doubts that there are immense pressures in some geographical areas unmatched by similar concerns elsewhere. Nevertheless, Grocott's work has enabled a fresh look at our first form of wastage, namely wastage in terms of wasted training.

While Grocott's arguments may hold for our first definition of wastage, they do not satisfy the second, in that for any move there is still the cost of recruiting and possibly retraining the new nurse. Of course, we must consider whether a stagnant workforce with no turnover might also be undesirable and if a certain amount of wastage should be tolerated, or even encouraged. Indeed, towards the end of the 1970s it was the concern about a stagnant workforce with no turnover which some (e.g. Redfern 1978) recognized as an equally serious problem. Hence, we need to consider the complex question of whether current levels of wastage are acceptable or whether they are a problem which needs management action.

Is there a wastage problem?

We have mentioned the dire warnings being expressed about the effect of the shortfall in 18 year olds on nursing recruitment. The problems associated with this, so-called, 'demographic timebomb' will be further amplified by the introduction of Project 2000 – where the aim is for learners to spend more time actually *learning*, as opposed to *doing* and to be supernumerary to the operation of wards. There is also evidence that regions and specialities are affected differently. As Pilkington (1989) points out, recruitment is a problem in some city regions such as London but in more rural areas the problem is often that there is insufficient finance to employ nurses.

However, not all authors think that the problems are as serious as these comments suggest. For example, Grocott (1989) has claimed that the number of learners is decreasing and yet the total workforce is increasing. From this, Grocott infers that *real* wastage must be decreasing in that the number leaving the profession is less than the number joining in. However, this inference may be too simplistic. For instance, part of the increase in nurse members may be due to the employment of more nursing auxiliaries who are recruited from a different pool from enrolled and staff nurses.

There have been many conflicting claims and arguments over the past decade about nursing wastage. The government's view of turnover/wastage among nurses remains complex and often contradictory. Only reluctantly during the latter part of the 1980s did the government begin to acknowledge a crisis in the health service of which nurses' concerns were a part.

Throughout the last decade, however, one consistent theme of the government has been in restricting the growth of the public sector and arguing that increasing costs in this sector have been damaging to the economy. As a consequence, there was no fundamental support or affinity with the difficulties and concerns of the nursing profession during the early days of the 'Thatcher revolution'. However, increasingly, since the mid-1980s the government has been forced to acknowledge that nurses' claims – in terms of both pay and other issues – cannot just be swept aside. While industrial action is a tactic which excites much controversy within the ranks of nursing (see Chapter 18 on 'Angels in Red? Patterns of Union Membership amongst UK Professional Nurses'), it is implicitly recognized by the government that industrial action by nurses may well receive sympathy and tacit support among the public in ways which most other public servants cannot – or have learned not to – expect. Pay, of course, was readily identified by government, opposition politicians, trade unions and the media as the main focus of concern. However, the range of issues which required attention soon emerged to run more deeply within the nursing profession than the familiar sore of low pay. More recently, the acceptance in large part of the recommendations of the UKCC's proposals on Project 2000 indicated that the government was willing to recognize that fundamental reorganization of the training and education of the nursing profession was required. The essential dilemma for the government remains that nursing 'wastage' and difficulties of recruitment in some district health authorities and regions – with the consequent effect of closed wards and reduced services – provide a ready and identifiable mark of failure which can easily be highlighted by the media and the political opposition parties. So the issue remains firmly on the agenda and many of the conflicting claims and arguments still have a strong currency.

In order to throw light upon some of the emerging conflicts and contradictions, the Review Body for Nursing Staff, Midwives, Health Visitors and Professions Allied to Medicine was set up in

1983 to publish a yearly report. It is interesting to summarize recent progress in the way that the Review Body has been able to obtain information. Although the quality of data being collected in improving, even the survey reported in 1990 was far from perfect.

In 1988 the Review Body reported on a survey of 40 district HAs (there are well over 250 in Great Britain) from which information was returned by 29 of them. Considering the vast differences between different areas of the country, this sample must be considered inadequate. For their 1989 report, responsibility for the survey passed to the Office of Manpower Economics. They surveyed all 222 HAs (or equivalent) in Great Britain and just under 200 replied. Although this response was a great improvement on the previous survey, analyses in the report were based on responses from only 95 of the HAs because a number of queries caused by the extra work involved in regrading nurses could not be resolved before the report was written. Finally, in 1990, survey returns were collected from 210 HAs, although only 182 were of sufficient quality to be used in the analysis (a further 52 of these could not be used for all analyses). Although we do not intend to go into much detail about the actual wastage figures, the main conclusions from the available data were that the overall staffing problem was being kept under control but that there were quite large variations in vacancy rates by region. In particular, the three-month vacancy rate for qualified staff in the London weighting zones was much higher than in the rest of Britain.

However, while we applaud the efforts made so far, we feel that the type of information collected by the Review Body is not sufficient to tackle the complexities of the wastage problem. Even within its own terms, there is still a need to ensure complete and accurate information from all of the HAs. However, the approach used has considerable limitations in the value of the information produced. Of equal, if not greater, importance is the need to look at wastage in a longitudinal rather than simply in a cross-sectional manner. That is, as well as quoting wastage rates at fixed points in time, we also need to know the turnover of nurses through time. For example, longitudinal analysis can show whether the workforce is largely static and whether it is a comparatively small proportion who leave rapidly or, alternatively, whether the employment time of all nurses in an organization is comparatively short lived. So, to take the example further, 25 per cent of a workforce may move every three months but the remaining 75 per cent of the workforce remains in post for many years. This is a very different pattern from all of the workforce moving after a year in post, and yet both organizations would return a yearly wastage rate of 100 per cent. The wastage figures may be the same, but the problems for the two organizations are very different. High turnover can be expensive in terms of time spent interviewing and training new staff as well as causing a disruption to the smooth running of patient care, but it is the *nature* of the turnover which can be crucial in trying to manage nurse wastage. A longitudinal approach would certainly give a better understanding of the ways in which nurses move in and out of the workforce.

Detailed longitudinal data such as these may seem difficult to collect but, in fact, HAs do have such data in their records. What is needed are systematic ways of gaining access to and using the available data (Barry *et al.* 1989). Of course, some types of information are not routinely stored and can be obtained only by asking nurses themselves. Sometimes progress can be made by combining the results of information which could be routinely published (but rarely is) with material from more specialized surveys. We report on such a study in the next two sections.

Estimating the nature of the problem

Grocott's recent work challenging whether there is indeed a wastage problem and proposing that, in fact, the total workforce is increasing is only the latest example of shifts in locating the nature of the problem.

Our own work developed as an implicit response to the view expressed in the second report of the Review Body for Nursing Staff, Midwives, Health Visitors and Professions Allied to Medicine (page 7) in June 1985 that '*in the management's view* only a very small proportion [of nurses] left the NHS for reasons of dissatisfaction' (our emphasis). This view did not seem to tally with other kinds of comments being made around that time. Our contribution has been to identify some of the recurring themes which emerge when you talk to *nurses* or ask them to respond to questionnaires. Mackay (1989) largely focused on the response to interviews. However, as part of this previous project a questionnaire was sent to all nurses in post in one health authority on

1 July 1986 and asked, among many other things, 'Will you leave this hospital within the next twelve months?' The possible reply options provided to this question were 'no chance', 'slight chance', 'definitely' or 'uncertain'. A documentary follow-up from the personnel records of this health authority over a three-year period charting the actual outcome for these nurses has produced some insights into the nature of the labour turnover problem for this health authority at least (Soothill *et al.* 1990).

In brief, the result showed that, after *one* year (which directly related to the question asked of the nurses), 52 per cent of those who said they would definitely leave had indeed done so. However, although nurses who expressed a slight chance of leaving came next in terms of percentage leaving (17 per cent), in practice this figure is little different from that of 'no chance' (6 per cent) and 'uncertain' (10 per cent) categories.

Interestingly, nurses who said they would definitely leave continued to have a much higher proportion of leavers in subsequent years as well. So, of those among the 'definitely' leaving group who were still there after one year, a further 33 per cent left within the second year; similarly, of those remaining after two years, a further 29 per cent left within the third year. The final outcome was that, by the end of three years, 77 per cent of those who thought they would definitely leave had indeed left. Hence, we can successfully identify a core group of 'leavers' who could be said to have a general propensity to leave, simply by asking whether they intended to leave.

In contrast, for the remainder, who ranged from saying that there was a 'slight chance', 'no chance' or were simply 'uncertain', the majority (72 per cent) were still in post, even after three years. Hence, overall these persons demonstrate a propensity to stay.

Having separated out the nurses into these two major groups of those, on the one hand, who are likely to stay (of whom around three-quarters do so even after three years) and those, on the other hand, who are likely to leave (of whom around three-quarters do so within three years), the crucial question for managers is the size of the respective groups. In other words, do they have vast numbers in the 'core leavers' group or, more hopefully for them, vast numbers in the 'core stayers' group.

For the health authority in the present study we fond that there were around 10 per cent in the 'core leavers' group (of whom 77 per cent actually left) while there were nearly 90 per cent in the 'core stayers' group (of whom 72 per cent actually stayed). This kind of distinction can lead to further analyses which attempt, for instance, to probe the differences between the 'core leavers' and 'core stayers' and, even more subtly, what causes those to stay in post who actually expect to leave and what causes those to leave who generally felt it likely they would stay (Soothill *et al.* 1990). Whether these figures on core leavers and stayers from our HA are typical values can be assessed only when comparable studies in other districts or regions are carried out. Nevertheless, it does show for this health authority something of the nature of their turnover problem. If they were able to take the analysis further to probe which specialisms have significant numbers saying they are likely to leave, then it could be worthwhile for an organization to carry out an in-depth study to assess what are the factors which produce such large numbers of 'core leavers' among certain groups. However, this raises issues of confidentiality and anonymity which need to be faced by managers in initiating, analysing and interpreting turnover data.

Elsewhere (Soothill *et al.* 1990) we have stressed that, as an independently financed research team from a university, we could assure the nurse respondents of anonymity and hence we maintain that the response to the question asking about leaving intentions was much more likely to be valid – or at least as genuine a response as the nurses could give at the time – than if a similar survey were launched by their direct employers.

Why do nurses leave?

While it is useful to know something of the nature of the turnover problem, it still fails to engage with what many regard as the crux of the issue, namely, why do nurses leave? Asking nurses why they are leaving is another delicate methodological problem regarding the quality of information one might receive. Many personnel departments of health authorities are improving the quality of their leaving interviews and, unlike previous times, making a much more significant effort to find out why their nurses are leaving. This is laudable and worthwhile, for many useful hints may emerge which in turn could lead to useful change. However, personnel managers must avoid deluding themselves that improving the procedures will resolve the issue entirely. In fact, many employees leaving an organization will feel they must construct a reason or set of reasons which avoid potential trouble for, after all, most will usually need in the future a reference from key members of the organization they are leaving. Others, with perhaps less caution, may emphasize a particularly upsetting incident which will suggest that the reasons for leaving are more of a personality clash than some more fundamental structural reason within the working environment which may have led to the incident occurring. The possibilities are enormous, but there are dangers in trusting entirely the responses formulated at a leaving interview conducted by the personnel department of an employing organization.

In 1989 we conducted a questionnaire and interview study at this same health authority. As part of the study, questionnaires were sent to 254 nurses who had left during the preceding three years. Of these, 90 were returned and fully completed. Although the response rate of 38 per cent might appear fairly low, considering the combination of the three-year time scale and the high mobility of nurses (particularly as many of them were previously living in nursing homes), we were fairly satisfied with this response. Elsewhere (Williams *et al.* 1991a,b; see also Chapter 13 on 'Nursing Wastage from the Nurses' Perspective') we have considered how nurses themselves feel about their situation and we shall concentrate here more specifically on the results which nurse managers should see as relevant, particularly as regards what might encourage nurses to return.

In the questionaire sent to leavers, one of the questions read: 'What caused you to leave the health authority on the last occasion?' Forty-one possible reasons were given and the nurse was asked to tick as many as applied. In addition, she was requested to indicate the three most important reasons. The most striking feature of the results is that the top three reasons – 'workload affects job', 'staff shortages' and 'underfunding' – all relate to the strains of working too hard and lack of resources. If this observation were generally true it would be ironic that keeping NHS expenditure down so as not to 'waste' money had the effect of increasing wastage which, in turn, leads to the need for more money to recruit and train new staff. That is, keeping expenditure down may be a false economy.

Another interesting point to come from our survey is that 'dislike pay' was only the eighteenth most popularly chosen reason, being ticked by just 13 nurses. Even more revealing is that only four nurses placed this reason as one of their top three reasons for leaving. Both of these statistics give greater strength to the argument that, while pay is of some significance, there are more important factors which influence nurses leaving – in particular, the perceived amount and stress of the workload.

More extensive analysis of the data reveals that, as expected, nurses are not a homogeneous group and that different types of nurse show great variation in their reasons for leaving. For example, nearly half of the nurses under 30 gave 'wanting to widen experience' as a reason for leaving, whereas this reason was given by only one-fifth of those over 30.

In the same questionnaire, we also asked nurses the question 'What would encourage you to return to the health authority?' Nurses had to give ratings of importance to 18 inducements to return. The top inducement turned out to be 'better management', which was placed as 'very important' by 78 per cent of the respondents. 'Increased salary' came only eighth on the list, with 'very important' being ticked by less than half of the nurses. Returning inducements such as 'better sports facilities' and 'more nursing accommodation' were two of the reasons felt least important, although even these were considered 'important' or 'very important' by more than half of the respondents.

The responses to our questionnaire reveal a certain amount of dissatisfaction amongst these nurses who have recently left. Their main reasons for leaving seem to have been related to working too hard and thus not being able to give the care that they wanted to. There was also a great tendency for nurses to complain about the quality of management. The overriding feeling was that management were aloof and did not want to 'get their hands dirty'. However, when talking to managers we were struck by the fact that they also found their work stressful and, indeed, concerned about future developments in the NHS. Thus, there seems to be a communication problem between managers and nurses which, if it could be resolved, would reduce many of the antagonistic feelings felt by nurses about management.

Discussion

In this chapter we hope to have demonstrated that nurse wastage is a complicated issue. The topic has attracted more interest from the government as it has been increasingly recognized that nurses' claims – in terms of both pay and other issues – cannot just be swept aside. Nurses continue to attract support from the general public and the spectre of closed wards and reduced services provides some readily visible – albeit perhaps inaccurate – indicators that nursing wastage and problems of recruitment in some district health authorities and regions may well be contributing to the difficulties. Sometimes, however, such expressed concerns may simply be a mask for lack of funds to recruit and retrain the appropriate staff.

Turnover/wastage among nurses may well have a particular poignancy for local managers of the health service. While trying to work within the financial constraints of government policy, a new set of conflicts and contradictions may emerge for managers. Obviously on a day-to-day basis it is more pleasant for those working at local levels to manage teams who have achieved an appropriate balance between a static and a liquid workforce, for it is much harder and more problematic to manage either of the two extremes. However, high turnover is not always regarded with quite the concern by managers as some might expect. Indeed, much of managers' rhetoric is, on occasions, to argue forcefully that there is no problem regarding turnover. They recognize that to say otherwise could be interpreted as reflecting adversely on their ability to manage.

However, nurse turnover produces hidden costs for management which are rarely fully recognized. It can be very expensive in money, time and energy. Recruitment, selection, orientating and retraining new staff are a high and largely hidden price to pay for a constantly moving workforce. Health service management – certainly traditionally (see Ackroyd et al. 1989 for a discussion of the 'custodial' role of health service management) – would tend to weigh the scales more to the desire to establish continuity by maintaining a stable workforce. But there is no doubt that in the 1980s the situation changed and the financial constraints are very real ones which have to be recognized by the general managers who have come into post since the first Griffiths Report reorganizing health service management. Hence, it is not really surprising that many nurses have felt betrayed by their management during the past decade. In brief, the rules have changed and the nurse has, as a consequence, felt increasingly isolated and neglected. The remedy is for managers to become much more interested in the needs and concerns of their nursing workforce. The actual or potential problem of nursing wastage is one such area where more focused attention is appropriate.

If managers are to have control over wastage it is vital that they are able to assimilate all the relevant information. In a small firm of business this would be relatively easy. However, in a large organization like a district health authority, managers cannot simply tour the shop floor; there is too much information to take in. However, with today's technology there is a ready solution. Namely, the computer.

The first hurdle to overcome is that managers should not be scared of computers. Even today many people see these machines as 'the Devil's work'. However, such attitudes must change if HAs are to be run effectively. However, only part of the problem lies with reluctant computer users. Other areas for concern are the inaccurate input and checking of data and the lack of user-friendliness and flexibility of information data bases.

The only way in which regulating bodies like the Review Body can gain information on wastage is from figures given by district HAs. It is important that these figures are as correct and relevant as possible. Presently, we suspect that this is not always the case. The HA where we have been studying has recently been making strenuous efforts to ensure that their data base of personnel records is up to date and free from errors. This is a huge task which would have been much easier if records had been conscientiously entered and checked in the past. We suspect that other health authorities have similar and possibly worse problems. For example, one HA recently had 100 nurses on their data base recorded as employed but who had in fact left the HA!

There are also technical issues to be considered. For example, when trying to link information on nurses – perhaps their current post with their previous career history – problems can be caused by people changing their name or with different numbers of initials being used in the two information sources. Similar problems in the matching of immigration records are discussed by Copas and Hilton (1990).

In summary, managers should have full knowledge and understanding of the way that wastage occurs in their HA. For example, is there a high level of turnover amongst some nurses and less amongst others, or is there a steady turnover amongst all nurses? There should be greater recognition that there are a number of aspects of wastage that managers can control. For example, the provision of creche facilities may encourage mothers with young children to remain in nursing; increased availability of job-share and part-time working would help many nurses; and, perhaps most importantly, managers could communicate better with nurses so that they are aware that mangers also face problems of stress and overwork. However, there are some aspects of wastage that managers cannot and, perhaps, should not control. For example, nurses may want to travel for extensive periods or experience the challenge of working at a new HA. Turnover, for reasons such as these, can help keep nurses' enthusiasm for their work. In brief, turnover is not always negative.

Hence, we conclude on an optimistic note by observing that there are some aspects of running a health authority that managers should be able to control, while recognizing that there are other aspects that they cannot and perhaps should not. The main problem is that the potential areas for understanding and control are not always being managed successfully at present.

Acknowledgement

The authors wish to thank the Leverhulme Trust for their financial support.

References

Ackroyd, S., Hughes, J. and Soothill, K. 1989. Public sector services and their management. *Journal of Management Studies* 26(6): 603–19.

Barry, J. T., Soothill, K. L. and Francis, B. J. 1989. Nursing the statistics: a demonstration study of nurse turnover and retention. *Journal of Advanced Nursing* 14: 528–35.

Bartholomew, D. J. 1976. The statistical approach to manpower planning. In D. S. Bartholomew (ed.), *Manpower Planning*. London: Penguin Books.

Copas, J. and Hilton, F. 1990. Matching algorithms for immigration records. *Journal of the Royal Statistical Society* A, 153(3): 287–320.

Dickson, N. 1987. Best foot forward. *Nursing Times*, 7 January, 83(1): 40–1.

Grocott, T. 1989. A hole in the black hole theory. *Nursing Times*, 11 October, 85(41): 65–7.

Hancock, C. 1986. The staffing equation. *Nursing Times*, 20 August, 82: 40–2.

Mackay, L. 1989. *Nursing a Problem*. Milton Keynes: Open University Press.

Martin, J. P. and Mackean, J. 1988. *Can We Keep Nurses in the Health Service? A Study of Nurse Retention in Two Health Districts*. Institute of Health Policy Study, University of Southampton.

Pilkington, E. 1989. A growing sick list of morale. *Guardian*, 29 November.

Price Waterhouse. 1988. *Nurse Retention and Recruitment: A Matter of Priority*. Report commissioned by Chairmen of Regional Health Authorities in England, Health Boards in Scotland and Health Authorities in Wales.

Redfern, S. J. 1978. Absence and wastage in trained nurses: a selective review of the literature. *Journal of Advanced Nursing* 3: 231–49.

Review Body for Nursing Staff, Midwives, Health Visitors and Professions Allied to Medicine (1985). *2nd report on nursing staff midwives and health visitors*, Cmnd. 9529. London: HMSO.

Review Body for Nursing Staff, Midwives, Health Visitors and Profession Allied to Medicine (1988). *5th report on nursing staff midwives and health visitors*, Cm. 360. London: HMSO.

Review Body for Nursing Staff, Midwives, Health Visitors and Professions Allied to Medicine (1989). *6th report on nursing staff midwives and health visitors*, Cm. 577. London: HMSO.

Review Body for Nursing Staff, Midwives, Health Visitors and Professions Allied to Medicine (1990). *7th report on nursing staff midwives and health visitors*, Cm. 935. London: HMSO.

Soothill, K. L., Barry, J. T. and Williams, C. 1990. *Words and Actions: A Study in Nurse Wastage*. Working Paper No. 9, Lancaster University, Department of Applied Social Science.

Waite, R., Buchan, J. and Thomas, J. 1989. *Nurses in and out of Work*. IMS Report No. 170, Brighton: Institute of Manpower Studies.

Williams, C. W., Soothill, K. L. and Barry, J. T. 1991a. Love nursing, hate the job. *Health Service Journal*, 14 February, 101(5238): 18–21.

Williams, C. W., Soothill, K. L. and Barry, J. T. 1991b. Targeting the discontented. *Health Service Journal*, 21 February, 101(5239): 20–1.

CHAPTER SEVENTEEN
Nurse supply modelling
David Worthington

Introduction

Nursing's 'demographic timebomb' has been clearly identified as a major problem for health service managers to solve (see, for example, Hancock 1986). The problem is essentially that, whilst there is no anticipated drop in the demand for nurses (indeed service plans and Project 2000 proposals may well mean as increased requirement), by the early 1990s the pool of school leavers from whom most nurse trainees are recruited will have fallen by about 35 per cent.

There are two other major sources of nurses which, although they complicate the problem, may well also contribute to its solution, namely the retention and return of previously qualified nurses.

In this context, nurse workforce planning is a vital activity for the health service, and is one that has gathered considerable momentum recently. However, serious interest is still relatively new and nurse workforce planning is evolving in the face of real practical problems.

In reviewing the current situation the NHS Management Board (1987: 1 and 3) emphasized the dual role of demand and supply modelling in strategic planning. It noted the wide variety of methodologies in use and provided guidance on 'minimum expectations on the use of manpower planning methodology'. This included the proposal that 'use of common methodologies should be the long-term aim', but recommended for the moment that:

a.   there should be a supply model in use in each region which does not have to be the same in every region;

b. there should be a demand model for strategic planning purposes in use in each region which should be common to each district in the region, but may differ between regions.

The purpose of this chapter is to introduce nurses and prospective nurses to the concept of nurse supply modelling in the context of nurse workforce planning. The next two sections explain the general concept of nurse supply modelling and then describe some of the major issues which impact on its practical application. We then go on to identify the possible practical roles of the present generation of nurse supply models, and finally we describe key areas of concern for the future.

Nurse supply modelling

The nature of nurse supply models

The general purpose of nurse supply models is to allow a manager to investigate the supply consequences of possible management actions. Such a 'model' is in fact almost always a piece of computer software which allows the user to input data that correspond to the management actions. The model then predicts the consequences of those actions using mathematical relationships that are designed to reflect what is known about the dynamics of the situation.

However, as in many other fields, nurse supply models are unable to incorporate the actual operational decisions that may be under consideration. For example, if management wishes to examine the effects of reducing wastage on the supply of nurses, a supply model could be reasonably expected to calculate the effects of different wastage rates. However, it would be very unlikely to show the effects of actual management actions, for example opening a creche. Current supply models, in the main, consider management actions only indirectly in terms of the rates that they will cause rather than the detail of how those rates will be achieved.

The problems involved in modelling in any greater detail in a systematic way make the current approach appropriate. However, this leaves a certain amount of responsibility with the manager to judge what rates can be achieved and how. This may of course lead to some other modelling exercises; however, in general these are better kept separate from the main supply model.

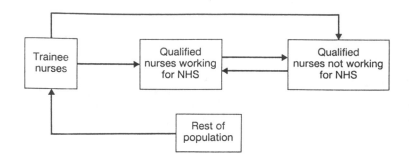

Figure 17.1 The basic structure of nurse supply models

The structure of nurse supply models

In general terms nurse supply models all have the same basic structure, as shown in Figure 17.1. The situation is modelled in terms of a number of stocks and flows. For example, at the national level the four most important stocks are; qualified nurses working for the NHS, qualified nurses in the UK who are not working for the NHS, trainee nurses and the rest of the UK population. In the main, these stocks change owing to flows between them, e.g. qualified nurses leaving the NHS or trainees newly recruited from the rest of the UK population. If the starting stocks are known and future flow rates can be predicted, then a supply model should be able to predict future stocks reasonably accurately.

Whilst Figure 17.1 summarizes the main principles of nurse supply models, it does not itself represent a realistic model. For example, because flow rates will usually depend on the ages and grades of the nurses involved, most practical models subdivide the major stocks by age groupings and by grade. The resulting model is still a network of stocks and flows, and hence the principles are unchanged. However a realistic model will normally be much more complex than in Figure 17.1.

Whilst models along the lines of Figure 17.1 are usually too simple to be of practical value, it is also important to avoid over-complicated models. In reviewing manpower planning models in general, Edwards (1986: 45–6) suggests that 'simple techniques should be used. . . . . The aims should be to encourage interaction with the models to gain an understanding of the quantitative aspects of the manpower system; none of these is beyond the capabilities of a good spreadsheet package (with grapics) . . .'

Types of models

Different supply models are appropriate in different circumstances. The circumstances can be reflected in terms of the time scale under consideration, the level within the organization (e.g. hospital, region), or simply the data that are available.

One important distinction is between 'prescriptive' and 'what if' models. In the former, the model tells the manager what rates will be required to achieve chosen targets. In the latter, the manager chooses the rates and the model calculates the consequences. In the context of manpower supply modelling, 'prescriptive' models can be very thought provoking, and can generate some useful solutions. However, given the ingenuity of managers and the complexity of the problem, the flexibility of 'what if' models is probably more useful in the long term. They will usually require a greater degree of involvement from the manager, but should provide a better level of understanding and a higher level of credibility.

Manager participation

Management participation is a sound principle in any modelling work. In the context of nurse supply modelling it is clearly essential that managers are involved to offer their judgement on what rates might be achievable, and perhaps to accept responsibility for attaining those rates. For the successful use of nurse supply models, a three-way interaction is therefore desirable, involving the manager, the analyst and the model.

Whilst this model of usage is obviously preferable, it can be very time consuming and various shortcuts can be envisaged. For example, supply models have been designed that are intended to be sufficiently user-friendly for a manager to be able to use them directly without the need for an analyst. In other studies, 'one-way interactions' have been tried in which the manager tells the analyst the parameter values, but does not fully understand what the analyst and the model are doing with them. However, such shortcuts are very risky given the form of the models and the present lack of experience in running and interpreting such models that exists amongst NHS managers. For example, data problems often require the analysis or the model to make additional assumptions in order to obtain results. Many results from the model may be relatively insensitive to these assumptions; for others they may be critical. Such a judgement would usually require inputs and awareness from both analyst and manager. In fact, one of the major benefits of some supply models is that they can act as a catalyst between managers and analysts.

Data-imposed limitations

As with many other areas of modelling, data availability rather than the ability to manipulate them provides the major constrint on what is possible. Thus in some cases the absence of data means that particular desirable features have to be omitted from the model, whilst in other cases sampling errors associated with the available data make a high level of aggregation necessary. Both these problems tend to encourage models that are relatively simple and aggregated.

One particular implication of this form of constraint is that, whilst in theory stochastic models of manpower supply systems can be devised, it is very rare that such models can provide much more information than can be obtained from deterministic models.

Major issues for nurse supply models

The idea of using nurse supply models to investigate the supply consquences of alternative management actions is clearly good in principle. Indeed a number of such models are now available, and others are being developed. The Second Report of the All Wales Manpower Planning Committee (1987) provides a comparison of seven of these models.

However, if models of this sort are to be used properly, a number of important issues need to be appreciated. In particular, it is important that nurse managers recognize the potential and the limitations of the modelling process, the criteria that are likely to lead to successful applications, and the respects in which they need to be improved.

Participation rates vs wastage rates

Existing models are based upon one of two methodologies, i.e. 'participation rates' (PR) or 'wastage rates' (WR). It is important to understand the differences between these two methods, although, as will be argued later, they also have much in common.

Referring back to Figure 17.1, the major difference is essentially in how the flows of qualified nurses between 'working for the NHS' and 'not working for the NHS' are modelled. If we refer to the *net* flow from the former to the latter as the 'net wastage rate', then the two models estimate age-specific net wastage rates as follows:

WR model:
Net wastage rate of nurses of age *a* years
= wastage rate at age *a* − joining rate at age *a*

PR model:
Net wastage rate of nurses of age *a* years
$$= 1 - \frac{\text{participation rate at age } (a+1)}{\text{participation rate at age } a}.$$

Note that the following standard definitions are used:

$$\text{Wastage rate at age } a = \frac{\text{WTE leaving of age } a \text{ during year}}{\text{WTE in post of age } a \text{ at start of year}};$$

$$\text{Joining rate at age } a = \frac{\text{WTE joining of age } a \text{ during year}}{\text{WTE in post of age } a \text{ at start of year}};$$

Participation rate at age *a* =
$$\frac{\text{WTE nurses of age } a \text{ employed by NHS}}{\text{Total no. qualified nurses of age } a}.$$

(WTE = whole time equivalent)

It has been shown in Worthington (1988) that the calculations that the two types of model perform with these two different estimates are essentially the same. However, a major difference between their results can occur because the two estimates of net wastage rate can be very different, as explained below.

Long-term or short-term estimates of net wastage rates

In the WR model, wastage rates and joining rates are estimated from recent data on numbers of nurses leaving the NHS and joining the NHS, preferably by age and possibly by grade as well. The level of aggregation will be determined by the detail and amount of data available. If the amount of data is small a high level of aggregation may be necessary to reduce sampling errors. Thus for the WR model net wastage rates will reflect current trends, probably at most the trends of the last two or three years, depending on the amount of reliable data available. These current trends will obviously reflect recent opportunities for nurses outside the NHS, recent levels of morale within the NHS, recent attempts by the NHS to attract qualified nurses back into the NHS, recent policies within the NHS to reduce nursing numbers in some areas, etc. If in addition wastage rates and joining rates have to be aggregated across age groups and so are not age specific, they will also reflect the current age structure of the qualified nursing workforce.

The PR model, on the other hand, estimates net wastage rates from current participation rates. However, current participation rates are obviously a product of wastage and joining rates from the last 40 years or so. Again it is preferable to use age-specific rates if possible, otherwise the rate will also reflect the current age structure of the total qualified nurse population.

Thus one basis for choice between the two approaches that could be put, rather unfairly, to managers is whether they wish to assume recent trends or trends based on up to the last 40 years for the nurse supply planning period that they are considering. Without the aid of a crystal ball this is likely to be a very speculative choice, particularly if the planning period is more than a few years.

An alternative and more constructive idea is that promoted by Trent Regional Health Authority (RHA) (see, for example, Beaumont and Peel 1987), namely to offer the manager supply projections on the basis of both sets of estimates. This at least informs the manager about the possible degree of inaccuracy involved in the method. There is also perhaps the hope that the true future will lie somewhere between the two – although of course this is not certain. There is clearly a role for a modelling approach that will help the user to consider alternative realistic net wastage rates other than these possible extremes.

Participation rates can be misleading

One of the initially anticipated advantages of the PR models was that data on participation rates would help managers to identify the scope for attracting qualified nurses back to working in the NHS. For example, a 60 per cent participation rate might indicate another 40 per cent who might be attracted back to the NHS. However, because an unknown proportion of the qualified nurses identified as not working for the NHS have no wish to return to nursing within the NHS, the figures are misleadingly over optimistic.

Other wastage rate models

The discussion so far has concentrated on WR models in which age-specific WRs have been used, and these have been compared with PR models. In some models wastage rates are aggregated across all age groups, whilst others use grade-specific rather than age-specific wastage rates.

Because of the lack of age-specific WR data, some supply models simply use an average WR which they apply to all ages of nurses together. Thus whilst the age structure of the nursing workforce will in reality change, this will not be reflected in a changing average WR. It is possible that in some analyses this simplification will not introduce significant errors. However, example calculations carried out by the author for two district health authorities in the North Western RHA suggested that ignoring the age structure led to overestimates in workforce projections for 1997 of approximately 6 per cent and 13 per cent respectively.

Perhaps more fundamental is the point that it is only possible to test the sensitivity of results to this particular assumption by using a model based on age-specific rates. This is especially worrying in a context where possible supply strategies may involve deliberately changing the age structure of the workforce.

Other WR supply models deliberately choose grade-specific WRs instead of age-specific rates. These models highlight an important problem, namely that joining and leaving rates could depend on the grade structure of the nursing population as well as its age structure. Whilst the results from these models will complement results obtained from those previously described, if presented alone they must be treated with caution for a number of reasons. As noted above they omit the effect of changing age structure. They also have to make some quite complex assumptions about grade-specific wastage, joining and promotion rates, the debate initiated through Project 2000 about restructuring and redefining the roles of nurses can only serve to complicate this problem further.

Cross-boundary flows

Although Figure 17.1 describes the main stocks and flows, there are others which we refer to here as cross-boundary flows. At a national level, examples would be qualified nurses leaving the UK to work abroad, or qualified nurses coming from abroad to work for the NHS. The numbers will be relatively small, and if they need to be modelled at all can probably be represented by simple net flow rates into/out of the system. However, at the regional level, cross-boundary flows are relatively larger in size, and so may need to be modelled in greater detail. This is particularly so because, unlike international boundaries, the NHS has some influence on, and interest in, what happens on both sides of the regional boundaries.

At the district level, cross-boundary flows take on a greater importance again. They will affect recruitment of trainees, the wastage rates of qualified staff to other districts, and the recruitment of qualified staff from other districts. These extra flows can be incorporated into the supply models relatively easily. However, obtaining data on their current values can be quite problematic, and estimating future values is likely to be little more than wishful thinking. The crux of the problem is that recent values, if available, will reflect recent policies of the district (e.g. to reduce staffing levels in the face of economic constraints or to increase training school intakes in anticipation of new facilities), and also those of its neighbours. Simple extrapolation from recent values is therefore very unwise. However, to do more than this a district has to consult not only its own schemes but those of its neighbours as well. This is not an easy matter given the fluid nature of nurse supply schemes that are likely to exist. Clearly the situation requires district-level models that are carefully coordinated between districts.

Data requirements

All nurse supply models have some data requirements and even with an excellent model the popular adage 'garbage in, garbage out' remains true.

The basic requirement for all models is up-to-date numbers of staff in post, preferably by age and by care group, and possibly by grade. Even these very basic requirements have posed problems for nurse supply modelling in the past. This has been particularly so for national figures, as they are essentially the sum of local figures and hence need all local figures to be available and reasonably accurate.

WR models also require numbers of starters and leavers, again preferably by age and by care group, and possibly by grade. Here it is important to know starters and leavers by source and destination, as people who simply change job within the NHS should not be counted as either starters or leavers. At the time of writing, this information is not available for all regions, so any national figures in particular will be either approximations or aggregates or both. Some of the confusions that this can cause are well described by Grocott (1989).

One of the basic data requirements of the PR models is the total number of qualified nurses in the population, by age and by care group. The best source of this information at present is the 1981 census. However this obviously needs to be updated, which requires further approximations to be made. A second problem with thes data is in the allocation of nurses to care groups. Many nurses hold qualifications in more than one care group and the census records this information in two ways. It counts numbers of nurses by most recent qualification, and it counts qualifications. Unfortunately, neither of these counts is precisely what is needed: the former can seriously misallocate nurses between care groups; the latter will count actual nurses in more than one care group.

Some models also incorporate data on the pool of school leavers from which the bulk of trainee nurses are likely to be recruited. In others this is important background information for the manager in considering possible future recruitment rates. Again, only approximate figures are available at the time of writing.

In the context of data requirements, one advantage that some districts (and regions) will have is the quality and detail of data that they hold. Thus whilst the data available at national level are essentially the minimum of those available in all districts, clearly many districts (and regions) will have better data. Conversely, although data may be available in greater detail at district level, they will also be subject to greater sampling errors. Thus staff groups may have to be aggregated simply to reduce these errors rather than because of lack of detail in data collection.

Expertise

Ideally, a nurse supply model will be a user-friendly piece of computer software which can be used easily and interpreted safely by nurse (and other health service) managers. However, the nature of the nurse supply modelling process at the present time prevents this possibility. In particular, the need to make the best of available data and then interpret the results in the light of the approximations in the data and the assumptions of the model will almost always require some additional modelling expertise. This may in time come from nurse managers who have become involved in the supply modelling activity, but will for the moment in most cases require some external input.

Role of nurse supply modelling

Role of local models

Despite the reservations outlined earlier, nurse supply models can make important contributions to the nurse workforce planning activity at the local level. The value extracted will to a large extent depend on the quality of information and effort put into the exercise. Three types of use can be distinguished.

- as a management game:
- to improve understanding by providing 'ball-park figures;
- to identify management targets.

MANAGEMENT GAME

The process of using a nurse supply model requires nurse managers to provide relevant statistics on such items as: current in-post staffing levels; recent joining and leaving rates; and possible planned training, recruitment and retention rates. Running the nurse supply model will then demonstrate to those involved the important influences that such factors are likely to have on future staffing levels.

Thus, using such a model, even with inaccurate and incomplete information, will cause managers to recognize the important factors; to start to collect relevant information; and perhaps to go on to monitor key rates with a view to controlling them (and hence the workforce size) in the future.

'BALL-PARK' UNDERSTANDING

Even though data are known to be inaccurate and there is a possible debate about modelling methodology, nurse supply models can still provide very useful messages for management.

For example, Figure 17.2 shows the result of using two different models to forecast the future supply of registered mental handicap nurses in a district in the North West. Whilst the results of the two models differ and the target figures are only approximate, there is a clear message for local management that there is a potential overstaffing problem.

Similarly, as described in Worthington (1990), applying nurse supply models to individual districts in the North West has indicated that the likely impact of a 30 per cent decrease in the number of 18–19 year olds would not have as severe an impact on future workforces as is often anticipated. The model projected the effect to be a 5 per cent decrease in RGN workforces by 1997.

SETTING TARGETS

If data are reasonably reliable and the model sufficiently realistic, then nurse supply models can help managers to set targets for training, recruitment and retention. For example, one might re-run the mental handicap model used to produce Figure 17.2 with alternative training, recruitment and retention rates until the projected workforce coincided with the target. These rates could then be used as management targets.

For this particular practical problem the models and data were not considered to be sufficiently accurate, nor indeed were the

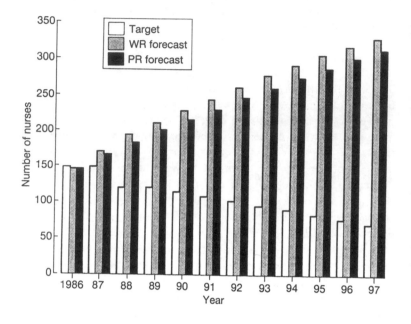

Figure 17.2 Forecast and target numbers of mental handicap nurses for an example district

targets. Hence no attempt was made to use the model in this way. Nevertheless with data improvements, increased knowledge of the plans of neighbouring districts and experience with the current model, this sort of exercise should soon be possible.

Role of national (and regional) models

Nurse supply modelling can in principle have similar value at the national (and regional) level as at the local level. However, many of the decisions that will affect the key rates in the models must be taken at district level, in the light of district circumstances, and many of them will be financed at districts' discretion. Moreover, the very different problems faced in different parts of the country mean that an average national (or regional) picture will hide many of the real problems that are at the local level, as well as some of the opportunities to solve them. It is thus important that any national (or regional) models are accompanied by district models that will enable local problems and opportunities to be identified and investigated.

The future

The major roles for nurse supply models have been outlined above. For them to succeed and to improve in these roles in the future there are three key areas of concern.

Data

As in many other areas of modelling, the most important improvements will be caused by the increasing availability of better-quality data. Accurate staff in-post figures by age and care group for all districts is the first requirement – and is already available in many parts of the country. Once age-specific WRs by care group are also available (which some parts of the country are already able to produce), WR models can then be used with reasonable confidence. However, this requires counts of joiners and leavers by source and destination respectively. In particular, joiners must distinguish internal flows within districts (which can be excluded), flows of qualified staff from other districts, appointments of previously qualified staff who have not been working in the NHS, appointments of newly qualified staff trained within the district, and appointments of newly qualified staff trained in other districts. Similarly, counts of leavers must distinguish internal flows within districts (which can be excluded), flows of qualified staff to other districts, and staff who leave the NHS. Clearly, if these data are collected by districts, simple aggregation will also provide the data required for regional and national models.

The UKCC live register is capable of providing reasonably up-to-date data on numbers of qualified nurses by age, by qualification and by district, which may help to improve the accuracy and value of PR models. Also the Nurses' Central Clearing House is starting to build up a data base on applicants to nursing schools that should shed greater light on future recruitment potential from and to individual districts.

In addition to these standard data sources, there is also an important role for local studies to improve understanding of the present situation and of possible future developments. For example, studies such as that of Barry, Soothill and Williams (see Chapter 16 in this volume) can provide insight into local wastage rates, into possible future levels and indeed into potential methods for controlling them.

Technical developments

A large number of nurse supply models have been developed over the last ten years or so. This has in part reflected a natural tendency for local managers to wish to develop models specifically for their local problem as they see it. For the future, a more coordinated development is probably preferable. This should not only be more efficient but also help to standardize and coordinate planning activities, particularly in adjacent areas.

Given the complementary nature of the WR and PR models via the concept of net wastage rates, a sensible technical development would be a single 'net wastage rate model'. Such model would offer maximum flexibility to the user, who could use the same model with input data expressed as wastage and recruitment rates or as participation rates, or in fact using any other parameters from which future net wastage rates can be derived.

There is also the need to develop models that will reflect changes caused by Project 2000 proposals. Because the effects are potentially quite complicated, there is a natural tendency to build complex models. This should be avoided if possible, as complex models usually have quite demanding data requirements which can cause a major stumbling block for the potential user.

Support

Alongside these information and technical developments there is also the need to support and develop further expertise in nurse supply planning. The data requirements described above must be clearly specified to districts and should be carefully monitored by 'experts', perhaps at region.

The process of nurse supply planning also needs to be supported and coordinated. Thus modelling in districts should actively involve local managers and nurse planning 'experts' who are able to advise on the use and interpretation of the models and are also able to coordinate the assumptions being made by districts, particularly about cross-boundary flows. Such coordinated activity may also help to find regional solutions to local problems.

There is similarly the need to coordinate regional planning to enable national solutions to be sought for the problems of individual regions.

Conclusions

Nurse supply modelling offers a powerful tool to nurse workforce planners. However, for it to be applied successfully, prospective users need to appreciate its potential and its limitations.

Nurse supply modelling is an approach that is continuing to develop. It should become increasingly successful as data improve, as better models are developed and as nurse workforce planners became increasingly familiar with the approach and become better supported in their planning activities.

Acknowledgements

Much of this material has stemmed from a project carried out on behalf of Operational Research Services, Department of Health and Social Security, during 1987. The work benefited greatly from a high degree of interest from a wide variety of health service personnel. Much of the writing of this report was carried out whilst the author was employed for five months at the University of Odense in Denmark.

References

All Wales Manpower Planning Committee. 1987. *The Second Report of the All Wales Manpower Planning Committee: Nurse Supply Modelling.*

Beaumont, K. and Peel, A. 1987. *The Trent Nurse Supply Model, User Guide.* Trent Regional Health Authority.

Edwards, J. S. 1986. Manpower planning in 1986. In V. Belton and R. M. O'Keefe (eds), *Recent Developments in Operational Research.* Oxford: Pergamon.

Grocott, T. 1989. A hole in the black hole theory. *Nursing Times,* 11 October, 85(41): 65–7.

Hancock, C. 1986. Project 2000 – The staffing equation. *Nursing Times*, 20 August, 82: 40–2.

NHS Management Board. 1987. Nurse manpower planning. Letter to regional, district and SHA general managers, 6 March, Annex A.

Worthington, D. J. 1988. *Nurse Manpower Planning (Supply Models and Quantitative Aspects of Recruitment, Retention and Return)*. Report for Operational Research Services, Department of Health and Social Security.

Worthington, D. J. 1990. Recruitment, retention and return: some quantitative issues. *International Journal of Nursing Studies* 27: 199–211.

CHAPTER EIGHTEEN

Angels in red? patterns of union membership amongst UK professional nurses

Paul Bagguley

Introduction

There is little doubt that nurses are represented by unions and quasi-professional organizations with quite different policies and strategies in the defence of their members' interests. This diversity is not a new phenomenon with the RCN (Royal College of Nursing) and with similar, but much smaller, quasi-professional organizations attempting to pursue a fairly orthodox professionalization strategy. In contrast, COHSE (the Confederation of Health Service Employees) organizes psychiatric nurses in particular in a more conventional trade union fashion (Carpenter 1988; Lewis 1976). The differences in strategic approaches were evident during the health disputes of the 1970s (Lewis 1976: 645–7), and have recently been brought to the fore again in disputes with management and government.

While the dichotomy between the RCN – as a semi-professional association – and more conventional trade unions remains evident, it should not be thought that the situation has remained unchanged and will not change in the future. Lewis documented the increased 'militancy' and 'shift to the left' in COHSE and NUPE (National Union of Public Employees) during the disputes of the 1970s (Lewis 1976). More recently, disputes over pay and regrading caused the RCN to reconsider the principled 'no-strike' policy. Despite the endorsement of the traditional approach within the RCN in a national vote, the major concern by the leadership about the dissidents in its ranks was evident.

The present study is not directly concerned with particular union reactions to the recent pay award. Ours is both a more general and fundamental set of questions. In brief, what are the patterns of organizational membership amongst UK professional nurses? What determines these patterns? What are nurses' assessments of their organizations' representations of their interests? Our interest goes beyond the simple descriptive level, however, for we wish to identify the possible sources of support for and opposition to various kinds of initiatives and developments in the coming decade. In particular we believe that two contradictory tendencies are emerging, which nurses' organizations will increasingly have to face up to. On the one hand, the semi-professional associations (especially the RCN) face an increasing 'legitimation crisis', where a significant minority of their members are dissatisfied with the organization's performance for reasons to do with the leaderships of the RCN and similar organizations being 'insufficiently militant'. On the other hand, the organization most likely to benefit from the 'fall out' of this legitimation crisis – COHSE – faces the decline of its traditional core membership base in the old mental illness and mental handicap hospitals as 'community care' policies are fully implemented over the next ten years.

In many respects the Committee on Nursing, chaired by Asa Brigss, is a benchmark of progress and change over the past couple of decades (Briggs 1972). At that time, as the *Project 2000* report of the UKCC (United Kingdom Council for Nursing, Midwifery and Health Visiting) has recently reminded us, 'nurses, midwives and health visitors seemed set for a major change . . . The air of gloom which Briggs had recorded in nursing seemed set to be dispelled' (UKCC 1987: 8).

While much has changed in the intervening period, the air of gloom has certainly returned. The most important proposals regarding the restructuring of nursing have come from the UKCC's Educational Policy Advisory Committee, *Project 2000*, in which they state that 'Project 2000's proposals, taken *in toto*, call for nothing less than a revolution in the usage of manpower [*sic*] in the NHS' (UKCC 1987: 66). The final practical outcome of Project 2000's proposals obviously remains uncertain, but the shortages of suitably qualified young women over the next ten years will be the crucial challenge facing management. It remains to be seen if the unions and professional associations will be able to influence the course of events during the ensuing period in favour of their members' interests. These uncertainties have been further compounded by the recent government initiatives for hospitals to 'opt out' of the NHS, and the related pressures towards local pay bargaining.

Previous studies of nurses and unions

Although Briggs provides a benchmark for analysis of the formal training and labour market situation in professional nursing, the report has little to say about trade unions and industrial relations. Generally its analysis, comments and recommendations were restricted to the role of the professional associations in relation to training and grievance procedures. There were no major discussions of what we are concerned with here – the pattern of organizational membership and attitudes towards organizations – nor were any major innovations in the Whitley Council system of negotiating recommended. What this does reveal, however, is that industrial relations were not perceived by policy makers as a major issue during the late 1960s and early 1970s (Briggs 1972).

Similarly, historical accounts of nursing and professional organizations and trade unions emphasize this formal organizational level (Abel-Smith 1960; Carpenter 1988). Their interest is in the political struggles between nurses' organizations, employers and the state, so they provide little or no detailed analysis of the determinants of organizational membership or hard data on nurses' attitudes to their organizations. The essays in Bosanquet (1979), although stimulated by the 1970s 'crisis' in health service industrial relations, focus on the formal legal, institutional and procedural aspects of health sector industrial relations in the UK. Dyson and Spray (1979), however, do provide some interesting data on the increasing involvement of nurses' professional associations in industrial relations issues. As we noted earlier, this is perhaps the major change since the early 1970s; the professional associations' response to the 'legitimation crisis' in relation to their members has been to become more 'trade unionist' in orientation.

There are more studies focusing on the central problems of

contemporary nursing from the point of view of health service policy makers – particularly the decline in suitable recruits – which unfortunately do not deal with organizational membership in any detail. Mercer's study was principally concerned with this issue in relation to labour turnover, but did not deal with organizational affiliations or their attitudinal correlates (Mercer 1979). More recently, a major study carried out for the RCN by Waite and Hutt (1987) of the Institute for Manpower Studies at the University of Sussex involved a national survey of RCN members analysing labour market and work dissatisfaction issues, but crucially failed to consider organizational membership and attitudes to organizations.

General accounts of the determinants of patterns of union membership emphasize aggregate factors such as the social composition of the workforce, industrial relations legislation and employer and union strategies (Bain and Price 1983; Winchester 1988). Since our level of analysis concerns variations amongst professional nurses within one particular district health authority at one point in time, these factors can for practical purposes be assumed to be constant.

Another body of literature explaining white-collar union growth in terms of proletarianization, however, demands some more attention since this model has been applied to nursing at similar units of analysis to our own by Bellaby and Oribabor (1977). Much of Bellaby and Oribabor's account consists of squeezing the formal empirical characteristics of nursing work and hospital organization into the abstract categories of Marxian theory. This provides an insightful rewriting of history as a conflict between professional and trade union strategies amongst nurses as responses to what Bellaby and Oribabor see as the long-run proletarianization of the profession. However, their anlaysis is limited to general hospital nurses, whilst most nurses who have traditionally been in trade unions have been in the mental illness and mental handicap sectors. Further, over the past 40 years or so nurses in these sectors have become professionalized rather than proletarianized, with the introduction first of pharmaceutical techniques and then of more sophisticated forms of psycho-therapy. The use of both of these techniques requires extensive professional training for the nurses involved (Carpenter 1988). Consequently it is clear that the proletarianization thesis does not hold for all professional nurses.

Bellaby and Oribabor's later work is, however, altogether more useful for our purposes, since they examined patterns of organizational membership at the level of an area health authority during the late 1970s. The major drawback of their later work is not only the small size of the sample ($N = 77$), but also the fact that it was drawn from only five wards (Bellaby and Oribabor 1980). In contrast, our data are from a much larger sample ($N = 435$) and are based on a one in three random sample of all professional and student or pupil nurses in one district health authority.

Despite this, Bellaby and Oribabor did come to some important conclusions. The first of these related to nurses' own stated reasons for joining a particular organization. This was especially important for membership of the RCN, which was seen as a defender of nursing standards. Secondly, the activities of local officers of organizations were seen as important for the growth of membership amongst the trade unions, and it was suggested that the RCN had not increased its membership owing to a lack of local activity. Thirdly, dissatisfaction with management, with which the RCN was identified, was leading nurses to join trade unions. Finally, they noted that the organization of work is a factor of some importance, since nurses in psychiatry, for example, were overwhelmingly members of COHSE (Bellaby and Oribabor 1980: 149–56).

In our view this last factor – what we term the institutional bases of organizational membership – is overwhelmingly important. Given our larger sample we are able to examine these issues more rigorously than Bellaby and Oribabor were able to do.

Background and sample details

The discussion below is based on an analysis of a postal questionnaire sent to nurses in 1986. One approach of the questionnaire was to replicate a number of questions from the research of, for example, the 1972 Briggs Committee (Briggs 1972; Birch 1975; Mercer 1979; Moores et al. 1983; and Latham 1985). Mackay has analysed the responses to questions concerning nurses' dissatisfaction with work, but has not considered union affiliation (Mackay 1988a,b, 1989).

Table 18.1 Union membership amongst professional nurses

Union	N	Per cent
RCN	220	54
COHSE	79	19
RCM	27	6
NUPE	18	4
HVA	6	1
Other	4	1
None	55	13
Total	409	98

Note: in this and subsequent tables percentages may not total 100 owing to rounding.

The research covered all categories of professionally qualified nurses and those training for such qualifications, using a one in three random sample of such nurses employed by the health authority on 1 July 1986. In total some 711 nurses were sent a copy of the questionnaire. Of the replies, 435 questionaires were suitable for analysis, and the response rate of 62 per cent can be regarded as satisfactory for a postal survey.

Overall patterns of union membership

The overall distribution of union membership amongst the nurses in our sample is presented in Table 18.1. Just over one half of our sample (54 per cent) named the RCN as their principal union organization. The Confederation of Health Service Employees (COHSE) had the next most sizeable membership with 19 per cent of respondents, whilst the National Union of Public Employees accounted for only 4 per cent of respondents. Other organizations (largely the Royal College of Midwives with 6 per cent and the Health Visitors' Association with 1 per cent) accounted for 9 per cent of respondents, whilst 13 per cent of the nurses in our sample were in no union organization. This compares with estimates of the national membership distribution in 1988 being: 57 per cent RCN, 26 per cent COHSE and 17 per cent NUPE (Beaumont and Elliott 1989: 123). Our sample apparently over-represents RCN membership, but this is likely to be due to the fact that COHSE and NUPE represent non-professional nurses, whilst our sample consists purely of professional and student nurses.

In comparison, Bellaby and Oribabor's sample seems quite exceptional with the majority of their professional nurses being members of the trade unions NALGO (37 per cent) and NUPE (29 per cent) (Bellaby and Oribabor 1980: 151). This partly reflects their narrow sampling base. In contrast, we are confident that our data enable us to give a much more informed account of the determinants of organizational membership among professional nurses.

It was felt during the design stage of the questionnaire that many nurses may be members of more than one union, and questions about this were asked. However, membership of more than one organization proved to be quite rare among the respondents in our sample. Only 3 per cent of the respondents indicated that they were members of more than one organization. Of these, dual membership was most frequent between the RCN and one of the organizations in the 'other' category – either the RCM (Royal College of Midwives) or the HVA (Health Visitors' Association) – accounting for one-third of those with dual membership. The vast majority of nurses, then, are at least formally committed to only one organization. In all the subsequent analyses we consider only the first named union.

Patterns of variation in union membership

In this section we consider variations in union membership in relation to a range of social and institutional factors. Only those tables which yielded statistically significant results are presented. Significant relationships were found with sex, age, nursing grade, hospital type and the number of career breaks from the NHS. We shall discuss the relevance of each of these factors in turn for patterns of union membership and potential tensions within nursing. We should note in passing, however, that cross-tabulations of union membership with a range of variables measuring dissatisfaction with various aspects of nursing such as pay, use of their nursing talents, opposition to community care developments, their general assessment of the hospital and lack of career opportunities did not yield significant results.

Table 18.2 shows how union membership varies by sex. The

Table 18.2 Union membership by sex.

	Sex		Total membership %
Union	Women %	Men %	
COHSE	75.9	24.1	19.3
	16.3	47.5	
NUPE	83.3	16.7	4.4
	4.1	7.5	
Other	100.0	0	9.0
	10.0	0	
RCN	93.2	6.8	53.8
	55.6	37.5	
None	94.5	5.5	13.4
	14.1	7.5	
Overall total	90.2	9.8	100.0
Total N	369	40	409
Missing information = 26			

Note: in this and subsequent tables the top line in each row refers to row percentages and the bottom line refers to column percentages.

overall predominance of women in the nursing profession (in our sample the ratio of women to men is 9:1) results in a majority of the membership of *all* organizations being women. The women are concentrated in the RCN (56 per cent of women), whilst men are disproportionately members of COHSE (48 per cent of all men). NUPE also has a higher proportion of men amongst its members than expected. All of the members of the 'other' organizations are women and this is largely owing to the predominance of midwives and health visitors in this category. Women are more likely than men to be in no union at all, but this relates to breaks in career (see Table 18.6 below).

It may be tempting to interpret these data in terms of the relative militancy/acquiescence of male and female nurses, with the more 'militant' male nurses thought to be more likely to join conventional trade unions affiliated to the TUC and willing to take strike action, rather than the 'anti-strike' RCN. This would be congruent with what was the 'conventional' view on working women's social consciousness and collective action, that women, being less committed to the labour market, are less likely to

Table 18.3 Union membership by age group.

Union	Age group				Total membership %
	Under 24 %	24–34 %	35–44 %	Over 45 %	
COHSE	19.0	34.2	26.6	20.3	19.3
	13.6	18.1	22.6	28.1	
NUPE	5.6	38.9	38.9	16.7	4.4
	0.9	4.7	7.5	5.3	
Other	10.8	40.5	24.3	24.3	9.0
	3.6	10.1	9.7	15.8	
RCN	36.4	35.9	17.7	10.0	53.8
	72.7	53.0	41.9	38.6	
None	18.2	38.2	30.9	12.2	13.4
	9.1	14.1	18.3	12.3	
Overall total	26.9	36.4	22.7	13.9	100.0
Total N	110	149	93	57	409

Missing information = 26

engage in trade union activity at whatever level (Brown 1976). However, in this instance we believe that the gendered pattern of union membership is largely to be accounted for in terms of the gender segregation of nursing jobs. The principal factor shaping these gender patterns of membership is, in our view, the specific work situation not gender per se. This interpretation is consistent with the conclusions of most other recent research on gender variations in attitudes to work (Dex 1988). We shall consider the issue of attitudes towards trade unions and professional organizations in more detail below.

Union membership by age group is shown in Table 18.3. The RCN has the youngest membership, whilst the 'other' group of unions has the oldest, containing large proportions of long-serving midwives and health visitors. In contrast, COHSE and NUPE have most of their members in the 25–44 age groups. Nurses who are not in any union are also largely to be found in these middle age groups. These age differences between the organizations are, in our view, shaped by the institutional factors of nursing grade and hospital, and it is to these that we now turn.

Table 18.4 shows union membership by nursing grade. Nursing grade correlates to some degree with age, so not unexpectedly the

Table 18.4 Union membership by nursing grade.

| Union | Nursing grade | | | | |
	Sister %	RGN %	EN %	Learners %	Total membership %
COHSE	25.3	25.3	36.7	12.7	19.3
	22.2	14.5	27.1	13.5	
NUPE	16.7	33.3	50.0	0	4.4
	3.3	4.3	8.4	0	
Other	40.5	40.5	8.1	10.8	9.0
	16.7	10.9	2.8	5.4	
RCN	21.4	31.8	23.2	23.6	53.8
	52.2	50.7	47.7	70.3	
None	9.1	49.1	27.3	14.5	13.4
	5.6	19.6	14.0	10.8	
Overall total	22.0	33.7	26.2	18.1	100.0
Total N	90	138	107	74	409

Missing information = 26

vast majority of learners (some 70 per cent) are members of the RCN. COHSE is most strongly based amongst enrolled nurses (ENs), with 37 per cent of its members being enrolled nurses. NUPE is another union which is strongly based amongst enrolled nurses with 50 per cent of its members amongst nurses on those grades. However, enrolled nurses as a whole are most likely to be in the RCN of which 48 per cent of them are members. 'Other' organizations, such as the Health Visitors' Association, are most strongly represented amongst the sister and RGN grades. While the RCN has membership levels of over 50 per cent among both sisters and RGNs, however, it still appear to receive its strongest support among learners with over 70 per cent of them in the RCN. Almost one half of non-union nurses (49 per cent) are RGNs, with 20 per cent of all RGNs not being in a union.

Patterns of union membership seem to vary most of all between hospitals and units where nurses work. This is shown in Table 18.5. COHSE has its highest levels of membership in hospitals A (the large district general hospital) and E (the mental illness/mental handicap unit), being particularly strongly based in the latter with 39 per cent of nurses there in COHSE. Similarly NUPE has almost two-thirds of its membership in hospital A

Table 18.5 Union membership by hospital.

Union	Hospital A %	B %	C %	D %	E %	SN %	Total membership %
COHSE	41.8	3.8	5.1	10.1	27.8	11.4	19.3
	19.3	11.1	12.1	13.3	39.3	14.5	
NUPE	61.1	5.6	5.6	16.7	11.1	0	4.4
	6.4	3.7	3.0	5.0	3.6	0	
Other	5.4	0	24.3	70.3	0	0	9.0
	1.2	0	27.3	43.3	0	0	
RCN	43.6	8.2	6.4	7.3	13.2	21.4	53.8
	56.1	66.7	42.4	26.7	51.7	75.8	
None	52.7	9.1	9.1	12.7	5.5	10.9	13.4
	17.0	18.5	15.2	11.7	5.4	9.7	
Overall total	41.8	6.6	8.1	14.7	13.7	15.2	100.0
Total N	171	27	33	60	56	62	409
Missing information = 26							

(61 per cent), but it has no members in the School of Nursing (category SN in Table 18.5). 'Other' unions are most strongly represented in the community (C) and midwifery/gynaecology (D) units, with no members at all in hospitals/units B, E and SN. Like COHSE and NUPE, the RCN draws the greatest proportion of its members from the large district general hospital (A), but it has the highest membership density in the School of Nursing. Hospitals A, B and C have the highest proportions of non-union nurses, while, in contrast, the mental illness/mental handicap units and the School of Nursing are the most densely unionized. Overall it seems to be the sheer size of the district general hospital that is very important in determining where large aggregate numbers of union members are to be found, although any particular hospital or unit will be disproportionately represented by one or two organizations.

The number of breaks from NHS employment seems to be related to union membership in an interesting way, as shown in Table 18.6. Overall it appears that the RCN tends to have lower levels of membership amongst those nurses who have returned to the NHS. In short, the RCN seems to lose members over time after they leave and then return to the NHS. This interpretation is

Table 18.6 Union membership by number of breaks from NHS.

| Union | Number of breaks | | | Total membership % |
	None %	One %	Two + %	
COHSE	55.7	26.6	17.7	19.9
	18.6	20.2	25.9	
NUPE	33.3	61.1	5.6	4.5
	4.1	7.5	0.0	
Other	52.8	36.1	11.1	9.1
	8.0	12.5	7.4	
RCN	72.4	16.2	11.4	53.0
	63.9	32.7	44.4	
None	32.1	47.2	20.8	13.4
	7.1	24.0	20.4	
Overall total	60.1	26.3	13.6	100.0
Total N	238	104	54	396
Missing information = 39				

reinforced by the data in Tables 18.3–18.5, where the RCN is shown to have a high density of membership among young trainee nurses in the School of Nursing. In contrast, older qualified nurses returning to the NHS are more likely to be members of other unions or to be in no union at all.

In this section we have shown that patterns of union and professional organization membership vary significantly in relation to gender, age, nursing grade, hospital or unit of employment and the number of breaks a nurse has had from the NHS. Overwhelmingly important in our view is the institutional basis of organizational membership as measured by the variables nursing grade and hospital. Organizations will build up over time a tradition of representation of particular hospitals and particular groups of nurses; for example, COHSE's representation of nurses in the mental illness and mental handicap sectors. Further, organizations will over time build up resources of organization in particular institutions in the form of experienced local activists and local branch committees which will be able to attract new members from amongst those starting employment there.

There remain, however, the issues of gender and age variations

Table 18.7 Attitudes towards union.

Attitude	N	Per cent
Anti-union	39	11
Satisfied	273	77
Low militancy	43	12
Total	355	100
Missing information = 80		

in organizational membership. The age variations we suspect are largely explicable by the concentration of younger nurses in the School of Nursing and the lack of young nurses among groups such as midwives and health visitors, who account for much of the membership of 'other' organizations. In relation to gender, men tend to be more frequently found among the sister and enrolled nurse grades than their overall numbers in nursing would suggest, whilst no men at all are found among midwives and health visitors in our sample. More significant are the patterns of gender segregation between hospitals, where 67 per cent of all male nurses are found in the mental illness and mental handicap units (Bagguley 1988). In our view, these patterns of variation in organizational membership by gender and age are largely effects of the institutional bases of the organizations and unions concerned.

Nurses' attitudes to their organizations

Nurses' attitudes towards their unions and professional organizations were measured by asking them whether or not they thought the union was looking after their interests, and, if not, why they thought the unions were not looking after their interests. The responses were coded into anti-union sentiments, pro-union satisfaction and pro-union, but dissatisfied, expressed in terms of the union not being militant enough. Table 18.7 shows that the vast majority of respondents were quite satisfied with their own union, and the remainder were fairly evenly split between those who were anti-union, feeling that the unions were too militant, or that their union was not being militant enough.

Surprisingly, of all the variables considered in relation to nurses'

Table 18.8 Attitude towards union by union membership.

Attitude towards union	COHSE %	NUPE %	Union Other %	RCN %	None %	Overall total %
Anti-union	13.2	5.3	15.8	50.0	15.8	11.0
	6.8	11.8	16.7	9.0	66.7	
Union alright	24.2	5.7	9.8	60.0	0.4	76.6
	86.5	88.2	72.2	75.7	11.1	
Union not militant enough	11.6	0	9.3	74.4	4.7	12.4
	6.8	0	11.1	15.2	22.2	
Total membership	21.4	4.9	10.4	60.7	2.6	100.0
Total N	74	17	36	210	9	346

Missing = 89

attitudes towards their union, only union membership itself produced a statistically significant result. The results are presented in Table 18.8. Two-thirds of those who were not in unions expressed anti-union sentiments, which is obviously consistent with their not being in a union. However, 22 per cent of these felt that the unions were not militant enough, but these results should be treated with *extreme caution*, given the low number of responses from non-union members. Of union members, NUPE and COHSE members were most likely to be satisfied with their unions, with over 85 per cent in each union feeling that their union looked after their interests satisfactorily. Members of the RCN were the most likely of union members to say their union was not representing their interests by reason of not being militant enough. Nevertheless, a clear majority of RCN members (over 75 per cent) felt that their union was adequately representing their interests.

Conclusions

The principal empirical findings of our work are as follows. First, there are significant gender differences in the membership of nursing unions. In particular, women are concentrated in the RCN, men are disproportionately members of COHSE. Lack of membership of unions was found to be related to age, nursing grade and career breaks. More specifically, middle-aged nurses, RGNs and those nurses who have had a break from NHS employment are more likely than other nurses *not* to be members of unions. However, we have argued that nursing grade and especially the hospital or unit where a nurse works are the most important factors shaping union membership. We contend therefore that the gender segregation of the workforce accounts for much of the apparent gender variations in union membership.

The only factor we identified which related to nurses' attitudes towards their unions was union membership itself. The first point to make is that a large majority of all nurses of all unions feel that their unions are looking after their interests. However, members of the RCN are more likely than members of other unions to feel that their union is not militant enough in representing their interests. In contrast, those who are not in any union are the most likely to express anti-union views.

Given the importance of institutional factors in determining nurses' membership of trade unions and semi-professional organizations, any forthcoming changes in the institutional forms of health care delivery could lead to significant losses of membership among professional nurses for particular organizations. On the ground, these shifts may well appear complex and confusing. The development of community care may be an important factor in this context, especially affecting COHSE. From another angle, the RCN, with the highest level of dissatisfaction with its performance among its members, may under some circumstances face potential losses to the unions. However, as Bellaby and Oribabor found in the late 1970s, this is not something new. None the less, if unions such as COHSE respond successfully to the threats to its membership levels by making significant inroads into the institutional bases of the RCN's support, then the next ten years could see major changes of membership and strategy among professional nurses' organizations.

Ackowledgements

The author was a member of the team of the Nursing Recruitment and Wastage project at Lancaster University financed by the Leverhulme

Trust. The team is grateful to the health authority concerned for their help and cooperation.

References

Abel-Smith, B. 1960. *A History of the Nursing Profession*. London: Heinemann.

Bagguley, P. 1988. *A Report of a Study of Turnover and Work Dissatisfaction amongst UK Professional Nurses*. Department of Sociology, Cartmel College, Lancaster University, Lancaster.

Bain, G. S. and Price, R. 1983. Union growth: dimensions, determinants, and density. In G. S. Bain (ed.), *Industrial Relations in Britain*. Oxford: Basil Blackwell.

Beaumont, P. B. and Elliott, J. 1989. Individual employee choice between unions: some public sector evidence from Britain. *Industrial Relations Journal* 22: 119–27.

Bellaby, P. and Oribabor, P. 1977. The growth of trade union consciousness among general hospital nurses viewed as a response to 'proletarianisation'. *Sociological Review* 25(3).

Bellaby, P. and Oribabor, P. 1980. 'The history of the present' – contradiction and struggle in nursing. In C. Davies (ed.), *Rewriting Nursing History*. London: Croom Helm.

Birch, J. 1975. *To Nurse or Not to Nurse: An Investigation into the Causes of Withdrawal during Nurse Training*. London: Royal College of Nursing.

Bosanquet, N. (ed.) 1979. *Industrial Relations in the NHS – the search for a system*. London: King Edward's Hospital Fund for London.

Briggs, A. 1972. *Report of the Committee on Nursing*, Cmnd 5115. London: HMSO.

Brown, R. 1976. Women as employees: some comments on research in industrial sociology. In D. Barker and S. Allen (eds), *Dependence and Exploitation in Work and Marriage*. London: Longman.

Carpenter, M. 1988. *Working for Health: the history of COHSE*. London: Lawrence & Wishart.

Dex, S. 1988. *Women's Attitudes to Work*. London: Macmillan.

Dyson, S. and Spray, K. 1979. Professional associations. In Bosanquet 1979.

Latham, J. P. 1985. Absence from work at the Royal Albert Hospital, Lancaster. Unpublished MA thesis, University of Lancaster.

Lewis, S. S. 1976. Nurses and trade unions in Britain. *International Journal of Health Services* 6(4).

Mackay, L. 1988a. Career woman. *Nursing Times* 84(10).

Mackay, L. 1988b. No time to care. *Nursing Times* 84(11).

Mackay, L. 1989. *Nursing a Problem*. Milton Keynes: Open University Press.

Mercer, G. 1979. *The Employment of Nurses*. London: Croom Helm.

Moores, B. *et al.* 1983. An analysis of the factors which impinge on a nurse's decision to enter, stay in, leave or re-enter the nursing profession. *Journal of Advanced Nursing* 8: 227–35.

UKCC. 1987. *Project 2000*. London: United Kingdom Council for Nursing, Midwifery and Health Visiting.

Waite, R. and Hutt, R. 1987. *Attitudes, Jobs and Mobility of Qualified Nurses: A Report for the Royal College of Nursing*.IMS Report No. 130. Brighton: Institute of Manpower Studies.

Winchester, D. 1988. Sectoral change and trade-union organization. In D. Gallie (ed.), *Employment in Britain*. Oxford: Basil Blackwell.

CHAPTER NINETEEN

Nurses and the prospects of participative management in the NHS

Stephen Ackroyd

Introduction

In many ways the management of public services is a different type of activity from management in most parts of the private sector. Because of the character of the relationship involved in the actual provision of public sector services, which is in most instances quite unlike that involved when services are supplied on the open market, management has grown up in response to quite different problems and pressures and takes quite different forms (Ackroyd *et al.* 1989). Moreover, the patterns exhibited by public sector management can be seen to be just as viable and efficient in their own context as private sector management often is when it coordinates and directs the supply of goods to the market. If this is so, it would be wrong to assume that the management found in public sector services is, or still less should be, an imitation of management in the private sector. Equally erroneous is the idea that the development of management must necessarily imply the extension of the market, privatization and the elimination of public service as traditionally understood (Hindess 1987).

From this general stance on public sector management the case of the NHS will be considered. The actual pattern of the development of management in the service will be traced and linked with ideas about the condition of general nursing in hospitals. First, however, it is necessary to develop the discussion of management in the public services more adequately, indicating the pressures that have given rise to the characteristic forms of public sector management. From this it can be argued that there are some directions in which public sector management can and should be developed so as to enhance and preserve what is distinctive and valuable in present services.

Different types of public sector management

Three types of public sector management can be identified in branches of the public services at the present time. These are: (1) centrally directed policy management; (2) producers' cooperative management, and (3) participative management. While current services often involve elements of all three types, it is argued that the participative management pattern actually does most to preserve and promote the best aspects of public service provision. In brief, the active encouragement of this pattern of management would be both desirable and beneficial as the core around which a distinctive and effective management for public services should be built.

Participative management in the NHS

It has to be admitted that, uniquely amongst British public services, the prospects for the development of participative management in the NHS are not particularly good. Essentially, the reasons for this are simple. First, there is the centralization of the system, of which the most significant aspect is the political control of NHS resources from the centre. This gives any government powerful leverage, encouraging tendencies towards the central direction of policy as well as the control and monitoring of activities, all of which may actually impede the effective delivery of care. Centralization also actively impedes public participation, which must be local as well as regional and national to be effective.

Participative management depends on admitting the general public to a share in policy-making. However, the second major factor limiting the possibilities for participative management in the NHS stems from the presence of three powerful but distinct occupational groups in the NHS – doctors, nurses and administrators – whose involvements and interest in the service are partly divergent. It is difficult for the public to share in policy-making in a situation where no one group has the ability to decide policy. In contrast, in education, social services and the police, there is only one relatively undifferentiated occupational group which, in effect, monopolizes the provision of a particular service and therefore controls it. This gives powerful support to tendencies towards the *producers' cooperative pattern* of provision of public services (Klein 1989), but also allows limited developments towards a more participative pattern. In such cases the management structures are exclusively staffed by members of the same occupation and this management tends to have the same basic services. In the NHS, the pattern of recruitment of managers is historically and currently quite different. Managers are recruited mainly from former administrators, while few doctors and nurses have been recruited to general management, especially at high levels. In fact, the management of the hospital services in Britain up to and after the formation of the NHS was essentially a *producers' cooperative* controlled by the doctors, with the nurses as junior partners responsible for much day-to-day management. By a process that will be traced here, the producer's cooperative style of management has passed into a system of more directed control in which former administrators (renamed managers) have much more power, ultimately deriving from their control of budgets.

The combination of centralization and occupational division has given the management of the NHS its quite distinctive qualities. In particular, it is perhaps the most overtly coercive of public sector managements, effecting control relatively crudely and often without much enthusiastic consent, mainly through the device of the control of budgets. In this arrangement, the nurses, who are the primary providers of actual medical care, are largely excluded from those aspects of management which set the general structure of resource allocation and which profoundly, if indirectly, affect both the quantity and quality of services provided. But this does not mean that the nurses have nothing to do with management and have been effectively excluded from all aspects of management. In the provision of hospital care, the tasks that nurses need to accomplish are many, and their resources limited, and only they are qualified, in conjunction with the doctors, to decide appropriate procedures and priorities in actual provision. Nurses not only 'man' but also manage the basic process of health care. As a matter of practicality, then, it is nurses who actually manage the final delivery of medical care. The outcome is that while managerial functions are not all in the hands of one managerial group, there is no uniformity of policy or outlook as a result. Hence, it will be argued that participative management is effectively prevented from developing in the NHS by the existence of other forms of management and of conflict between them. Indeed, arguably, the present condition of NHS management is actively damaging to the service. It will certainly be suggested that the way forward is to take active steps towards the development of participative management, in which the primary producers – the nurses – have a very much more active role.

Origin and character of types of public sector management

The origin of public sector services in Britain is extremely local. Such provisions as were first made historically for the relief of acute needs were made by the action and initiative of local people. Sometimes this was within the framework of national legislation, as in the case of early attempts to provide relief from poverty. But even here the services provided varied a good deal according to pre-existing standards of provision. The beginnings of medical services for the general public are in many ways a classic case of local initiatives being the basis of service. Early hospitals, first developed in a recognizably modern form in the early period of the industrial revolution (Abel-Smith 1964), as well as personal medical services which pre-dated the hospitals, were deeply rooted in localities. Costs of these services were borne by local people and the services were for the benefit of the local community. In many ways, the founding of the NHS in 1948 was not a departure from localism except in funding and administration. The founding policy of the NHS was personalized care – an individual provider treating an individual patient. Generally, the growth in the scale of public services resulting from the growth of population size and the concentrations of populations into urban centres did not produce any change from this basic plan. What did occur, however, was the rapid and extensive emergence of a more bureaucratized administration of services, in which extensive recording of aspects of provision developed. To some extent this was justified by the need for good clinical records, sometimes also by the perceived need for good housekeeping in respect of the escalating cost of provision.

It is important to distinguish this increasing administration associated with services from the active management of services. With administered services, clerical staff simply support the activities of professionals by keeping records and accounts and recording decisions. Policy decisions about physical development, expenditure on capital and consumable equipment, employment policy and employment decisions were all securely retained by professionals as extensions of their professional capacity. In the health service, a curious division of professional labour grew up between doctors and nurses, in that clinical and treatment decisions as aspects of care were retained by the doctors – together with control over all major expenditure and other policy matters – whilst the nurses developed a very extended responsibility for the actual day-to-day and hour-to-hour delivery of care (Abel-Smith 1960; Davies 1980). This role carried with it, as did that of the doctors, very real responsibility for many aspects that would be seen today as basic to management – for example, autonomy over the employment, training and use of staff, the cleaning and refurbishment of wards and office areas as well as responsibility for the quality of clinical routine. The matron of a hospital any time up to, and until 20 years after, the Second World War was primarily a line manager whose principal task was responsibility for most of the practical health care delivery within the hospital (Davies 1980). Although they did not think of their work in that way, management being a male occupation mainly restricted to factories, analysis of the actual activities of senior nurses shows how very large were the directing, controlling and organizing aspects of their occupation. During this period, with doctors and nurses sharing the bulk of the directive and organizing work, there was actually very little except record-keeping for administrators to do. Their numbers were few and their status low.

In most of the public sector services the rise of a professional managerial cadre – which even now shows very little independent development – can be traced to the emergence of increasing centralized government interest in local service provision. It is interesting that management, which in many people's thinking is automatically associated with the activity of the capitalist class, can be shown in the case of public services to arise largely in response to the activities of the central government.

In point of fact, however, this is an oversimplification because the development of private sector management itself, as a distinctive occupation and competence, was the product of the increasing separation of ownership and control in the maturing private enterprise economy. Management is a role which mediates between contending parties. Thus private sector management emerged with large-scale industry and grew up because of the need for coordination and planning of large-scale industry. The new managers were largely non-capitalist, that is property-less, professionals. True, they had a vested interest in the profitability and success of any busiess they were managing, but their concerns were not precisely the same as those of owner-managers. They had an interest, for example, in the longer-term development of an organization, for the specialization and development of the management profession, which owners may not have had. For career managers in private enterprise, shareholders and their representatives on boards of directors were increasingly just one of a number of groups whose legitimate interest in a firm had to be managed. Hence a case can be made that private sector management also first emerged as a role which mediates between different parties: owners, employees and customers.

In a similar way, the rise of public service management can be traced to the time when the government began to subsidize the activities of local authorities, and so acquired an interest, somewhat akin to that of a large shareholder, in the economical and efficient provision of services. However, early public services, even in their highly bureaucratized form, were administered rather than managed, in that such policy decisions as were made were largely determined by professionals whose expertise originated from their capacities as service providers: senior doctors, social workers and educators. Those who had no such occupational competences were regarded as administrative support staff. Administrators kept records of what was done and in other ways supported ongoing activity; that is all. The emergence of an active managerial function, in which separate attention is given to problems of the organization and coordination of services and the consideration of efficiency in service delivery, was slow to develop in these circumstances. To the extent that it did so it was largely an additional function acquired by professionals, that is, doctors and nurses, who had come to devote their time increasingly to administrative activity. For this reason, when it did emerge, the specialized management of public services was defensive in character.

Professionals managing the services which they had at some time practised naturally sought in some part to protect the autonomy of service providers and what they saw as the integrity of service provision. When a powerful and largely external agency, in the shape of the government, began to exert real control with the threat to reduce funding, the relevance of economy and efficiency began to be seen, but only within the assumption that the service should be preserved. Thus, to a large extent, early management was subordinated to professional expertise, and, to a considerable degree in many areas, still is. For this reason, this defensive condition of public sector management can be thought of as the expected style of public sector management in this country. This management orientation has been described elsewhere as 'custodial management' (Ackroyd *et al.* 1989). It is certainly true that managers in much of the public sector base their role not on a claim to managerial skill per se but on their professional skills and abilities as service providers. Chief constables and chief education officers are managers in the sense that they devote their time to organizational matters and are generally interested in performance, but they are equally if not more interested in maintaining customary types and standards of service provision. Because they have these matters at the centre of their concern, they can be thought of as custodians of the services they provide as much as managers of them. Equally, however, because this management is management of producers by producers, another name for this type of management is suggested by the work of Klein (1989) on the political history of the NHS, in which he describes aspects of organization as a 'producers' cooperative'. The idea of producers' cooperative management is perhaps most relevant to situations in which any collusive aspects of public sector service control predominate over either administrative or managerial functions. In fact this idea is perhaps more relevant to other services, as we shall see. The senior levels of educational administration, the police service and social services are still securely monopolized by people who began their public service as teachers, police constables and social workers, which is not the case in the NHS any longer. However, in the following, the terms 'custodial management' and 'producer's cooperative management' will be used as synonyms.

It will be argued that the label 'producers' cooperative' was appropriate to the hospital service in the early stages of its development, up to and including the period of local authority control before nationalization. It was still true in the early days of the development of the NHS. Here, however, the wealth and independence of the senior doctors, and the fact they shared their managerial role with senior nurses, weakened the security of specifically professional involvement in and therefore control over emerging managerial structures. The adoption of the unique form of a board of management for health authorities reflects the complex division of labour between professional groups in the service, and actually proved inimical to direct forms of local democracy.

In accounting for the rise of public service *management* – as a separate and more complex form of organizational coordination that public service *administration* – it is important to recognize that the interests of political paymasters in government and of the actual providers of services in localities do not precisely correspond. Very generally speaking, the former are interested in obtaining maximum benefit for minimum cost, whilst the latter has as its primary concern serving a particular community, by supplying what are seen to be their immediate needs. Whilst, from the point of view of the political centre, there must necessarily be some limit to state expenditure, from the point of view of service providers this is much less obviously true. In contrast, for professionals, what might be done for people is limited mainly by the applicability of their experience and knowledge. In most of its present forms, public service management can be seen as mediating between these two orientations and adopting charac-teristic strategies to do so. By various means and devices, the political centre may seek to reduce the cost of public service provision, but, because they cannot directly control the activities of service providers, by whose changed activity any economies will be made, it is difficult to translate their economizing intentions into real economies in provision. Moreover, in devising more economical and effective ways of delivering the same – or preferably better – levels of services for the same price, the political centre is almost entirely in the hands of the professionals themselves.

It is hardly surprising therefore that it has been government that has taken initiatives to impose what are taken to be the best innovations of practice by progressive localities on other authorities as well as taking other initiatives for dissemination of ideas and sponsoring research. This has often involved government directly and indirectly fostering the emergence of local management, because this is the agency through which such changes will be introduced. Indeed, much central government administration can now be seen to be implicated in the process of local management development. These processes of engineering change by administrative devices are just as important as straightforward ideological attempts to limit policy and provision of public services. However, the basic problem for government is that so much depends on basically qualitative judgements about the appropriateness of particular treatments and services which can only be made by public sector workers themselves. Doctors have for many years successfully claimed the right to be the only party whose judgement is relevant to clinical decisions. In effect, the degree of customary control over 'clinical' decision-making is one of the main concerns of public sector management and an indicator of their custodial orientation. In a similar way, but with less conviction and less complete success, educators, social workers and policemen have made similar claims. To the extent that government has been the leader in forming policy and effectively ensuring that localities follow such directions, we may refer to a different kind of public sector management which we label 'centrally directed policy management'. In doing so, no implication is made that management of this type is simply the tool of government policy or that elements of custodial control have entirely disappeared.

One variant of centrally directed policy is to make the supply of services responsive to consumer demand. Apart from the ideological preferences some governments may have for this, such a policy recommends itself as a way of making services in some degree responsive to the preferences of recipients. However, there are other ways of making sure that the interests of the public are taken into account. In recent decades, an identifiable consumer interest in patterns and standards of service has emerged. This can vary between increased willingness to complain, to express dissent either personally or through complaints machinery such as tribunals. Most significant, perhaps, is the increasing organization of public opinion through pressure groups and even mass movements expressing interest in the effects of public service provision. In many ways these are significant developments because public opinion of this kind constitutes, potentially, an alternative basis on which appropriate levels and kinds of service provision might be judged. As such, public opinion stands as a clear alternative to the principle of economy, with which the political centre tends to operate, and which tends to dominate in the centrally directed mode of public sector service management. Similarly, it is an alternative to the idea that the principles underlying professional judgement should be the supreme point of reference concerning the nature and types of service offered, which is the operative idea behind the producers' cooperative pattern of management.

It is an arresting idea but none the less probably true that, for much of their history, public sector services were provided substantially in ignorance of what their recipients thought about them. This applied not only to the standards of services, but to the provision of services as such. In a sense, the police are the public providers whose activity marks the extreme of this approach. Members of the public area, in certain circumstances, likely to get the attention of the police 'service' whether they want it or not. In much the same spirit – at best paternalistic and at worst authoritarian – other public services operate. So, for example, within the NHS the real therapeutic benefits of proffered treatments are often not fully discussed with patients. Indeed, there is no escaping the conclusion that public sector services have always had a coercive element (Pinker 1971).

In a democratic and increasingly individualistic age, paternalism and authoritarianism are questioned and resisted. As a result, public services have developed the capacity to take public opinion into account. To the extent that they appear to do so, they can acquire increased legitimacy and security. In this sense, pressure groups and other devices by which public opinion can achieve expression so as to be taken into account by service providers are the equivalent to the feedback given to producers by consumer demand in the private sector. Indeed, it seems clear that, unless such devices are fostered, public sector services will disappear. What will be left will be services provided only on the market, whose level of provision is regulated by the price mechanism, together with a residue of overtly coercive state functions the impact of which is regulated directly by political power.

The significance of the development of organized public opinion about public services can hardly be exaggerated. This is because it offers a way in which the effects of public services and the needs and desires of the public can be more effectively reconciled. This is vital. Only by aligning more closely the needs of people as they perceive them with what the public services actually provide can the future of public services be effectively guaranteed. Where public opinion is taken into account, viable and responsible public sector services can survive and develop. Management which recognizes the need for this may be called 'participative management'. Elements of it are recognizable in all contemporary public sector services, but their survival depends on the willingness of managers to take participation seriously. Whilst in many ways the NHS has shown considerable development of public sector management, its capacity for participative management is weak.

Three types of hospital management and the role of the nurse

In this section the three patterns of public sector management distinguished in the last section will be applied more systematically to the case of the hospital service in the NHS. Broadly speaking it will be argued that the service has followed a particular path between the three patterns of management discussed earlier, and has done so for reasons that can be quite clearly identified. The consequences of change for the status and role of nurses have been profound, and we need to trace out these connections.

Briefly, the pattern of change has been as follows. A very full development of *producers' cooperative management* occurred in the early years of the development of the modern hospital service. Up to the end of the first decade after the formation of the NHS the hospital consultants were the dominant group in the hospital service, but the producer's cooperative gave over very rapidly to a full development of *centrally directed policy management*. In the first arrangement, the nurses, as the junior partner to the hospital doctors, had a considerable role in management and considerable occupational prestige. This was to some extent reflected in the adoption of a highly hierarchical form of occupational organization which copies the professional hierarchy of hospital consultants. However, the emergence of centrally directed policy management had the effect of changing the status of the nurse, by reorganizing the functions of management and placing effective power in other hands. Nurses now found themselves relatively powerless to change their situation. Unlike other public services, the NHS has been firmly locked into the centrally directed mode.

The progressive exclusion of the nurses from any managerial functions other than routine supervision of junior nurses, and particularly from effective policy in the use of resources, is the key to understanding the fall in the status of the profession, the loss of morale and the rise of aggressive trades unionism. The rapid movement of some other public sector services towards a more decentralized form of organization, which has been associated with managerial autonomy and public participation in management, has not been in any significant degree observed in the NHS. Without much understanding of the importance of participative management in public service, central government has used centralization as a platform on which to develop a management with a market orientation, and has developed a managerial function which concentrates power in the hands of a specialized cadre of non-professionals. In this situation, nurses are substantially deprived of participation in management, but are exposed to the rising demands of the public. Nurses today have to deal with insurgent public opinion without any possibility of mobilizing management to recognize their problems or those of the public concerned. Very wide-ranging adoption of participative management and participative structures is needed in order to deal with the growing alienation of the nurse (with other health service workers) from their organization *and* from the general public. First, however, we need to identify in more detail the distinctive path followed by the NHS and its importance for nurses.

Producers' cooperative management: nursing as an elite profession

Until the formation of the NHS, and for more than a decade thereafter, the emergent form of public sector management in the hospital service was the *producers' cooperative*. The hospital consultants were securely in charge of the medical services provided by hospitals in which they worked, and nurses, as junior partners with the doctors, completed the monopoly of control of the clinical services provided (Abel-Smith 1964). It is true that their control was not absolute, in that they had to operate within a political structure, in the shape of either a local authority committee from 1930 or a regional hospital board after the start of the NHS. None the less, the power and influence of the consultants was considerable; they were often the single most concerted voice on the hospital boards, and had an important presence at regional level. But the point to note is not simply their formal power, but the fact that their professional standing commanded great respect. In decisions about what should be done, and how monies should be divided between heads, a good deal of deference was extended to medical opinion. True, in order to gt their way and to achieve their ends, there had to be a degree of professional solidarity amongst consultants. Agreements between consultants had to be secured, but where this occurred, professional control of the hospitals was almost absolute.

Nurses had every reason to consolidate a professional alliance with doctors. Nurses had historically identified closely with the doctors and modelled aspects of their professional organization on medicine (Davies 1972). The steep hierarchy in nursing – hierarchy based on academic knowledge and ability as much as practical skill – is a key indicator of the extent of the traditional identification with the medical profession. Also, along with this copying of forms of organization, it is important to emphasize the symbiotic relation (of mutual dependence) between doctors and nurses in the division of labour for the provision of care. The work of doctors in dealing effectively with large numbers of patients was enormously facilitated by the understudy and support role taken by the nurses. Nurses were very much subordinated to medical control, taking over all of the routine and most of the distasteful aspects of care, but they also obtained involvement in significant aspects of management. Indeed, in career terms, in the first half of the present century nursing was one of the very few professions offering the possibility of the progression to positions of considerable power and influence specifically to women. Of course, nursing hierarchies were steep and the number of elite positions – as the matron of a major hospital, for example – very few, but symbolically the existence of these positions was arguably much more important than their numbers.

If the tradition of managerial power for senior nurses has not persisted, one important legacy of this period for the nurse has remained. This lies in opportunities for education. One aspect of this is the high level of specialist training that the able and energetic and able recruit to nursing could expect to obtain. The high level of education of many recruits to nursing in the post-war years, and the highly formalized character of knowledge on the subject, allowed the emergence of degrees in nursing studies. Nurses were often very much better qualified academically than many of their administrative counterparts. Nevertheless, the position of nurses in the professional division of labour depended very much on the continued power and influence of the doctors.

The great problem with the producers' cooperative as a form of management has been the extent to which it may serve the interests of the producers – as opposed to those who consume the production – more than it should. It is not easy to provide a built-in regulatory mechanism to operate when there is abuse of professional power. It would be wrong to assume, however, that only the market can constitute a mechanism to ensure the provision of excellent service. As evidence of this, it is clear that the post-war period produced some of the finest and largest hospitals in Europe and possibly the world. Renowned centres of specialist treatment such as Christies, Addenbrookes and the Brompton hospital attracted first the specialized staff and then the level of capital equipment and consumable funding allowing them to rise to importance. Nor were centres of excellence confined to specialist centres; many London and provincial urban hospitals became deservedly renowned for the range of services provided. Sadly, however, the producer's cooperative form of organization will, of course, protect the inadequate to the same degree that it can empower the excellent. Indeed, the justification of centralized control, the next stage in the development of hospital management, was partly in trying to limit the wide variations in levels and standards of service throughout the country.

The rise of centralized control: nursing as a costly factor of production

The deal struck with the reforming post-war Labour administration by the hospital consultants as a condition for their participation in the NHS was, as is well known, extremely beneficial to them. It left many of the consultants with a high and secure income, and the majority of senior consultants with the option of being employed only part time within the new structure. This contractual arrangement certainly enhanced the professional prestige of consultants, and so, in the short term, enhanced their political standing as independent advisers. However, indirectly and in the longer term, the influence of the professionals within the hospital structure was fatally compromised. It led senior doctors progressively to reduce their interest to strictly professional issues and to be concerned about resource questions only in so far as they directly affected their ability to perform their own specialist aspects of care.

To an extent this development is attributable to the very success of the early NHS hospitals. Under the producers' cooperative, hospitals had become large and expenditure huge. As managers everywhere in the world have discovered, logistical problems grow disproportionately with scale. Coordination becomes a pressing issue. In short, the practical division of labour worked out by the doctors and nurses was not equal to the new tasks now placed upon it. Bureaucracy, the extensive record-keeping and accounting work of the hospital administrators, burgeoned, and this development was not entirely without function or obvious benefit. Hence, we must add to the idea that senior doctors had less financial and political stake in controlling the hospitals, the idea that a quantum growth in the scale of the managerial task which faced them made the control of hospitals increasingly difficult. In these circumstances, senior doctors relied more and more on administrators for support. In this set of related processes, nurses, as the weaker dependent part in the old professional alliance, lost both function and status.

Introducing a national system of hospital provision, the NHS involved a quantum increase in administrative functions and overhead. The advent of the NHS added new tiers of bureaucracy. Some of this would be concerned with monitoring the costs of the service, comparing the activities and costs from region to region, and imposing policies for public health on localities. But for a long time, this increased administration had few recognizably *managerial* attributes. There was a delay before administrative practice began to acquire significant managerial aspects and to become the main organizational device for coordination and control of the service.

It is common for descriptions of the management of the NHS in the 1970s and into the 1980s to stress the plurality of kinds of practice in the service. Smith (1978), for example, stressed the simultaneous existence of three domains – management, professional and political – and suggested that each was extremely influential in affecting practical outcomes. He suggested, however, that no one of these domains could be dominant and that the NHS was a strange hybrid type of organization which did not fit the available theoretical accounts of organization. Similarly, Davies and Francis (1976) suggested that neither a pure professional model of the hospital as an organization nor a bureaucratic model would do as a basic description. In their different ways these writers suggested that the hospital service of the time was best understood as an overlapping set of processes in which specifically managerial functions were dispersed amongst a number of groups. In fact, it was possible to interpret this as a process of transition from an organization controlled by professionals to one in which bureaucracy was very much more in evidence. Crudely expressed, the pattern of change was that administrators – through their tie with the central bureaucracy and overall knowledge of expenditures – were gaining an increasing control over resources. In the emergent arrangement, the senior doctors retained some control over decision-making through a power of veto, while the nurses in practice organized and managed the delivery of care.

At this point, however, administrators were increasingly seeing themselves as managers in the sense of having strategic control of the organization and giving direction to other groups of employees, particularly nurses, technicians and ancillary staff. Nurses fought a tentative rearguard action over their exclusion from the executive aspects of management, retaining formal recognition of their function as controllers of the activity of other nurses. By the use of the 'management team' concept and other devices, they tried to perpetuate a version of the producer's cooperative form (cf. Bellaby and Oribabar 1980). The point to make, however, is that in the process of the emergence of a more centrally directed kind of management, in which strategic control was seen as the core function and the control of costs became the key means of exerting control, the actual managerial role which nurses continued to discharge was, not lost, so much as devalued and overlooked. The perceived importance of their functions was vastly weakened by the absence of control over resources. The progressive alienation of senior nurses from what was now seen as basic managerial practice, increasingly consolidated in the hands of administrators turned managers, has had a number of identifiable effects.

One of the most obvious early indicators of the exclusion from key aspects of management was a drop in morale amongst nurses. It is no accident that the classic study of occupational morale by Revans (1964) took place in the 1960s amongst nurses in a hospital. Since that time, concern for the morale of nurses has been recurrent (Ackroyd 1987; Mackay 1989). Perceiving the problem of low morale amongst hospital staff to be more than a matter of psychology, Revans conducted with others a series of studies of communication in hospitals. There is some substance to the suggestion that hospitals suffered from problems of poor communication and indeed still do. It would seem that these problems are more than just the results of being made a large-scale operation. The plurality of hierarchies in which the professionals have a separate pattern of relationships and norms of conduct from the bureaucrats and administrators is compounded by the fact that they are actively in contention with each other over aspects of organizational control. Conflict over te day-to-day control of hospitals obviously has many implications for the effectiveness of communications within them. Another indication of the same tension is the increasing split between the collegiate or 'quasi-professional' form of trades unionism embodied in the highly traditional RCN, and the rise of more militant radical trades unionism in COHSE and other unions (see also Chapter 18 in this volume).

Nurses have been extensively researched since the 1960s. Research that has looked at the way that nurses in hospitals actually organize themselves has shown that they are extremely resourceful and independent. They fit very well with what have been described as autonomous or self-managing work groups. Nurses achieve remarkable levels of care in the face of undermanning and other shortages (Anthony and Reed 1990; Strong and Robinson 1990). It can be argued that the system of self-management evolved by the hospital nurse in recent decades is remarkably effective in the routine accomplishment of care. In a sense, of course, nurses have not relinquished managerial functions but have simply been excluded from those aspects of management which have become its key aspects under the regime of *centralized policy management*.

It is tempting to suggest that what occurred during the 1960s and the 1970s was the proletarianization of the hospital nurse. The gradual subordination of nurses in hospitals to the administrative cadre is a reality which ought to be acknowledged. But control of the nursing profession has many features that are not symptomatic of classic proletarianization. There is no effective direction of labour to specific tasks or close supervision of quantities of work done, as in the 'scientific management' applied in many industrial situations. In fact, the direct control of nursing in anything like the fashion used in scientific management would be very difficult to contrive by those who have no direct experence or detailed knowledge of the work. The pressures of work in hospitals are often considerable, but they are not externally imposed. There is a good deal of self-pacing of work activity in nursing, with periods of remission from intense work. There is also considerable variety of task, and team work and other forms of cooperation are everywhere apparent. Regular movements between intense work pressure and relative inactivity seems to be symptomatic. There is also some evidence that absenteeism and other kinds of time indiscipline are much higher in nursing than would be tolerated in private enterprise. On the other hand, it would be difficult to exaggerate the extent to which the hospital nurse has been marginalized and ignored in the organization of hospital care. To those who have acquired executive power in the hospitals, the nurse has become merely a costly and potentially troublesome factor of production, a fact that can hardly have greater symbolical importance.

The prospects for participative management in the NHS: nursing as skilled public service

It is a considerable paradox of contemporary management that private and public sector management are moving in opposite directions. In the private sector, radical initiatives are being taken to increase the team-working and cooperative capacities of employees in a situation where they have scarcely existed, whilst, at the very same time, public sector management often works on the assumption that they must achieve exclusive power and control over work performance in the manner assumed to be operative in the private sector. Public service managers often assume that they must learn from the private sector and, working on an outdated model of practice, are at best overlooking and at worst dissipating the results of generations of practical team-working and cooperation.

Another way in which public and private are directly opposed is in attitudes towards centralization. The private sector is trying to decentralize, pushing out all managerial functions except those elements necessary for strategic control to the periphery and reducing the size of units that can be autonomous, whereas the public sector – particularly in the NHS – seems to be obsessed with centralization. Large-scale and excessively bureaucratic organizations cannot be responsive to the public interest, and therefore decentralization of management in the NHS is a necessity. This cannot be done effectively without the participation of the main occupational groups and of the general public in policy-making. The nurse, as the person who shapes the interface between the organization and its clientele, must become the key contributor to a new system of cooperative management.

A case can be made that the private sector has as much to learn from public services as the other way about. This is because the way many public sector services are organized depends very much on the skills of highly knowledgeable and experienced people, people used to adapting themselves to giving high-quality services in difficult circumstances. In short, some of the key ingredients of participative management seem actually to be already present in our mature social services such as the hospitals. This pattern of provision recommends itself for two reasons. First, it is highly appropriate to the provision of care in circumstances where the public is increasingly vigilant about the treatment being given. Secondly, this pattern actually conforms with many attributes now taken to be indicative of best practice in many parts of the private sector. The government has its own reasons for wanting a version of private sector management style to be adopted in the NHS. Hospital managers have been only too happy to take their cue from the Griffiths Report (1983) and are attempting to model their practice on this outmoded caricature of what modern management is actually like. But as nurses know well, and their actual practice clearly shows, nursing is not a tin of beans, and the retailing of baked beans and the provision of health care are by no means the same thing. More recent recommendations than

Griffiths about the management of health care, for example in the government proposals for self-managing hospitals, are more obviously appropriate to the dilemmas of the health service at the present time, and should be looked at more carefully, and preferably not through ideological lenses (cf. Strong and Robinson 1990). There is much in such proposals that constitute opportunities for a responsive and caring hospital service fully within the public sector.

Nurses occupy a key position in the delivery of health care between any executive management and the patient. In a situation where the actual experience of care is a crucial one for the perpetuation and development of the service, management cannot proceed without the participation of such crucial people. Nurses are in a position to make or break the NHS as a social service. Equally, managers are in the position to ensure the making of the service rather than the breaking.

References

Abel-Smith, B. 1960. *A History of the Nursing Profession*. London: Heinemann.

Abel-Smith, B. 1964. *The Hospitals 1800–1948*. London: Heinemann.

Ackroyd, S., Hughes, J. A. and Soothill, K. L. 1989. Public sector services and their management. *Journal of Management Studies* 26(6).

Ackroyd, S. 1987. *Report of the Exploratory Study of Nurse Morale in the Acute Unit of Lancaster District Health Authority*. Occasional Paper, Department of Behaviour in Organisations, University of Lancaster.

Anthony, P. D. and Reed, M. I. 1990. Managerial roles and relationships in a district health authority. *International Journal of Health Care* 2.

Bellaby, P. and Oribabor, P. 1980. Determinants of occupational strategies adopted by British hospital nurses. *International Journal of Health Services* 10.

Davies, C. 1972. Professionals in organisations: observations on hospital consultants. *Sociological Review* 20.

Davies, C (ed.) 1980. *Rewriting Nursing History*. London: Croom Helm.

Davies, C. and Francis, A. 1976. Perceptions of structure in NHS hospitals. In M. Stacey (ed.), *The Sociology of the NHS*. Sociological Review Monograph 22, University of Keele, Staffs.

Griffiths Report. 1983. *NHS Management Inquiry*. London: DHSS.

Hindess, B. 1987. *Freedom, Equality and the Market: Arguments on Social Policy*. London: Tavistock.

Klein, R. 1989. *The Politics of the NHS*, 2nd edn. London: Longman.

Mackay, L. 1989. *Nursing a Problem*. London: Open University Press.

Pinker, R. 1971. *Social Theory and Social Policy*. London: Heinemann.
Revans, R. 1964. *Standards for Morale*. London: Oxford University Press.
Revans, R. 1974. *Hospital Communication – Choice and Change*. London: Tavistock.
Small, N. 1989. *Politics and Planning in the National Health Service*. London: Oxford University Press.
Smith, G. W. 1978. Towards an organisation theory for the NHS. Unpublished Organisational Development Conference Paper.
Strong, P. and Robinson, J. 1990. *The NHS: Under New Management*. London: Oxford University Press.

Index

Absenteeism 59, 69, 215, 262, 327
Accountability 89, 92, 97, 106, 124,
    127–8
  and performance indicators 114–35
  and resource allocation 121
  'consumer' 134
  future patterns 131–4
  in society 115
  of management 118
  'split' 131
Adaptive partnership 253–4
Administrators 315–16, 326
  and management recruitment 312
  and senior nurses' qualifications 323
Advertising 41–55
  an ethical issue 3, 42
  and health care environment 44–9
  and informed choice 49
  by pharmaceutical companies 43, 52
  definition 42
  doctors' services 45
  misleading 42–4
  social and political context 46
Advocacy 158–76
  and Project 2000   96, 103, 109
  definition 171–2
  ethical understanding of 175
  environment for 173–5
  nurses' role 11, 171–3
American Nurses' Association,
    identification of essential
    components of nursing 198
Angels, media representation of nurse
    20–1
Attitudes 139–41, 145, 154
  aspect of nursing care 204, 210
  doctor–nurse 2, 13–14
  of nurses' to work conditions 56–7,
    217
  to nursing related to age 60–2, 68–9
Authoritarianism, and supply of
    services 319
Autonomy, interpretation of 255
  in nursing research 250, 254–5
  managerial 321

nursing 162–4, 208, 326
  personal 47–9, 53, 96, 107, 155,
    176, 203–4
  professional 92, 98
Auxiliaries, attitude to 'extra' work
    234–5
  and patients 234–8
  and Project 2000   231, 240
  care of the elderly 231–43
  caring for people at home 237–8
  job 232–4
  job satisfaction 237, 243
  'learning the ropes' 238–40, 242–3
  refusal of training 239
  supervision of 240–2

Bedford Fenwick, Mrs. 57
Behaviour 105–10
  and qualitative research 249–50
  and quantitative research 246–8
  in mental illness 149–50
  maladaptive 138
  role 167
Behavioural therapy 149–50
Beliefs 139–41, 145, 154
  doctrine for 199, 202
'Biological reductionism' 93
Body language, and stress 189
Briggs Report on Nursing (1972) 58,
    294, 297
  and caring aspect of nursing 198
  and industrial relations 295
  and wastage rates 119
Budgets 116–18, 312, 316, 322
Bureaucracy, in NHS management
    324–6, 328

Care/caring
  and carative factors 200
  and cure 205–6
  and technology 200
  conceptions of 196–211
  context of 201–2
  defining 199–201, 211
  'duty to' 198

Care/caring—*cont.*
environment 197, 205–6
for carers 210
frameworks 202–3
humanistic approach 203
in context of nursing 196–9
in Intensive Care Units 206, 211
lay and professional 197
model 200–1
personal cost of 209–11
reciprocity of 203–5
roles 199–201
special skills of 197
transcultural aspects 199
see also Nursing care
Career structure 58, 120–1
and wastage 217–19, 222
see also Grading
Carry On films, media representation
of nurse 23–4, 33
Casualty, media representation of nurse
31–2
Centralization 311–12, 321, 323
and development of local
management 318
and specialist treatment centres
323–7
attitudes to 328
Child-care facilities, relevance to
wastage 60–1, 65, 70, 218, 274
Commonsense knowledge, and
auxiliaries 233–4, 237–8
and psychiatric nurses 139, 145, 154
'distancing tactics' 182
Communication, doctor–nurse 4
and 'good nurse' 6
in hospitals 326
interpersonal 105, 107–9
non-verbal 189
nurses–persons with cancer 182,
184–5
skills 203
and Project 2000   103
specialist 185, 193
training in 184
student–nurse–patient 104
Community services 4
restructuring of care 123–4
White Paper 29
Compliance and conformity, in nursing
165–7
Hofling's studies 166
in organizations 169
Milgram's studies 165–6

Computer technology, in nurse supply
modelling 277, 286
and wastage monitoring 261, 273
in workforce planning 259
Confederation of Health Service
Employees (COHSE) 293, 298,
300–4
Confidentiality and anonymity, in
research on wastage 269
Consumer, choice in health care 45,
132
and complaints machinery 318–19
demand and supply of service
318–19
interests of 44–6
of public services 106
oriented service 110
pressure groups 319
satisfaction and performance
monitoring 134
Consumerism, and Project 2000
108–9
and wastage 226
Coping mechanisms 109–10, 183
Cost-Benefit Analysis (CBA) 117
Cost-related indicators 123
Counselling 107, 203
lack of education for role 193
Credit Accumulation Transfer Scheme
(CATS) 97

Death, and concept of persons 83
Decision-making 11, 38, 164
and performance indicators 129–30
and stress 165
by medical profession 159
clinical 318
freedom in 174
management 325
Defence mechanisms, and stress 187,
192
'Determinism' 152
Doctors, deal with government 323–4
and logos 52
'good' 8–10
management role 311–12, 314,
316–18, 322–4
resistance to nursing autonomy 163
role 11–13
Dr. Kildare, media representation of
nurse 22
Drugs, in mental illness 148

Economic and Social Reearch Council
5

Economy, Efficiency and Effectiveness (the three 'Es') 118, 127
Education, continuing/post-basic 92, 97–100, 102
and exploitation of labour force 91
and performance indicators 114–35
curriculum 108
distance learning packages 98
learning programmes 98
parity with other students 95
pre-registration 103, 108
protected learning in clinical setting 94–7
regional 121–2
transfer to universities and polytechnics 164
Education advisory groups (EAGs) 119, 130
abolition of 121
Electroconvulsive therapy (ECT), nurses' stand against 165, 173
Empathy skills 110, 203
English National Board 97
and performance indicators 114, 125
internal review 121
Management of Change open learning package 128
Ethical education 87, 175
Ethical issues 127, 133, 155–6
in nursing, advertising and sponsorship 41–55
in nursing research 250–1, 253–7
Ethics, health care 97, 251, 255
in psychology 155
professional 175

Family, and persons with cancer 190, 192
Feedback, and innovations in organizations 174–5
Fee-splitting 53
Financial Management Initiative 118–19, 131, 134
Freedom, and advertising 47
at work 173–4
in nursing research 249, 257
'Free-will' 152–3
Funding/resources, and public sector management 316
and wastage 219–21
see also Budgets

Grading 34, 120–1, 123, 266
and trade union/professional organization membership 301–2

Griffiths Report 272, 328–9
Guillebaud Committee 116–17

Health authority, board of management 317
Health care
nurses' role in delivery of 329
nurses' role in management of 312–13
Health disputes 29, 293, 295
Health Visitors Association 298–9
Henderson, Virginia 161, 197, 201
Hierarchy, in nursing 164–5, 173
and management of hospitals 321–3
and organizations 169–71
plurality of in hospitals 326
Holistic care 102, 104, 202
for persons with cancer 192

Image 19–20
of nurse 52–3, 160–1
male 160
of nursing 35
Informed consent 47, 49
in nursing research 250, 255–7
Intelligence, concept of in mental illness 140–2, 144
International Council of Nurses, role of nurse 162
Interpersonal skills 9, 102–4, 108–10
and caring frameworks 202–3
Izsak and Medalie's psychosocial assessment scale 186

Job appraisal 120
Job-share 274

Lancaster University, interpersonal relationships research 4–9
Language, meaning and use of in psychiatric nurse study 139, 150
and wastage 214–15, 228
Latent class analysis 3, 62–3
Leadership style, and innovations in organizations 174
Local Government Finance Act (1982) 118
Local training committees (LTCs) 121

Management, centralization 311, 318, 327
and nurse supply modelling 276–91
centrally directed policy 311, 320–1

Management, centralization—*cont.*
  'custodial' 316–17
  development of profession 315–16
  exclusion of nurses from 312, 321
  Griffith's Report 272, 328–9
  health service 272, 310–29
  hospital 313, 320–7
  local 318
  participative 260, 310–29
  policy decisions 314
  political control of 311, 317–20, 322
  private sector 315
  producers' cooperative 311–12,
    316–17, 320–3
  public participation in 321
  'team' 325
Manpower planning 276, 278–9
Matron 23–4
  role in hospital management 314,
    322
Media, and change within nursing 33
  and recruitment 56
  definition 17
  functioning and location in society
    26–7
  portrayal of nurses on television
    29–32
  representation of nurse 2
Media Watch, media representation of
    nurse 16
Medical model, and nursing 92–4
Medicine Now, media representation of
    nurse 32
Mental illness, broad conceptions of
    146–7
  definition 138
  emotional problems as feature of
    151–2
  professional conceptions and related
    issues 138–54
  psychiatric nurses perception of
    139–41, 153
  psychological features of 147
  treatment 147
Mentally ill individual, psychiatric
    nurses perceptions of 140–1
  punishment for 147–8
Mind, nature of 84
Monitoring, performance and quality
    132–4
  resource usage 123
Morale, loss of due to exclusion from
    management processes 321, 326
  low 93–4, 96–7, 215, 227–8, 282

National Association of Local

Government Officers (NALGO)
    299
National Caring Conference (1981)
    199
National Health Service, and cost
    effectiveness 116
  and participative management, *see*
    Mangement, participative
  divison of labour and occupational
    groups within 311, 314
  industrial relations within 294–5
  Management Board 276
  political control of resources 311,
    317
  recruitment of managers 312
  reorganization (1974) 117
  retention and return of qualified
    nurses 58–62, 64–7, 276, 282–3
  wastage 214–17, 261–74
National labour force planning bodies
    125
National Union of Public Employees
    (NUPE) 293, 298–304
Nightingale, Florence 1, 29, 70, 163
  and caring function of nurse 205
  and non-nursing duties 57
  and performance indicators 116
  definition of nursing as women's
    work 6, 159–60
Nurse(s),
  and higher education 97–9
  and logos 41, 43, 49–50, 52
  and medical profession 163
  and sexual availability 23, 28
  as angel 20–1, 27, 29, 36
  as battle-axe 23–4, 26
  as handmaiden/non-entity 21–2,
    29–30, 36
  as patient's advocate 171–3
  as sex symbol 23, 26, 30–1, 36
  autonomous professional 11, 111,
    162
  depiction of in First World War 21
  exclusion from management 312,
    321
  'good' 6–8, 20, 159, 168
  public image of 16, 25, 33, 215
  representation of by media 2, 16–39
  role 11–12, 18, 158, 160, 162, 201
    extended/expanded 206–9
    in primary health care 32
    in public sector management
      312–14, 320–7
    re-evaluation of 37
  self-image 26

status of 27
stereotyping of 17–24
Nurses' Central Clearing House 289
Nurse supply modelling 276–91
  manager participation in 279–80
  nature and structure of models
    277–9
  role of 286–9
  types of models 279
Nurse workforce planning 259, 276–7,
  290–1
Nursing
  and social influence 165–71
  as female occupation 24, 159
  as profession 51–2
  changing the image of 32–7
  control of 327
  definition of 161
  diagnosis 12, 207
  essential components of 198
  glamorization of 36
  hierarchy 164–5, 173
  needs of older female employees 58
  political awareness in 171, 175
  public image of 17, 25, 33–4, 37,
    101, 161
  role of in health care system 18, 160
  secondary job status 23, 25, 28, 34,
    57
  skills 34, 36, 102–3, 197
  specialism 201–2
  status in society 2, 16–17, 26, 33,
    101
  uniqueness of 92, 198, 207
Nursing care 155, 164, 197, 202–4,
  245
  and auxiliaries 233
  outcomes 197
  plans 233, 241
  prescribing 11, 158
  theory 172, 197
Nursing curriculum, communication
  skills 184–5
  ethics 87
  patient advocacy 172–3
Nursing models 155, 197, 202
Nursing process 155, 162
  assessment phase and stress 181,
    185–6
  philosophy 191
Nursing research, considerations of
  personhood 245–58
  ethical issues 250–1, 253–7
  process 250

Nursing theory 197, 203–4, 208

Office of Manpower Economics 266
One Flew Over the Cuckoo's Nest,
  depiction of nursing 24
'Opting-out' of hospitals 29
Option appraisal studies 121
Organizations, conformity within
  167–71
  and hierarchies 169–71
  innovations within 173–5
  nurses' role in 167–71
  reduction of variability, instability
    and unpredictability of human
    acts within 169
  rules of conduct within 169

Participant observation 252–3
Paternalism 47–9, 57, 96
  and ethical issues 251
  and supply of services 319
Patient education, and auxiliaries 233
Pay 3, 25, 56, 59–60
  and changes in nursing structure 34
  and conditions 27, 217
  and media 22
  and regrading disputes 293
  and wastage 219, 265
  special responsibility 69
Pay Review Body 120, 227–8
Peer review 133
Performance indicators 89
  and changing patterns of
    accountability in nurse education
    114–35
  cost-based 128
  definition of 125–6
  for ENB 125
  in planning and decision-making
    129–30
Person-centredness 107, 161, 172
Personhood, and birth/pre-birth 83, 86
  and death 83, 86
  and partnership 157
  central to nursing 249
  conceptions of 75–81, 83–5
  ethical and educational issues 85–7
  features and content of persons 84
  in nursing research 245–58
  models of 76–81
  persons and non-persons distinctions
    83
  status in mental illness 139–40,
    142–3

Personality disorder, psychiatric nurses perception 143–6
Phenomenology 248–50, 252
Planning Programming and Budgeting Systems (PPBS) 117
Plowden Committee 117
Policy making 27, 321
  and participative management 311, 328
Preventitive medicine, and advertising 46
Primary nursing, and auxiliaries' work 233
Professional 'burnout' 69, 210
Professional judgement 132, 318–19
Professionalization 34–5, 95, 199, 208
Programme Analysis and Review (PAR) 117
Project 2000   34, 120, 131–2, 156, 265
  and Briggs Report 119, 294
  and cost-appraisal 120, 123
  and interpersonal/therapeutic skills 101–11
  and nurse education 91–100
  and nurse supply modelling 290
  and trained staff 97–9
  replacement of auxiliaries by support workers 231, 240, 243
  restructuring of higher education and community care 123–4
  usage of manpower in NHS 294
Psychiatric nurses, perception of mental illness 138–54
  professional education 153
Psychological care, of persons with cancer 181–93
  review of literature 182–5
  role of nurse 182
Psychological morbidity, in persons with cancer 182–3, 185–6
Psychology, counselling 107–10
  humanistic 106, 108
  perceptual 106–7
Psychological Adjustment to Illness Scale, and persons with cancer 185–6
Public expenditure 115
Public Expenditure Survey Committee (PESC) 117
'Public Image of the Nurse' campaign 16
Publicity 44, 47, 49, 54
Public opinion, and supply of services 319–21

Public sector services, growth of 115, 265
  management 310–20
  national legislation 313
  performance 116–18
  rise of professional managerial cadre 314–15, 321
Punishment, in mental illness 141, 143, 147–8, 150–1, 154
  in Milgram's studies on obedience 166

Qualitative research 248–50
Quality assurance 211
Quality of care 105, 111
  and auxiliaries 242
  and patient advocacy 175–6
'Quality Strategy' 128–9
Quantitative research 246–8

Recruitment 35–6, 58, 68, 101–2, 265, 272
  and nurse supply modelling 289
  availability of qualified staff 130
  'demographic timebomb' 58, 263–4, 276, 296
  DOH campaign 36
  funding 264
  of men into nursing 36
Registered General Nurse (RGN), academic weighting 97
Registration, of nurses 57
Relationships
  auxiliary–patient 236–7
  causal 246
  doctor–nurse 1, 4, 31–2, 159
  interpersonal 169–70
  interprofessional 4, 93
  nurse–patient 11, 103, 165, 173, 198, 201, 210
  primary and secondary 202–3
  power 10–11, 19, 25, 51–2, 93, 236
  professional–client 52–4, 134
  therapeutic 103, 107
Resource allocation 122, 132, 324–6
  and performance indicators 130–1
  doctors involvement 324
  nurses exclusion 312, 321
  political control of 311
Resource Allocation Working Party 117
Respect, for persons 250–1, 255
Responsibility 106
  and job appraisal 120

and mental illness 141–2, 144, 152, 154
Retirement 216, 223
Review Body for Nursing Staff, Midwives, Health Visitors and Professions Allied to Medicine 216, 265–7, 273
Role(s), behaviour 167–9
blurring of nurse–doctor 10
care giver and receiver 199–200
extension/expansion of nurses' 103, 206–9
men as healers 28
models 104
inappropriate 231
nurses' 102, 199
re-evaluation of learners 93
re-evaluation of nurses' 37
Royal College of Midwives (RCM) 298–9
Royal College of Nursing (RCN) 95, 293, 299–304
'no-strike' policy 293, 300
nursing standards 129, 162, 297
survey of members on labour market/work dissatisfaction 296

Sanity and rationality, in mental illness 141–2, 144
Schizophrenic individual, psychiatric nurses perceptions of 142–3, 151
Screening, and advertising 46
Self-actualization, and nursing models 203
Self-care 191, 203
Self-help 110
Semantic Differential Scaling Booklet 139
'Significant learning' 108
Socialization 167
girls/women in society 27
in training 5, 8, 164–5, 168
nurses 27–8, 164
professional 102, 105
Social phenomena 248
Social reality 249, 252
Sponsorship, commercial 41, 54
Staff development programmes 110
Staff shortages, politics of 228
and provision of efficient service 227, 326
and wastage 58, 68–9, 218, 220, 225
Standards 58, 128–9, 175–6
edcuational 129

Standards of Nursing Care, Rcn report 162
Statutory bodies, DOH review 122–3
Stereotypes 2, 5, 17–24
and role reversal 31
historical basis of in nursing 28–9
ideology behind 18–19
sex 20
Stitching Up the NHS, media representation of nursing 29–30
Strategic planning 133
demand and supply modelling 276–7
Stress, adaptation to 189–90
and body language/non-verbal cues 189, 192
and social support network 174
and wastage 219, 223, 271
assessment of 181, 191–2
associated with life events 190
concept/definition of 186, 191
'general adaptation syndrome' (GAS) 187
in persons with cancer 181–93
models of
humanistic/transactional 181, 191–2
response-based 186–9
stimulus-based 189–90
nurses vulnerability to 109, 164–5, 184
physiological response to 187–9
Stressors 187, 189–90
Strikes/industrial action 21, 29, 265
Student–staff ratios (SSRs) 122–3
and resource allocation 131
as a performance indicator 127
Supervision, of auxiliaries 240–2
of learners 110
Support, for cancer nurses 193
lack of education for role 193
of persons with cancer 183–4, 192
peer 110
psychological and emotional 109
social network 174
Support worker 156
in care of the elderly 231, 243
Survey, differing expectations of nursing in NHS held by nurses 59–70
Synapse, media representation of nurse 16

Teamwork 11, 13, 109
and wastage 221–2

Technology, effect on care 200, 211
  and extended role of nurse 208–9
  see also Computer technology
'Therapeutic' skills 105, 108
The Young Doctors, media
  representation of nurse 23, 30–1
Trade unions/professional
  organizations 36, 259–60,
  293–307
  interest in 321
  nurses' attitudes to 295, 301, 305–6
  patterns and variations in
  membership 298–305, 326
  reasons for joining 297
  role in training and grievances 295
Training 25, 28, 34–5
  and education 95
  and emergence of degrees in Nursing
  Studies 323
  in-service 110
  specialist 323
  see also Education
Truth-telling, misleading
  advertisements 42–4
Turnover 266–7, 269
  hidden costs to management 272
  high 261, 267, 272
  positive aspects of 264, 272, 274
  rate 35, 273
  see also Wastage

United Kingdom Central Council
  (UKCC) 3, 48–9
  and logos on uniforms 50
  and role of nurse 162
  and wastage study 91–2
  Code of Professional Conduct 41,
  46, 51–3
  live register and nurse supply
  modelling 289
  policy reviews 124

Uniforms, depersonalization of nurse
  167, 169
  logos on 41, 43, 49–50, 52, 54
University of London Institute of
  Education, performance indicator
  project 114, 119

'Value for money', in NHS 116, 132
Value judgements 145
Values 127, 139–41, 154
  and caring 200, 210
  and qualitative research 249
Vocation 7, 56–70, 217
Volume planning 117

Ward closure, reduction of services 272
Ward reports, and auxiliaries 233, 241
Wastage 57, 92–4, 96–7, 156, 259
  and nurse supply modelling 282–4,
  290
  and performance indicators 118
  current attitudes 225–9
  from nurses' perspective 214–29
  identifying the problem 215–16, 261,
  264–7
  management of 261–74
  natural 216
  political dimensions 216, 228
  positive aspects 264, 272, 274
  reasons for 64–7, 216–23, 265, 267,
  269–71
Whitley Council 295
Witches and nursing 28
Women's Issues, media representation
  of nursing 25, 38
Workforce, increase 262–3
  stagnation 264
Working for Patients 123, 134
Wood Report (1947) 118–19

Zero-Based Budgeting 117